1995

······························

HMOs
AND THE
ELDERLY

······························

HMOs
AND THE
ELDERLY

EDITED BY
HAROLD S. LUFT

Health Administration Press
Ann Arbor, Michigan   1994

98 97 96 95 94   5 4 3 2 1

Library of Congress Cataloging-in-Publication Data

HMOs and the elderly / Harold S. Luft, editor.
    p.   cm.
"Conference on HMOs and Alternative Delivery Systems and the Elderly . . . held in San Francisco on November 17 and 18, 1992"—Pref.
    Includes bibliographical references and index.
    ISBN 1-56793-021-2 (alk. paper : softbound)
    1. Health maintenance organizations—United States—Congresses.
2. Medicare—Congresses. 3. Aged—Medical care—United States—Congresses.
I. Luft, Harold S. II. Conference on HMOs and Alternative Delivery Systems and the Elderly (1992 : San Francisco, Calif.)
    [DNLM: 1. Health Maintenance Organizations—economics—United States—congresses. 2. Medicare—organization & administration—congresses.
3. Quality of Health Care—United States—congresses. W 275 AA1 H6773 1994]
RA413.7.A4H56   1994   362.1'0425—dc20   94-28777 CIP

The paper used in this publication meets the minimum requirements of American National Standard for Information Sciences—Permanence of Paper for Printed Library Materials, ANSI Z39.48-1984. ∞™

Health Administration Press
A division of the Foundation of the
    American College of
    Healthcare Executives
1021 East Huron Street
Ann Arbor, Michigan 48104
(313) 764-1380

The Association for Health
    Services Research
1350 Connecticut Avenue, NW
Suite 1100
Washington, DC 20036
(202) 223-2477

Contents

153, 169

Acronyms and Abbreviations

AAPCC   adjusted average per capita cost: the amount paid by HCFA to HMOs each month for beneficiaries enrolled in the Medicare risk program

ACG   ambulatory care group

ADL   activities of daily living

AMI   acute myocardial infarction

BDMS   Bureau of Data Management and Strategy

CMP   competitive medical plan: HMOs that are not federally qualified for other organizations

COPD   chronic obstructive pulmonary disease

CPS   current population survey

CVA   cerebrovascular accident

DCG   diagnostic cost group

ESRD   end-stage renal disease

FFS   fee-for-service

GA   geographic adjuster

GHAA   Group Health Association of America

GHPO   Group Health Plan Operations

HCFA   Health Care Financing Administration

HCPP   health care prepayment plans

HMO   health maintenance organization

IADL   instrumental activities of daily living

ICU   intensive care unit

IPA   independent practice association

MCD   Medicare Capitation Demonstration
MI   myocardial infarction
MSA   metropolitan service area
MSA   Metropolitan Statistical Area

NLTCS   National Long Term Care Survey
NMCE   National Medicare Competition Evaluation

OACT   Office of the Actuary
OCCPP   Office of Coordinated Care Policy and Planning
ORD   Office of Research and Demonstrations, HCFA

PGP   prepaid group practice
PPS   prospective payment system
PRO   peer review organization
PSA   prostate-specific antigen

RBRVS   Resource-Based Relative Value Scale
RIND   reversible ischemic neurologic deficit

SEGA   six-equation group adjustment model
S/HMO   Social/Health Maintenance Organization
SNF   skilled nursing facility

TEFRA   Tax Equity and Fiscal Responsibility Act: legislation that went
           into effect April 1985 authorizing the Medicare risk program
TIA   transient ischemic attack

URHIMRS Medicare master beneficiary file
USPCC   United States Per Capita Cost: the national average per capita
           reimbursement for Medicare-covered services

Preface

This conference began with an interest expressed by Dr. Robert Gumbiner, who chairs the FHP Foundation board of directors. Dr. Gumbiner and other members of the board were particularly interested in up-to-date research on comparisons of quality, acceptability, and appropriateness of care provided to Medicare beneficiaries in HMOs and fee-for-service settings. Although the underlying set of questions one might ask about these issues is relatively straightforward, health services research has come a long way in the past decades in terms of the level of sophistication in addressing these questions. For example, credible assessments of quality of care should include both outcome and process measures and, if random assignment of health plans is not an option, substantial effort is required to assure comparability in case mix. Likewise, measures of enrollee satisfaction as well as cost and utilization have to take into account the fact that people may select HMOs based on factors that can also influence their satisfaction and use of services. While these problems are daunting, they have been addressed to various degrees in the existing literature, so state-of-the-art new research must include these methodological enhancements.

From a policy perspective, solid methodology is necessary to avoid incorrect conclusions based on inappropriate data or analyses. For example, earlier studies of risk differences among plans focused on the prior use of people who switched plans, yet it is now known that these "switcher" studies provide biased estimates of the medical care that people *would have used* had they stayed in the original health plan. That is, people sometimes change, or refuse to change, plans because they are anticipating a need for medical care in the near future. New studies using old methods would therefore be less than fully credible.

A second issue relating to credibility from a policy perspective is replicability, which seeks to address the policymaker's concern about how sure one can be in interpreting findings. Perhaps the best way to assure replicability is to undertake multiple studies on the same question, preferably with different data sets, HMO locations, and independent investigators. In this way one can attempt to avoid having a series of results that all suffer from the same biases of method or interpretation. Consistency in findings is reassuring; differences may be enlightening if one can identify the underlying reasons for these differences. That is, the apparently conflicting results may be explained by other factors that aid in understanding the overall situation.

Generalizability addresses the policymaker's concern about the broad applicability of a study's findings to a wide range of real-world situations, not just the specific cases under study. One of the most important studies relating to HMO performance was a segment of the RAND Health Insurance Experiment. This study was particularly valuable because it involved the random assignment of persons to specific health plans, one of which was an HMO. This random assignment, combined with extensive measures of risk factors and health status both at the beginning of the study and at subsequent junctures, made this a "gold standard" in terms of research design. Unfortunately from a policy perspective, the data refer to the mid-1970s, only one HMO was involved, and the nature of the experiment excluded the poor and elderly. Further, the HMO that was studied, Group Health Cooperative of Puget Sound, is a large, mature, and highly regarded consumer-controlled staff model plan. Thus, when policymakers wanted to know about the performance of newer HMOs with different organizational and historical characteristics, much conjecture, but little evidence, was available.

After extensive discussions concerning the complexity and cost of undertaking new policy-oriented research to fill the gaps in the existing literature, and the desirability of assessing the findings of multiple projects, not just a single study, a different strategy was developed by the FHP Foundation board. A grant was made to the Institute for Health Policy Studies, University of California, San Francisco, to support a "Conference on HMOs and Other Alternative Delivery Systems and the Elderly." The purpose of this conference was to bring together the best researchers in the nation who were working on projects in this subject area. The meeting would allow a vigorous exchange of ideas. Both papers and commentaries would be published so that the findings would reach as large an audience as possible. The conference was held in San Francisco on November 17 and 18, 1992.

The project was designed with incentives to elicit the best new work, not just rehashes of old studies or thoughts put down during the flight to the meeting. In most instances, the research findings in this book have not been published elsewhere; one paper was published earlier.

There is constant tension between the desires of researchers to design a clean, methodologically sound study using the most advanced techniques and the desire of policymakers for clear, concise results that take into account the constraints and demands of the "real world." To address this tension, we invited two discussants to focus on each pair of papers. One discussant was drawn from the research community and one from the HMO or policy community. The discussion that followed each segment of the conference was transcribed to provide the reader with the feeling of being in attendance.

Harold S. Luft

Acknowledgments

This conference and volume would not have been possible without the generous support of the FHP Foundation and the assistance of many people. I am particularly grateful to Dr. Robert Gumbiner, Chairman of the Board of the Foundation for his interest in initiating this conference. Both Dr. Gumbiner and Harriet Wilder of the Foundation board attended the meetings and offered helpful insights. Sandra Lund Gavin, Executive Director of the Foundation, was extremely understanding in dealing with all of the contingencies inherent in this undertaking. I would like to thank all of our authors and commentators for providing manuscripts that met our goals: state-of-the-art and policy-relevant papers and responses. In addition, their comments throughout enriched the meeting considerably.

Without our expert and dedicated staff at the Institute for Health Policy Studies, neither the conference nor this volume would have been possible. Nancy Ramsay coordinated all of the activities involved and edited the manuscripts for final publication. She helped make the manuscripts uniformly comprehensible to the interested, but not necessarily expert reader. Holly Wong handled all the complex logistic and financial arrangements for the meeting (including a last-minute cancellation by our initial hotel) with grace, good humor, and efficiency. Lucy Marton and Pamela Weatherford mastered the challenges of converting manuscripts from a babel of word processing languages and machines to the Macintosh Word and then to PC-based WordPerfect for publication. Without them we would still be cutting and pasting with scissors and glue.

I am also indebted to the capable and helpful staff at Health Administration Press for ensuring that the original conference proceedings became a book. Sandy Crump guided us each step of the way with patience and encouragement that were both greatly appreciated.

List of Contributors

Authors

Randall S. Brown, Ph.D.
Mathematica Policy Research, Inc.
Princeton, NJ

David M. Carlisle, M.D.
University of California,
Los Angeles

Dolores Gurnick Clement, Ph.D.
Virginia Commonwealth
University
Richmond, VA

Robert Newcomer, Ph.D.
University of California,
San Francisco

Sheldon M. Retchin, M.D.
Medical College of Virginia
Richmond, VA

Louis F. Rossiter, Ph.D.
Medical College of Virginia
Richmond, VA

W. Pete Welch, Ph.D.
The Urban Institute
Washington, DC

Catherine Wisner, Ph.D.
Group Health Foundation
Minneapolis, MN

Discussants

Joseph R. Antos, Ph.D.
Health Care Financing
Administration
Baltimore, MD

Jon Christianson, Ph.D
University of Minnesota
Minneapolis, MN

Mark C. Hornbrook, Ph.D.
Kaiser Permanente
Portland, OR

Sheila Leatherman
United Health Care
Minneapolis, MN

Jan Malcolm
Group Health Incorporated
Minneapolis, MN

Susan E. Palsbo, Ph.D.
Group Health Association of
America
Washington, DC

Thomas Rice, Ph.D.
University of California, Los
Angeles

Patrick S. Romano, M.D., M.P.H.
University of California, Davis

Haya Rubin, M.D., Ph.D.
Johns Hopkins University
Baltimore, MD

Edward Wagner, M.D.
Group Health Cooperative
Seattle, WA

Introduction

Harold S. Luft

The performance of health maintenance organizations (HMOs) and similar plans in providing care for the elderly has recently taken on new importance for several reasons. One arises from continued change in the Medicare program for the elderly and disabled. These changes have affected physician payment in particular, and they may make the transition to HMOs more attractive for some physicians and patients. A second factor is that, after decades of debate and little evidence about their performance, HMOs are the subject of a new set of studies that shed light on a wide range of questions. Many of these findings are reported in this volume for the first time.

Perhaps the most important reason for renewed interest in HMOs and the elderly is the current opportunity for major systemwide changes in the U.S. health care delivery system. While many would agree that Medicare can still be improved, it comes the closest to universal coverage in the United States, at least for the population aged 65 and over. Further, while many current ideas for reform rely on managed competition, one major criticism of this approach is that it has never really been tried. Formulating a major restructuring of the system based on an untested hypothesis is an invitation for disaster, but the Medicare program has had contracts with HMOs for years, and this has led to development of a number of key features that will be needed in a managed competition environment. These include risk-adjusted premiums, enrollment mechanisms, and attempts to monitor and assure quality. As will be seen in the work that follows, the current forms of these approaches are far from perfect. However, examining how they work, where they succeed, and where they fail can help identify issues for consideration in the design and implementation of current health care reform.

HMOs and the Elderly

The papers from the conference focus on a wide range of issues associated with HMOs and other alternative delivery systems, on the one hand, and the elderly, on the other hand. However, these questions, broad as they are, must be examined in the still broader context of this country's social, medical, economic, and political environment. In particular, Medicare, as administered by the Health Care Financing Administration (HCFA) is by far the dominant payer in this setting. To a substantial extent, Medicare legislation and HCFA regulations determine the nature of the health insurance market for the elderly. That is, HCFA pays HMOs a monthly premium (the adjusted average per capita cost, or AAPCC) for their Medicare beneficiaries. HCFA sets the AAPCC according to a formula that takes into account the age, gender, disability insurance status, Medicaid eligibility, and nursing home status of the beneficiary and the local fee-for-service costs in the county (Palsbo 1992). Several papers presented at this conference address problems with HCFA's approach in setting the AAPCC, but the key point for the current discussion is that it reflects a nonnegotiable rate set by HCFA for HMOs wishing to be in the Medicare risk market.

There are, however, other mechanisms that HMOs can use for contracting with HCFA. For example, plans can opt for cost-based reimbursement or the health care prepayment plan (HCPP) model, both of which limit the risk that plans bear and may lead to higher payments. In fact, as of November 1992, only 95 of the 177 prepaid contracts reported by HCFA were on a risk basis. These contracts accounted for two-thirds of the total Medicare enrollment of 2,334,669 in "coordinated care" (a somewhat broader concept than just HMOs) (Horwitz 1992). Nevertheless, nearly all of the research and discussion focuses on enrollees in the risk-contracted plans.

The multiple means by which plans can "enter the Medicare market" have several other important implications, especially if one wishes to view this research as possibly informing the larger health policy reform debate. First, many HMOs, including some large plans, do not have risk contracts with HCFA, even though they may have large numbers of Medicare beneficiaries who have "aged into" coverage after having been enrolled in the HMO through their employer. These HMOs just appear to HCFA as fee-for-service providers in terms of their billing arrangements, and by converting the standard HMO policy into a Medicare supplemental plan, copayments and deductibles for the beneficiary are essentially eliminated. Thus, just as beneficiaries have a choice of being in an HMO or using FFS providers, HMOs have a choice of being prepaid in terms of their relationships with HCFA. In both instances, it is reasonable to assume that decision makers (beneficiaries or HMOs) make choices they think are best for themselves, thereby creating the possibility for biased selection.

Biased selection causes problems from an analytic perspective because differences in cost, use, or other assessments of various options may reflect not the effects of differences in health plans, but the attraction of different people into the various plans. It is important to note, however, that opportunities for biased selection are shaped by the rules and practices of the market. For example, the ability of Medicare beneficiaries to change health plans every month, unlike the typical annual open enrollment seasons for employees, enhances the opportunities for biased selection by enrollees. Likewise, the ability of an HMO to decide whether or not to enter the Medicare market, and the type of contract options available, make selection by plans more likely.

One must also remember that the Medicare market is but one segment of the overall health care market. Some health plans market coverage largely to Medicare beneficiaries, while others focus largely on the employed or Medicaid populations, with Medicare as a sideline. In some parts of the nation, such as south Florida, the large retiree population has a major influence on the overall health care market. Likewise, the structure of the local provider system may be an important component of HMO performance. For example, if there is a surplus of hospital beds in an area, then HMOs may be able to negotiate better rates with hospitals and other suppliers. The opposite effect has also been noted in which hospitals in areas with a higher proportion of HMO members tend to slow their rate of growth in costs relative to those with a lower local HMO market share (Robinson 1991). Furthermore, these "feedback effects" may be felt in various ways in addition to their bearing on prices and costs. That is, if local competition among HMOs leads to pressure on hospital costs and possibly physician fees, these providers may react by attempting to increase volume. (This question of supplier-induced demand is hotly contested in the research literature, and is well beyond the scope of this book. While its importance is controversial, it must be considered a possible effect.) If such responses occur, then overall costs of care provided for patients in the fee-for-service sector may increase and this, in turn, will tend to increase the payments available to HMOs through the AAPCC. This complex set of interrelationships is important both because it reflects the environment in which HMOs must operate, and because it foreshadows the challenges facing researchers in this field.

Assessing the Evidence

Interest in the use of HMOs and similar alternative delivery systems stems largely from the possibility that such programs may be able to provide medical care coverage at lower cost than the traditional fee-for-service system. The question of cost, however, is complex because there are many perspectives from which to measure cost. Economists often focus on cost from society's perspective. That is, what is the value of the resources used in a certain endeavor compared to their value in their best alternative use? In the health care context, this is a difficult standard since some would argue that certain resources are overpaid in the medical care system due to entry barriers. For example, many allege that the pharmaceutical industry has been able to earn above-average profits for long periods of time (Miller and Luft 1993). Likewise, some argue that physicians receive a higher return on their educational investment than do other professionals. Thus, if one were to undertake an analysis of "true economic costs," one would need to develop adjusted measures of the values of the various inputs.

While the above distinction may seem a bit arcane, it becomes important when comparing medical care delivery systems. For example, part of the earnings of physicians in independent practice is a return on their capital investment. If physicians choose to work for HMOs on a salaried basis and purchase stock in their companies, then comparisons of physician incomes in fee-for-service practice and HMOs will be skewed. As another example, most HMOs and other alternative delivery systems are in an expansion mode, while fee-for-service in the same areas is declining. Thus, HMOs are attempting to borrow money or attract capital by being profitable, and conventional providers may even be using up capital by investing less than their assets are depreciating. This means that HMOs may charge premiums that are higher than one would expect in a steady-case state. Unfortunately, developing consistent medical care input prices and costs of capital has not been undertaken in any studies to our knowledge. Thus, comparisons of the proverbial "bottom line" may be more misleading than helpful.

Stepping back a bit, we can ask the question, If one accepts the prices of medical care inputs as given, are some delivery systems more efficient than others at combining these inputs to produce a given set of outputs? This notion of efficiency incorporates important assumptions that may not be evident immediately to the casual observer. In theory, one would like to compare the inputs used by various systems to achieve the same outputs. Most people would agree, at least after some thought, that hospital stays and physician visits are simply intermediate inputs used to achieve a certain level of health status. (Other inputs would include preventive measures to keep people healthy.) From this perspective, the estimation of the relative efficiency of delivery systems should begin with attempts to measure the output of such systems, that is, their ability to improve or maintain the health status of their enrollees.

Except in rare experimental situations, such as the RAND Health Insurance Experiment (Newhouse et al. 1993), people are not randomly assigned to health plans, so one must assess carefully the health status of people upon entry to the delivery system: some delivery systems may attract healthier enrollees, some of them less healthy enrollees. Ideally, one would have precise tools for measuring a population's health status upon joining a health care system and then, subsequently, for measuring the effects of the system on that population's health status. Unfortunately, such precise tools either are not yet available or are not easily applied to large populations.

Many of the most clinically important medical interventions are used for the small number of people who experience significant health problems. Some observers are concerned that HMOs or similar alternative delivery systems may be quite capable of "caring for" the vast majority of people with minor illness, but will be less able to treat people appropriately when they need care the most, such as after a heart attack or stroke. This concern leads to a different type of analytic approach to assessing quality, one in which attention is concentrated on the treatments offered and outcomes achieved in different practice settings for subpopulations of patients with specific illnesses. Thus, despite an initial interest in costs and efficiency, health economists are quickly drawn into the complex field of health status and outcome measurement. Furthermore, outputs of the medical care system are more than just aspects of health status, in the same way that outputs of airlines are more than just transportation. Most travelers will agree that, while safety and on-time arrival are important, if those characteristics are roughly similar across carriers, one probably will begin to focus more on the quality of the inflight meals, interactions with airline personnel, and other "softer" measures of satisfaction.

Cost-effectiveness can be examined from various perspectives. As just indicated, economists typically take a societal perspective and attempt to estimate the resource costs associated with achieving certain outcomes. However, in a policy context, other perspectives may also be relevant (Luft 1976). For example, a narrower view of the effectiveness of HMOs with regard to the elderly takes HCFA's vantage point and asks whether the total of government payments for Medicare beneficiaries has become higher or lower since the introduction of HMOs. This immediately gets into the complex set of issues around copayments and deductibles in the Medicare program, the role of supplementary insurance coverage, and the method HCFA uses to determine payments to HMOs. Furthermore, even HCFA's focus can be broad or narrow. For example, one may ask what HCFA's payments are to HMOs relative to the fee-for-service costs of those beneficiaries, or one can take a broader view and ask whether the presence of HMOs actually influences the fee-for-service costs of Medicare beneficiaries not in the HMOs.

Conference Outline

The papers presented at the conference were grouped into four pairs, reflecting four major aspects for assessing performance of HMOs and other alternative delivery systems for the elderly. These major topic areas are (1) overall costs and use of services; (2) satisfaction with access and quality of services received; (3) quality of care for specific conditions; and (4) effects of HMOs on costs for fee-for-service (FFS) and costs to HCFA.

The preceding discussion outlined the need for a multifaceted approach to examining the performance of complex systems, such as HMOs and other alternative delivery systems, operating in a larger FFS environment with a major government agency as the primary payer in the market. The first two papers (chapters), "The Effects of Medicare HMOs on the Use and Cost of Health Care," by Randall S. Brown and Jerrold Hill, and "The Twin Cities Medicare Health Plan Market: Choice, Cost, and Health Status," by Catherine Wisner, Roger Feldman, and Bryan Dowd, provide overall assessments on both national and local levels.

The Brown and Hill paper examines the use and cost of services for a large random sample of Medicare beneficiaries in 75 risk contract HMOs across the nation. This study incorporates information drawn from interviews with nearly 13,000 individuals combined with their Medicare claims data. The great strength of the design is that, by focusing on a random sample of all beneficiaries enrolled in HMOs, findings can be interpreted on a programwide basis. This is in contrast to many earlier studies of Medicare contracts with HMOs in which one could argue that the plans studied were not representative of the "universe" of plans. The combination of interview and claims data means that the authors can use more sensitive measures of risk factors derived from the survey to assess the importance of selection while having the more precise measure of costs derived from the claims data.

As always, research designs involve trade-offs. The Brown and Hill paper offers national breadth, but even a sample size of 13,000 is not large enough to assess the performance of individual HMOs. Thus, for a consideration of how health plans operate in the context of a competitive local market, one needs a narrower focus. Wisner, Feldman, and Dowd offer such a view with their examination of the Twin Cities Medicare health plan market. For example, they are able to provide a history of HMO development and expansion in the Minneapolis–St. Paul Medicare market. They combine interview with claims data to develop models that account for nonrandom plan choice. They are also able to examine some effects of plan choice on health status, findings that are relevant to the group of papers in Part III. By focusing on a circumscribed market, Wisner, Feldman, and Dowd are able to discuss the choices faced by individuals and ways in which these alternative options may affect the overall pattern of use and cost.

The commentators provide different perspectives on these two papers. In the first part of Chapter 3, Tom Rice discusses some of the differences between the two papers and then goes on to list their implications for the AAPCC, an issue dealt with in more detail in the last group of papers. Then, as a senior vice president of government relations and public programs in one of the Twin Cities HMOs, Jan Malcolm offers a health plan view of both studies and provides grounding for their findings.

The two chapters in Part II are papers that offer a similar split in perspective as they focus primarily on enrollee satisfaction. In fact, "Satisfaction with Access and Quality of Care in Medicare Risk Contract HMOs," by Dolores Gurnick Clement, Sheldon Retchin, and Randall Brown, is the second of three papers based on the large-scale TEFRA Evaluation contract carried out by HCFA, Mathematica Policy Research, Inc., and the Medical College of Virginia. (The Brown and Hill paper is also part of that study.) The authors are thus able to draw upon the large-scale national survey of enrollees in HMOs and, for comparison, beneficiaries with fee-for-service providers in the geographic areas. In this paper the focus is on satisfaction with various aspects of access and quality of care in risk contract HMOs. Clement and colleagues are able to contrast the overall assessments of FFS and HMOs, after taking into account various enrollee risk factors.

The paper by Robert Newcomer and associates, "Satisfaction in the Social/HMO Demonstration," reports on the findings drawn from Medicare beneficiaries enrolled in four demonstration plans in Brooklyn, Minneapolis–St. Paul, Santa Barbara, and Portland, Oregon. These plans include, in addition to the standard HMO benefits, a set of long-term care benefits and services of particular importance to the frail elderly. The underlying notion of the Social/HMO (S/HMO) is that, by combining a full range of services in a single organization, the health plans can more effectively serve the elderly with special needs. Given the additional services offered by S/HMOs, selection is expected to be a major problem in evaluating differences in the assessments of enrollees and those still in fee-for-service. As was the case in the Wisner, Feldman, and Dowd paper, the limited sample of sites (even though these four are the only S/HMOs in the nation) allow Newcomer and colleagues to examine in much more detail the differences in assessments among the four plans, rather than focus just on FFS versus S/HMO.

Haya Rubin offers a commentary on measures of satisfaction concentrating on patient judgments of HMOs and managed care. Sheila Leatherman, Deborah Chase, and Cynthia Polich provide a commentary that addresses the issues raised by the two papers and goes beyond them to question the role of satisfaction surveys in assessing the effectiveness of various managed care systems. This assessment brings to bear their experiences in policy and evaluation for a large, multistate HMO.

The papers assessing quality of care take a procedure-specific approach. This allows careful selection of comparable patients in various settings followed by a detailed examination of services provided and patient outcomes. It offers a focus on both process and outcome measures, and it also permits an investigation of the appropriateness of some of the interventions. As part of the TEFRA evaluation, Sheldon Retchin, Dolores Clement, and Randall Brown chose colon cancer and stroke as their two tracer conditions. Their chapter, "The Care of Patients Hospitalized with Strokes under the Medicare Risk Contract Program," reports on the findings of the latter group. Unlike the other two papers from this evaluation, the study design focused on a subset of all TEFRA HMOs, but the 19 plans included are representative of the universe of plans contracting with HCFA.

David Carlisle focuses the analysis of his research group on nearly 1,500 patients with acute myocardial infarction (heart attack) enrolled in three HMOs, along with a comparison group of beneficiaries in fee-for-service settings. While prior confidentiality agreements preclude identification of the three HMOs, Carlisle's study design makes it possible to examine not only the HMO versus FFS comparison, but also variability across the three plans. This helps us remember that HMOs, like hospitals and other organizations, are not all alike.

In his role as discussant, Patrick Romano raises a series of questions concerning the methods and approaches undertaken by the authors in their assessment of quality. Edward Wagner expands the discussion to ask, "Can we move beyond the question of whether HMOs are harmful to health?" In doing so, he also focuses on some of the differences in the use of various interventions as indicated in the two papers, thus drawing together issues of utilization of services and appropriateness in the context of quality.

The final set of papers moves to a more global view. W. Pete Welch's chapter examines overall Medicare costs for markets across the nation to determine whether increased HMO market share is associated with higher costs to HCFA, or lower costs. That is, the standard payment to the HMOs set by HCFA, the adjusted average per capita cost (AAPCC), is supposed to be 95 percent of the FFS cost in the area. However, if selection occurs such that HMOs actually enroll lower-risk people, this

5 percent discount could easily be wiped out. On the other hand, if the presence of HMO competition leads to cost-containing changes in behavior by physicians in FFS, then the savings to HCFA from the growth by HMOs could exceed the simple 5 percent discount.

Welch's analysis focuses on the AAPCC, but some of the other authors in this series, such as Brown and Hill, suggest that the AAPCC may be flawed. Louis Rossiter, Herng-Chia Chiu, and Sheau-Hwa Chen examine this question in "Strengths and Weaknesses of the AAPCC: When Does Risk Adjustment Become Cost Reimbursement?" They argue that alternative approaches may be both more accurate and fairer.

Commentator Jon Christianson agrees that the two papers raise important questions concerning the setting of payments to HMOs by HCFA and that the current approach has significant flaws. Susan Palsbo's discussion returns us to the reality that not all HMOs choose risk contracts with HCFA. That is, the AAPCC is a fixed price, and if the HMOs feel it is too low, or too risky, they can choose to contract on other bases or to forgo the Medicare market entirely. This reminds us that the whole system is intertwined and narrow analyses are particularly vulnerable to error.

The final two discussants, Joseph Antos and Mark Hornbrook, provide summaries of all of the papers, commentaries, and discussion around the table during the two-day conference, and Mr. Antos offers a prescription for future research on the subject.

References

Horwitz, R. Medicare Coordinated Care Contract Report: Data as of 1 November 1992. Washington, DC: Health Care Financing Administration, Office of Prepaid Health Care Operations and Oversight, Office of Operations, 1992.

Luft, H. S. "Benefit-Cost Analysis and Public Policy Implementation: From Normative to Positive Analysis." *Public Policy* 24, no. 4 (Fall 1976): 437–62.

Miller, R. H., and H. S. Luft. "Assessing the Assumptions Behind Health Reform Projections: Cost Savings Due to HMOs." Washington DC: Report prepared for the Office of Technology Assessment, U.S. Congress, 1993.

Newhouse, J. P., and the Insurance Experiment Group. *Free for All?: Lessons from the Rand Health Insurance Experiment.* Cambridge, MA: Harvard University Press, 1993.

Palsbo, S. J. *The AAPCC Explained.* Washington, DC: Group Health Association of America, 1992.

Robinson, J. C. "HMO Market Penetration and Hospital Cost Inflation In California." *Journal of the American Medical Association* 266, no. 19 (20 November 1991): 2719–24.

Part **I**

Costs and Use of Services

Chapter 1

The Effects of Medicare Risk HMOs on Medicare Costs and Service Utilization

Randall S. Brown and Jerrold W. Hill

The rapid rise in Medicare costs since the program's inception in 1966 has led the Health Care Financing Administration (HCFA) to look for ways to bring these costs under control. Between 1968 and 1980, Medicare costs per beneficiary rose by 13.1 percent per year, compared to an annual increase of 7.5 percent in the consumer price index during this period. A key feature of the program that is often blamed for the escalation in costs is the lack of incentives for physicians to provide cost-effective care for Medicare patients. In fact, physicians can increase their income and reduce the likelihood of malpractice suits by overprescribing tests and office visits. Beneficiaries have little incentive to pressure physicians to hold utilization down, because HCFA bears the bulk of the cost of Medicare-covered services, and nearly 80 percent of beneficiaries have supplemental insurance (or Medicaid) to cover the cost of deductibles and copayments.

HCFA has sought to reverse these incentives by involving health maintenance organizations (HMOs) in the provision of services to Medicare beneficiaries. For each beneficiary enrolled in its Medicare risk plan, participating HMOs receive a fixed monthly payment equal to 95 percent of an actuarial estimate of the amount that HCFA would expect to spend in reimbursements for that beneficiary had he or she obtained Medicare-covered services from providers reimbursed on a fee-for-service (FFS) basis. HCFA therefore has expected to save 5 percent, and has anticipated that HMOs would prosper as a result of having both the incentive and the organizational structure to provide care more efficiently. Beneficiaries who enroll in an HMO no longer face Medicare's deductibles or coin-surance, but they are required to obtain all of their Medicare-covered services from the HMO. HMOs offer this coverage for rates below those charged by Medigap insurers for comparable or inferior coverage, in order to entice beneficiaries to join the HMO.

Our purpose here is to assess whether HMOs do indeed provide services more efficiently than the FFS sector, and whether the Medicare risk program saves money for the Medicare program. It is important to bear in mind, however, that HMO effects on the service use of enrollees have no bearing on whether the program saves money for Medicare. The savings or the cost to Medicare depends solely on how accurately the payment mechanism predicts what Medicare *would* have spent for enrollees had they not joined the HMO. It should also be noted that our focus is on measuring program effects on costs to the Medicare program, rather than any effects on the cost of overall resource use.

The Medicare Risk Program and Its Expected Effects

HCFA was experimenting with introducing HMOs to the Medicare pro-gram in several demonstration programs prior to utilizing the Medicare risk program in April 1985. The experiments were initiated in 1980, after early options for HMOs to participate in Medicare failed to attract many HMOs (because HCFA set limits on HMO profits but not on losses). The first demonstrations, the Medicare Capitation Demonstrations, tested various reimbursement options in eight HMOs that began operating in 1980 and 1981. The second demonstrations, the Medicare Competition Demonstrations, tested a program similar to the current risk program in 26 HMOs that began enrolling members between 1982 and 1984. This ended in April 1985, when legislation authorizing the current Medicare risk program (the Tax Equity and Fiscal Responsibility Act or TEFRA) went into effect, and most of the demonstration plans signed risk con-tracts at that time in order to continue serving Medicare members.

Size and scope of the Medicare risk program

By June 1992, 83 HMOs were participating in the Medicare risk program, operating in 28 states and serving almost 1.4 million beneficiaries (about 4 percent of the Medicare beneficiaries in the United States). Since the beginning of the first full year of the program, January 1986, the number of beneficiaries enrolled has grown steadily, to nearly three times its 1986 size. However, the number of active plans, after having grown rapidly from 71 to 134, has fallen by over one-third from that peak.[1]

The risk program currently includes a variety of plans whose enrollment size, model type, tax status, chain affiliation, market areas, and other characteristics are quite diverse. These differences could have significant effects on the efficiency of the HMOs and on the cost savings to HCFA. Table 1.1 displays the distribution of active risk plans (those that have enrolled members) and enrollments, for 1986 through 1992.

Current risk plans tend to be independent practice associations (IPAs) and for-profit organizations, and most have been enrolling Medicare members since 1988 or earlier. IPAs are HMOs that contract with individual physicians to provide services. Group model HMOs are those that contract with physician groups to provide services to enrollees; staff model HMOs hire their own physicians. IPA and group model plans typically have various financial incentives, based on utilization rates, to encourage physicians to practice cost-effective care; staff model plans pay their physicians a salary. IPAs comprise over half of the risk plans currently, but they account for only about 40 percent of total program enrollment. For-profit plans account for about 60 percent of both plans and enrollments. Plans in TEFRA since 1987 account for over 90 percent of total 1992 enrollments in the program.

Although risk plans are located in all areas of the country, they are most prevalent in the Pacific and Midwest regions. However, distribution of enrollments is much more skewed—the one-fourth of plans that are located on the West Coast account for over 45 percent of total enrollments, reflecting the much larger average size of these plans. The risk program is dominated by HMOs in two market areas that together have 12 plans and account for over 53 percent of total risk program enrollments. The three largest plans alone (all located in either Miami or Los Angeles) account for over one-third of total program enrollment.

Determination of payment rates

The most critical feature of the risk program for assessing its effects on cost or savings to HCFA is the payment methodology, the adjusted average per capita cost (AAPCC). The amount paid to HMOs each month for beneficiaries who enroll is determined based on the enrollees' age, sex, reason for entitlement (age or disability), place of residence (in a nursing home or not), Medicaid eligibility, and county of residence. The rate is arrived at by actuarial calculations performed by HCFA and provided to HMOs in the fall prior to the year the rates become effective. The calculations involve projecting the national average per capita reimbursement for Medicare-covered services (the USPCC or United States per capita cost), multiplying this rate by a geographic adjustment factor reflecting historic differences across counties in average reimbursements, and

Table 1.1   Characteristics of Active Medicare Risk Plans

Characteristic	Percent of Plans				Percent of Enrollment			
	1986*	1988	1990	1992	1986	1988	1990	1992
Total Number of Active Plans	71	122	94	81	71	122	94	81
Total Number of Enrollees					467,381	981,145	1,091,635	1,379,667
Model Type								
IPA	49.3	54.9	54.3	56.8	53.3	52.8	37.2	40.2
Group	26.8	29.5	30.9	27.2	32.2	35.0	26.9	23.7
Staff	23.9	15.6	14.9	16.0	14.5	12.1	36.0	36.1
Tax Status								
For-profit	43.7	38.0	52.1	58.0	54.1	40.1	58.1	63.7
Nonprofit	56.3	62.0	47.9	42.0	45.9	59.9	41.9	36.3
Region								
New England	15.5	13.1	9.6	7.4	8.2	6.5	4.1	3.6
Mid-Atlantic	11.3	13.1	11.7	11.1	4.4	6.2	7.2	6.4
South Atlantic	9.9	12.3	13.8	12.3	35.3	19.5	19.5	20.7
Midwest	35.2	32.0	25.5	21.0	30.9	29.5	17.2	11.7
South Central	4.2	6.6	7.5	9.9	0.3	0.7	1.7	3.2
Mountain	8.5	8.2	13.8	13.6	3.4	6.3	7.7	9.1
Pacific	15.5	14.8	18.1	24.7	17.6	31.3	42.6	45.3
Year Began Enrolling under TEFRA								
1985	91.6	41.0	38.3	34.6	98.9	64.1	63.4	61.6
1986	8.5	44.3	27.7	19.8	1.1	28.9	16.1	15.4
1987	NA‡	13.1	16.0	13.6	NA	6.7	14.4	14.4
1988	NA	1.6	12.8	13.6	NA	0.3	1.6	3.5
1989	NA	NA	2.1	1.2	NA	NA	3.8	3.1
1990	NA	NA	3.2	4.9	NA	NA	0.7	1.6
1991	NA	NA	0	11.1	NA	NA	0	0.5
1992	NA	NA	0	1.2	NA	NA	0	†

Source: Office of Prepaid Health Care, Monthly Medicare Prepaid Plan Reports, January 1986, January 1988, January 1990, and January 1992.

* Data for each year reflect the program experience as of January for active plans (those with enrollees).

†Less than 0.1 percent.

‡Not applicable.

finally multiplying by a demographic risk factor, reflecting the expected differences in reimbursements among beneficiaries who differ on the foregoing personal characteristics (see Palsbo 1989, for a more detailed explanation).

The AAPCC methodology has been criticized widely, for a number of reasons. The most serious problem with the AAPCC for generating savings for HCFA is that the demographic factors used to vary the capitation rate to HMOs for particular individuals fail to control adequately for differences in health care needs between those who enroll and those who remain in FFS. Eggers (1980), Eggers and Prihoda (1982), Brown (1988), and Hill and Brown (1990) have all shown that the AAPCC adjustment factors fail to explain fully the *pre-enrollment* differences in reimbursements between those who enroll in HMOs and those who do not. Other critiques of the AAPCC have focused on problems with the geographic adjusters, including (1) wide disparities among seemingly similar areas and even among adjacent counties within a metropolitan area, and (2) erratic movement of the AAPCC rates for counties from one year to the next. Data on nursing home residence and Medicaid eligibility variables have also been criticized as being inaccurate.

Expected effects of the risk program

As indicated earlier, HCFA's expectations were that (1) the Medicare risk program would save money for Medicare by paying HMOs 5 percent less than Medicare would have spent for Medicare, and (2) Medicare risk plans would reduce service use. The expectation, based on various studies of HMOs serving nonelderly members, was that HMOs would reduce hospital use by eliminating unnecessary admissions, shortening stays, and substituting less expensive types of care (office visits, prescription drugs, home health care, and skilled nursing facilities) for hospital care where possible. Reductions in hospital use were expected to arise from the incentive to control costs, from HMOs' proved ability to coordinate patient care, and from their emphasis on the use of preventive care to identify problems early. Because of the expected substitution effects of other services for hospital care, there were no clear expectations concerning whether total use of these other services would be increased or decreased by HMOs.

Evidence from the Literature

Previous evidence from the literature, including evaluations of the early demonstration programs for Medicare risk plans, suggests that HMOs do indeed reduce hospital use by reducing admissions and shortening lengths of stay, but other studies indicate that the Medicare risk program actually increases costs to Medicare rather than reducing them, despite paying only 95 percent of the estimate of what reimbursements would have been for enrollees under FFS. However, limitations of both types of prior studies (reviewed further on) prevent them from providing comprehensive and reliable answers to questions about the effects of the risk program. Further, a number of the studies were conducted prior to full implementation of Medicare's prospective payment system for hospital services, which shortened average lengths of stay for Medicare patients treated on a FFS basis.

Effects of HMOs on use of medical services

Virtually every study of HMOs, whether for the Medicare or non-Medicare population, has shown that HMOs decrease hospital use. Early studies of HMOs serving the non-Medicare population, reviewed by Luft (1981), showed reductions of 10 to 40 percent in hospital days. However, as Luft notes, many of these studies had limited data to control for possible differences in health status of HMO members and non-members, and thus the results may be biased. Two more recent studies provide somewhat stronger evidence of HMO effects on hospital use. Manning et al. (1984), using data on individuals who had been randomly assigned to HMO or non-HMO options, estimated that the HMO participating in the RAND Health Insurance Experiment reduced hospitalizations by 40 percent. However, the study included only one HMO, and the results may be biased due to the sizable rate of refusal to participate among those assigned to the HMO option (although the authors control for health status measures). Dowd et al. (1991) also have stronger control variables than earlier studies and use a more sophisticated econometric model to estimate that HMOs in the Minneapolis area reduced hospital days by about 30 percent. Only one study (Nelson and Brown 1989) has examined the effect of HMOs on hospital use for Medicare members. Using data from nine HMOs participating in the Medicare Competition Demonstrations, the authors estimated that hospital admissions were reduced by 14 to 28 percent relative to FFS levels. Again, however, very limited control variables were available, and the data on hospital use were obtained from different sources for the enrollee versus nonenrollee samples, which could also produce biased estimates.

While these studies have focused on total hospital days or admissions, two more recent studies (Stern et al. 1989, and Bradbury, Golec, and Stearns 1991) have investigated the effect of HMOs on hospital length of stay and have found that HMOs reduce stays by 14 percent on average. The results are noteworthy in that they show an HMO impact on length of stay after controlling for diagnosis, health risks, and severity of illness.

However, both are based on a small number of HMOs and hospitals. Other studies (Dowd, Johnson, and Madson 1986; Johnson et al. 1989; Yelin, Shearn, and Epstein 1986) show mixed results, with HMO patients having shorter lengths of stay for some diagnoses but not for others. All of these studies are based on the non-Medicare population.

Although the bulk of the evidence to date suggests that HMOs reduce hospital days through reductions in either admissions or length of stay, or both, the impact of HMOs in the current Medicare risk program may be considerably smaller. Rates of hospitalization and average lengths of stay among Medicare beneficiaries in the FFS sector declined during the 1980s (ProPAC 1991, 87–88), resulting in a decline of one-third in the number of hospital days per 1,000 beneficiaries between 1980 and 1989. The decline in length of stay is attributable at least in part to the introduction of PPS, which gives hospitals an incentive to reduce lengths of stay. Whatever the reason, the decline in hospital use rates in Medicare's FFS sector makes it more difficult for Medicare risk plans today to achieve reductions in hospital use of the magnitude estimated in some of these previous studies.

Studies of the effects of HMOs on use of physician services are much rarer, in part because the data are more difficult to obtain. Dowd et al. (1991) find no significant HMO effect on physician visits. McCombs, Kasper, and Riley (1990), in examining two of the Medicare Capitation Demonstration plans, found that one plan reduced Part B services substantially relative to Part B services provided by Medicare FFS providers, while the other increased these services by a large percentage. However, this study had very limited control variables to account for possible differences in health care needs between the HMO members and the FFS comparison group. To the extent that HMOs' reductions in hospital use are achieved by substituting outpatient care for inpatient services, there may be little savings in total resource use.

Finally, we are not aware of any studies of HMO effects on the use of home health services or skilled nursing facilities. For most HMOs, such estimates would be of little value, since non-Medicare members rarely need these services. However, interviews with Medicare risk plans suggest that for some plans, utilization rates of these services are among the biggest cost control problems that they face.

Effects of Medicare HMOs on costs

The relevant literature for estimating the savings or cost to HCFA of the risk program is that dealing with "biased selection." While not providing a direct measure of the costs or savings to HCFA, measures of the extent of biased selection provide some guidance concerning the likely direction and rough magnitude of savings. If beneficiaries who enroll in Medicare risk plans are healthier, after adjusting for demographic risk factors, than those on whom the reimbursement rates are based (the nonenrolled beneficiaries in the area), the HMO is said to have experienced favorable selection. If this occurs, the AAPCC will overestimate the FFS costs that would have been incurred for the enrollees, and HCFA will not realize the intended 5 percent savings. Favorable selection could occur either because beneficiaries who are in poor health may be less likely than healthy beneficiaries to be willing to change from their usual physician to an HMO physician, or because HMOs market in ways that attract (by design or chance) healthier than average beneficiaries (HMOs are not allowed to screen applicants). Conversely, if enrollees have poorer than average health, after accounting for differences in demographic risk factors, selection is said to be "adverse," and HMOs will receive even less than the intended 95 percent of the FFS costs that Medicare would have incurred. Adverse selection can occur if beneficiaries who are most in need of health care are attracted by the more comprehensive coverage offered by HMOs.

Previous evidence suggests that although a few Medicare risk plans have had adverse or neutral selection, the great majority experience favorable selection. Three types of measures of biased selection have been used in the literature, each involving a comparison of HMO enrollees to nonenrollees in the same geographic area, controlling for differences between the two groups on AAPCC risk factors: differences in pre-enrollment reimbursements, differences in mortality rates, and differences in self-reported health status measures. The most extensive and recent study of prior reimbursement differences was conducted by Hill and Brown (1990), who found that for the 98 Medicare risk plans with 1,000 or more enrollees in 1989, prior reimbursements for enrollees (weighted by length of time enrolled) were about 23 percent below the adjusted mean reimbursements for nonenrollees. The enrollee-nonenrollee difference was negative and significantly different from zero for nearly two-thirds of the plans. For the remaining one-third, only about six plans had enrollee-nonenrollee differences greater than zero, and none of these differences was statistically significant. These results were similar to those obtained by Brown (1988) for 17 demonstration plans and by Eggers and Prihoda (1982) for four of the earliest demonstration risk plans.

Mortality rate comparisons revealed differences of comparable magnitude. Both Brown (1988) and Riley, Lubitz, and Rabey (1991) found that mortality rates were 20 to 25 percent lower among beneficiaries enrolled in Medicare risk plans, after controlling for enrollee-nonenrollee differences in factors included in the AAPCC payment rate schedule.

Finally, Brown et al. (1986), Lichtenstein et al. (1989), and Hill and Brown (1992) all find that, at the time of enrollment, Medicare beneficiaries who enroll in risk plans are significantly more likely than nonenrollees to be able to perform routine daily activities without assistance, and are less likely to rate their health as poor. Enrollees also were less likely than nonenrollees to say that they worried more about their health than did other people their age.

Despite the decidedly consistent evidence that HMOs experience favorable selection, the previous studies suffer from a number of limitations and do not provide an estimate of the amount that the risk program costs or saves HCFA. All of the studies (except Hill and Brown 1992) suffer from the problem that they are based on predictors of enrollees' likely health care needs only at the time they enroll. These differences may disappear as enrollees "regress toward the mean" of all beneficiaries over time. That is, enrollees may join the HMO at a time when, as a group, they are healthier than average; but this group will later tend to have average health care needs much more similar to the overall average for beneficiaries. Under this argument, these differences between enrollees and nonenrollees overstate the differences between the groups that will exist after the beneficiary has been enrolled for a few years.[2] Mortality differences are less subject to this criticism, but fail to reflect differences in health status between enrollees and nonenrollees for the 95 percent of beneficiaries who do *not* die in a particular year. While enrollee-nonenrollee differences in the various measures are sufficiently large that regression toward the mean is unlikely to change the conclusion that the AAPCC overestimates the FFS cost that HCFA would have incurred, the estimates do probably overstate the error in the AAPCC.

Nelson and Brown (1989) provide the only direct measure of the savings or cost to HCFA for Medicare risk contracting, based on their findings for 17 Medicare Competition Demonstration plans. The authors estimate that HCFA paid 15 to 33 percent more in capitation payments than it would have paid in FFS reimbursements for enrollees during their first two years in a risk plan. However, these estimates were obtained by assuming that the ratio of enrollee to nonenrollee reimbursements during the pre-enrollment period for enrollees would have persisted during the two years after enrollment. Thus, these estimates also probably overestimate the cost to HCFA.

Data and Methodology

Estimates of the effects of the risk program on both costs and service use were obtained from regression analyses conducted on detailed survey data obtained on nearly 13,000 Medicare beneficiaries, about half of whom were enrolled in Medicare risk plans and half of whom did not enroll but resided in the same counties as enrollees. This large sample size was chosen in order to ensure a high probability of detecting effects on hospital admissions of 10 percent or larger (approximately the low end of the range of previous estimates of HMO effects on hospital use).

Sample and data used in the analysis

The analysis sample consists of 6,476 beneficiaries who were enrolled in a Medicare risk plan and 6,381 beneficiaries who did not enroll but resided in the same counties as enrollees. The enrollees were a random sample of all beneficiaries who (1) as of April 1, 1990, were enrolled in one of the 75 Medicare risk plans that contained 1,000 or more members at that time; (2) had been entitled to Medicare Part A and Part B for at least one year; and (3) had been enrolled for at least three months. These eligibility criteria encompassed about 88 percent of the total number of beneficiaries enrolled in Medicare risk plans as of April 1, 1990, according to HCFA's Group Health Plan Operations (GHPO) file of all beneficiaries ever enrolled in Medicare plans. Thus, the sample, equal to about 0.6 percent of all enrollees at that time, should be representative of Medicare risk plan members. Enrollees in small plans (1,000 to 7,500 members) were oversampled (a minimum sample size of 40 enrollees per plan was targeted), and those in the four largest plans were undersampled, so that the sample could be weighted to give equal representation either to each enrollee in the program or to each plan in the program without a significant loss in precision. Over half of the resulting enrollee sample had been enrolled in the Medicare risk plan for at least three years at the time of the interview; only 11 percent had been enrolled for less than one year.

The nonenrollee sample, selected from beneficiaries who were not members of an HMO between April 1989 and the date of interview, was drawn to match the distribution of enrollees across zip codes in the 44 market areas where the HMOs were operating. This design eliminated differences between the two groups that could arise from variations in practice patterns and service environment across regions or cities. Nonenrollees, like enrollees, were required to have been eligible for Medicare Part A and Part B for at least one year prior to the April 1990 start date of the survey.

The telephone survey, conducted between April and October 1990 for both groups, gathered data on the recent utilization of Medicare-covered services by sample members and on the characteristics that might affect their utilization. The latter included measures of health (their ability to perform routine activities, self-reported health status, and history of serious illness), access to care (income and insurance coverage), and propensity to use care (relative worry about health, inclination to avoid doctors, and having a usual place of care). Utilization measures included dates of hospital and nursing home admissions during the year preceding the interview, lengths of stay, number of visits to physicians during the past one month, three months, and twelve months, and number of home visits by nurses and home health aides during the three months preceding the interview. Survey data on sample members were supplemented with Medicare claims data for 1989 for nonenrollees, and with HCFA data on sample member deaths during the nine-month period subsequent to the interview.

The survey data reveal many significant differences between enrollees and nonenrollees (Table 1.2). Enrollees are younger, and much less likely to reside in a nursing home, to be disabled, or to be on Medicaid—all characteristics for which AAPCC rates are lower. However, enrollees also are much healthier on every other measure of health status, and they indicate a lower propensity than nonenrollees to seek care (worry less about health, more likely to avoid doctors, less likely to have had a usual place for care prior to enrolling).[3] Enrollees also have significantly lower average incomes (about 12 percent less), however, suggesting that they may have had less access to health care than nonenrollees if they had not joined the HMO.

The mean values for several characteristics of nonenrollees show a close match with national estimates from other sources, increasing our confidence in the quality and representativeness of the data. For example, 73 percent of nonenrollees have Medigap coverage, 5 to 6 percent reside in nursing homes, and about 5 percent died within the nine months following the interview (or between the April 1 sampling date and the date a proxy respondent completed the interview in their stead). Nine percent say that their health is poor, consistent with data from the National Health Insurance Survey. The survey also finds that nearly one-third of beneficiaries have a history of serious illness (cancer, heart disease, or stroke), and that over 91 percent have a usual place of care.

Methodology

Our most reliable estimates of program effects on both costs and utilization were obtained from simple regression and probit models. More sophisticated econometric methods were tested but yielded estimates that were either very unstable or very similar to those of the simpler models.

Table 1.2   Beneficiary Characteristics Included in Models Predicting FFS Costs and Utilization (All Variables Are Binary except Income and Number of Impairments)

	Enrollee Mean	Nonenrollee Mean	Enrollee-Nonenrollee Difference
AAPCC Risk Indicators			
Disabled (under age 65)	.028	.077	−.050***
Ages 65–69	.227	.217	.010
Age 70–74	.309	.270	.039***
Age 75–80	.223	.188	.034***
Age 80–84	.129	.134	−.005
Age ≥ 85	.085	.114	−.028***
Male	.442	.417	.025***
Medicaid	.024	.093	−.070***
Nursing home resident	.018	.058	−.040***
Health Status			
Poor health	.058	.095	−.037***
Number of impairments on activities of daily living	.130	.307	−.178***
Number of impairments on instrumental activities of daily living	.673	1.101	−.428***
History of cancer, heart disease, or stroke	.276	.329	−.053***
Died within nine months of interview date	.046	.054	−.008*
Preferences for Seeking Care			
Worry about personal health more than others	.178	.211	−.033***
Avoid doctor if a problem arises	.274	.256	.018***
Have a usual place of care (prior to enrollment for enrollees)	.850	.914	−.063***
Medigap Coverage	NA	.723	NA
Other Personal Characteristics			
Race (percent not white)	.079	.069	.010**
Income	$17,679	$20,148	−$2,469***
Education			
College degree	.120	.155	−.035***
High school graduate, no college degree	.557	.561	−.004*
Sample Size	6,475	6,107	

*Significantly different from zero at the .10 level, two-tailed test.
**Significantly different from zero at the .05 level, two-tailed test.
***Significantly different from zero at the .01 level, two-tailed test.

Estimating impacts on service use

Impacts of the Medicare risk program on the following survey measures of utilization were obtained: number and probability of hospital admissions, hospital days, number of physician visits, probability of frequent visits, probability of having a SNF (skilled nursing facility) stay and having home health visits, and the number of SNF days and home health visits. These services are the principal types of care covered by Medicare.

To estimate the impacts, these outcome variables were regressed on all but one of the control variables included in Table 1.2, plus a binary variable equal to 1 for enrollees and 0 for nonenrollees. Market area characteristics for the city in which the beneficiary resided were also included, to capture differences in practice patterns and service availability across areas (physicians per capita, hospital beds per capita, etc.). The only variable in Table 1.2 that was excluded from the model was the Medigap coverage indicator, because we wish to compare the utilization of HMO members to that of *all* beneficiaries in FFS (since some but not all enrollees would have purchased Medigap coverage had they not enrolled in the HMO). For binary outcome measures (for example, whether admitted to a hospital), probit models were used to estimate impacts. For other outcomes, ordinary regression models were used initially.

Two problems with these specifications were that (1) all of the utilization variables were truncated at zero, and (2) HMO enrollment may be endogenous. HMO enrollment is endogenous if there were unmeasured beneficiary characteristics that influenced both actual service use and the likelihood of being enrolled in a risk plan, such as strength of tie to a particular physician. If such factors exist and are not captured by our included variables, our estimates of HMO effects will be biased. The fact that the utilization variables are truncated at zero indicates that a Tobit model or other method of dealing with such variables should be used to avoid negative predicted values. Thus, other models were investigated to account for these potential problems.

A model to control for potential bias due to self-selection. Maddala's (1983) variant on Heckman's (1978, 1979) selection bias correction procedure was first used to assess whether the estimate from the simple models was biased by self-selection of beneficiaries into and out of HMOs. Under this method, a probit model was first estimated to predict the probability of being enrolled in an HMO, given beneficiaries' personal characteristics and two additional identifying variables: the number of Medicare risk plans in the market area and the average premium charged by these plans. The probit coefficients were then used to construct an additional variable (λ) for each sample member, equal to a constant times the conditional expected value of the error term in the utilization equation, given that the individual chose to enroll or not enroll:

$$\lambda = f(xb)/F(xb) \qquad \text{for enrollees,}$$

$$= -f(xb)/[1 - F(xb)] \quad \text{for nonenrollees,}$$

where x is the set of explanatory variables in the probit enrollment model, b is the estimated probit coefficients, $f(xb)$ is the normal density function, and $F(xb)$ is the normal cumulative distribution function (the predicted probability of being in an HMO), both evaluated at the point xb. The new variable λ was then included as an additional regressor in separate utilization equations estimated for enrollees and nonenrollees. Inclusion of the additional term in the utilization equations eliminates any (asymptotic) bias in our estimates due to correlation between the disturbance terms in the enrollment decision and utilization equations. Tests of the statistical significance of the coefficients on the λ term provide evidence concerning whether such correlation, if any, is large enough to create serious bias in our estimates.[4]

Estimates of the model, including the selection bias term, suggested that estimates from the simpler model are not biased by self-selection of beneficiaries (see Hill et al. 1992, for details). The probit model of enrollment contained a number of statistically significant coefficients, including those on the two variables assumed to influence enrollment but not utilization. Thus, the model is identified. However, we could not reject the hypothesis that the coefficients of the λ terms in both enrollee and nonenrollee equations were equal to zero. Furthermore, addition of the selection bias terms had little effect on the coefficients on the other explanatory variables. Thus, we concluded that our estimates from the basic model are not biased by beneficiaries' selection of HMO or FFS care. This finding is likely due to the detailed set of health status and attitudinal variables that are included in the regression model and are found to be highly significant. These variables appear to have captured any important differences between enrollees and nonenrollees that could create bias. However, it is also possible that the model of HMO enrollment provides too little variance in predicted probabilities to capture any biases, despite the statistically significant identifying variables.

Truncation of the utilization variables at zero. The second potential problem with the simple regression model, failure to take into account the truncation at zero of the utilization measures, could also lead to invalid or inefficient estimates of program effects. To investigate this issue we reestimated the utilization equations for the number of hospital and SNF admissions, the number of visits to a physician, and the number of visits by home health nurses and aides, using the two-part model and "smearing" adjustment developed by Duan et al. (1983). Under this model, a probit equation is first estimated to predict the probability of any service use, followed by a regression model to predict the amount of the service used, conditional upon use being greater than zero. The expected value of utilization for any individual is then constructed as the product of the predicted probability of having some use and the predicted amount of use, conditional upon use being greater than zero. The regression model is typically estimated with the dependent variable expressed in logarithmic form, in order to better represent the usually skewed distribution of service use or costs and to reduce the influence of inordinately large values on the results.

Again we found results that are similar to those obtained from our simpler regression models, with one exception. The predicted effect on SNF days was markedly closer to zero when the two-part model was used (−1.3 percent) than in the basic model (−24.4 percent). However, in neither case was the estimated effect statistically significant. Thus, we chose to rely on the simpler regression model estimates for our basic findings, given their greater simplicity and ease of obtaining standard errors (see Hill et al. 1992, for estimates and further explanation).

Models for estimating impacts on cost to HCFA

To estimate risk program effects on costs to HCFA we first estimated a FFS reimbursement equation on *nonenrollees* in the sample, then used it with *enrollee* characteristics to project the average reimbursement per enrollee that HCFA would have paid for these individuals had they remained in the FFS sector. We then compared this estimate to a projected average AAPCC capitation payment for the enrollees.

Predicting fee-for-service reimbursements for enrollees. To estimate the amount that HCFA would have reimbursed providers for services to enrollees had the enrollees not joined a risk plan, we first regress Medicare reimbursements for 1989 on characteristics of the beneficiaries (those contained in Table 1.1) and a set of binary site variables for the 44 market areas, using only the sample of nonenrollees (since reimbursement data do not exist for enrollees). Separate regressions are estimated for Part A and Part B reimbursements.

Mean values for enrollees on each characteristic were then inserted into the estimated equation to obtain the hypothetical FFS reimbursements for enrollees had they stayed in FFS. It was necessary, however, to estimate the value for two of the enrollee characteristics before constructing means—whether the enrollee would have had Medigap coverage and whether he or she would have had a usual source of care—since these characteristics were obviously not observed. We obtained these values by estimating probit models for these two characteristics as functions of other beneficiary characteristics, using data for nonenrollees; then we obtained predicted probabilities for each enrollee from the estimated models. Hill et al. (1992) provides the estimates of these models.

Alternative models tested. As we did for the utilization models, alternative models were estimated to determine whether a correction for selection bias was required and whether the two-part model provided better estimates of costs than our simpler regression model. We again found that the selection bias term for nonenrollees was not statistically significant in the reimbursement regression. Furthermore, including the appropriate selection bias term when projecting reimbursements for enrollees yielded estimates that were obviously not credible.[5] Hence, we concluded that the estimates from the ordinary least squares regression model were superior.

The two-part model estimated on the nonenrollee sample was also found to be inferior to the basic regression model. This assessment was based on simulations performed with the estimated model, which showed that it frequently overpredicted reimbursements for the test samples by sizable margins. Because the ordinary least squares regression model performed much better in these simulations, we rely on that model in projecting what FFS reimbursements would have been for enrollees.

Methodology for predicting payments. Finally, to estimate the savings or costs to HCFA, we compared the projected FFS reimbursements for enrollees to what HCFA paid in capitation rates. However, it was necessary to estimate these capitation payments rather than use the actual amount paid, because the FFS reimbursement projections were based on a model estimated for the year prior to interview, when all of the nonenrollees were alive (HCFA data on reimbursements for 1990 were found to be incomplete). Thus, comparing AAPCC payments, which are designed to reflect the average cost to HCFA for all beneficiaries (including those who will die during the year), to projections based on reimbursements for only the survivors would greatly overstate the cost (or understate the savings) of the program. Hence, we estimate a capitation payment model by regressing reimbursements for nonenrollees on the AAPCC factors and site indicators only, then use this model to project the implicit AAPCC capitation payment for enrollees, based on their risk indicator variables.

This approach—estimating capitation payments—has two additional advantages over using actual payments, even if this option were feasible. The first advantage is that the actual capitation payment could be a poor estimate of actual reimbursements for the particular sample of nonenrollees that we have or for the particular year (1989) that we are examining, even though it has been found to predict average FFS reimbursements nationally with reasonable accuracy in most years (Gruenberg, Pomeranz, and Porrell 1988). In this case, differences between capitation payments and projected FFS reimbursements would not provide an estimate of costs to HCFA that is representative of the "typical" situation. AAPCC projections are likely to have been especially prone to error for 1989, because the Medicare Catastrophic Coverage Act had just gone into effect and projected effects of the expanded coverage on Medicare costs were likely to have been inaccurate. By estimating the capitation equation using ordinary least squares with binary variables for site, we are implicitly assuming that the AAPCC correctly predicts the average reimbursement for the nonenrollees in each market area, as it is intended to do. Any difference between predicted FFS reimbursement and predicted capitation payments for enrollees, both based on the equations estimated on nonenrollees, must then be due solely to failure of the AAPCC factors to account for other characteristics that influence Medicare reimbursements, and not to errors for the particular year examined or for the particular set of nonenrollees sampled.

This feature of using an estimated AAPCC rate generates the second advantage to this approach: the ability to identify exactly *why* the AAPCC overpays or underpays HMOs for the persons enrolled. Unlike impact estimates obtained by comparing a "treatment" group to a "control" group, in which the effect is essentially any between-group difference in the outcome measure that cannot be explained away by the statistical model and available control variables, the impact under our approach is due to observable characteristics and the effects of these characteristics on Medicare reimbursements. That is, our FFS reimbursement equation is simply:

$$Y = X_a b_a + X_o b_o + u \qquad (1)$$

and our capitation equation is:

$$Y = X_a c_a + e \qquad (2)$$

where Y is 1989 Medicare reimbursements,[6] X_a contains the variables included in the AAPCC rate structure (including binary site variables),[7] and X_o contains the "other" variables from our survey that are likely to affect Medicare reimbursements but are not incorporated in the AAPCC. Enrollees mean values for X_a and X_o are substituted into these two equations to obtain predicted FFS reimbursements and predicted capitation payments (.95 times the predicted AAPCC rate), with the difference between the two estimates measuring savings or costs to HCFA. The savings or costs are determined only by the estimated coefficients and the characteristics of enrollees. As we shall see further on, the total difference between the predicted capitation payment and predicted FFS reimbursement can be allocated among the variables in X_o, based solely on their effects on reimbursements (b_0) and the failure of the X_a variables to capture the differences between enrollees and nonenrollees on these X_o variables.

The Impacts of the Risk Program on the Use of Services

We first examine program effects on hospital use, since that is the most costly service provided and the one that HMOs typically cite as the most critical to control in order to prosper. We then examine impacts on physician visits, home health use, and SNF use.[8]

Estimated effects on hospital use

HMOs did not reduce rates of hospitalization, but did reduce the number of hospital days (and average length of stay) by about 17 percent, from a projected value of 1,839 to the observed 1,530 days per 1,000 member years (Table 1.3). This finding that HMOs have no impact on the hospitalization rate contrasts with the sizable reductions found in previous studies of the impacts of HMOs on hospital use among the non-Medicare population, and with the few studies on the Medicare population. However, as noted earlier, these previous studies were subject to serious weaknesses, due to the limited data on characteristics of enrollees and nonenrollees for use as control variables, or were for an earlier time period. Our estimated impact of HMOs on the hospital admission rate would be much larger and statistically significant (2.7 percentage points, or about 15 percent of the mean) if we used only AAPCC factors as control variables, rather than our more comprehensive set of characteristics (not shown here; see Hill et al. 1992, 110). Furthermore, general medical practice has responded to financial incentives to eliminate discretionary hospital admissions, which is not reflected in earlier studies of HMO impacts. Admission rates for Medicare FFS patients declined by 25 percent between 1985 and 1989. Thus, the ability of HMOs to secure further reductions in admission rates may be quite limited for Medicare members and perhaps non-Medicare members as well.

Table 1.3   Estimated HMO Impacts on Hospital Use

	Sample Size (Enrollees/ Nonenrollees)	Enrollee Mean	Nonenrollee Mean	Unadjusted Enrollee- Nonenrollee Difference	HMO Impact
Probability of one or more hospitalizations	6,457/6,071	0.150	0.186	−0.036*** (19.4)†	−0.009 (−5.7)
Hospital stays/1,000 beneficiaries	6,457/6,071	218	269	−51** (19.0)	6 (2.8)
Hospital days per 1,000 beneficiaries	6,457/6,071	1,530	2,490	−960*** (38.6)	−309* (−16.8)
Average length of stay	969/1,117	7.25	9.46	−2.21*** (23.4)	−1.44* (−16.6)

*Significantly different from zero at the .10 level, two-tailed test.
**Significantly different from zero at the .05 level, two-tailed test.
***Significantly different from zero at the .01 level, two-tailed test.
†The numbers in parentheses are HMO impacts expressed as a percent of the expected service use for enrollees had they remained in the FFS sector, which we estimate here by the enrollee mean for service use in the HMO sector minus the HMO impact. Thus, for hospital days per 1,000 beneficiaries, we have $-309/(1,530 - [-309]) = -.168$, or −16.8 percent. Impacts on the probability of a hospital admission were estimated with a probit model. Impacts on other outcome measures were estimated using ordinary least squares.

The 17 percent reduction in hospital days and average length of stay is quite consistent with recent findings in the literature for the non-Medicare population (14 percent reductions cited in Stern et al. 1989, and Bradbury, Golec, and Stearns 1991), and with our findings from examination of hospital records for stroke and colon cancer patients (18 and 23 percent reductions, respectively) for the quality-of-care component of our evaluation of the Medicare risk program (Retchin et al. 1992). The reduction in hospital length of stay is particularly impressive, given the incentives under Medicare's prospective payment system to shorten stays in the FFS sector.

Effects on use of physician services

In contrast to the effects on hospital use (but consistent with expectations and previous estimates), HMOs *increased* the proportion of beneficiaries receiving some physician services but *decreased* the proportion receiving extensive services. Medicare risk plans increased the likelihood of having at least one visit to a physician during the year by about five percentage points (from 84 to 89 percent). Enrollees were also six percentage points more likely to have received a physical examination in the past year than were comparable nonenrollees (Table 1.4). However, enrollees were significantly less likely to report frequent visits to a physician (12 or more a year). The results are consistent with the financial incentives facing both enrollees and HMO physicians. In most Medicare risk plans, beneficiaries face little or no copayment for primary care visits, and are typically offered preventive care as part of their benefit package. Thus, because enrollees face few or no financial barriers to receiving care from their primary care physicians, we would expect that they would be more likely to have some physician visits than would nonenrollees. However, HMO physicians—in particular, those under capitation or profit sharing—have a financial incentive to reduce the number of visits per patient and to see more patients. Thus, we observe no difference in the average number of visits in the past month (about 0.6 visits per beneficiary) and a small but statistically significant reduction in the proportion of beneficiaries with frequent visits (one or more per month on average).

Impacts on skilled nursing facility and home health care use

HMO effects on the use of SNF and home health care are consistent with the general pattern of equal or greater access to services but lower intensity of utilization.

1. Medicare risk plans increase the likelihood of receiving care in a SNF but not the number of days.

Medicare risk plans increased the likelihood of receiving care in a skilled nursing facility by 0.3 percentage points (Table 1.5). This increase is statistically significant and large in percentage terms but small in absolute magnitude, since only 0.8 percent of enrollees in the sample received care in a SNF over the past year. The estimate is consistent with the expectation that HMOs may reduce the length of stay in an acute care hospital by substituting SNF care for inpatient care. However, HMOs deliver the same or *fewer* SNF *days* per beneficiary: the estimated effect is negative but not statistically significant. This result, as with the results for physician visits, suggests that HMOs increase the frequency of SNF use but reduce the intensity of use.

2. Enrollees are equally likely to receive home health care as comparable nonenrollees, but have fewer visits overall.

HMOs have no impact on the likelihood that HMO enrollees receive home care by a skilled nurse, therapist, or home health aide (Table 1.5).

Table 1.4 Estimated Effects on Physician Visits

	Enrollee Mean	Nonenrollee Mean	Enrollee-Nonenrollee Difference	HMO Impact
Whether had one or more visits, past four weeks	.335	.345	−.010	.019** (6.2)
Number of visits, past four weeks	.596	.690	−.106***	.026 (4.6)
Whether have at least occasional doctor visits (1 or more a year)	.889	.876	.013	.052*** (6.2)
Whether have at least periodic doctor visits (3 or more a year)	.584	.582	.002	.060*** (11.5)
Whether have frequent doctor visits (12 or more a year)	.126	.181	−.055***	−.016** (−11.4)
Whether had physical exam, last year	.704	.682	.022***	.058*** (9.0)

*Significantly different from zero at the .10 level, two-tailed test.
**Significantly different from zero at the .05 level, two-tailed test.
***Significantly different from zero at the .01 level, two-tailed test.
†The numbers in parentheses are HMO impacts expressed as a percent of the expected service use for enrollees had they remained in the FFS sector, which we estimate here by the enrollee mean for service use in the HMO sector minus the HMO impact. Sample sizes range from 6,384 to 6,427 for enrollees and from 6,013 to 6,028 for nonenrollees.

However, enrollees received 50 percent fewer home health visits from either nurses or aides than did comparable nonenrollees. The results suggest that Medicare risk plans are not substituting home health care visits for acute care hospital days, although it is possible that such substitution does occur but that the increase is offset by reductions in home health admissions for other cases. The large reduction in visits per recipient may be due in part to HMOs not matching the rapid increase in home health visits per episode that occurred in the FFS sector during 1989. Between 1987 and 1990, the number of home health visits per episode of care nearly doubled in the FFS sector, due to a change in the interpretation of Medicare rules (see Brown et al. 1992). HMOs may not have fully adapted to this change by 1989, or may not view the expanded use as necessary, in most cases, for adequate patient care.

Table 1.5   Estimated Impacts on SNF Days and Home Health Visits

	Enrollee Mean	Nonenrollee Mean	Enrollee-Nonenrollee Difference	HMO Impact
Percent with one or more SNF stay last year	0.8	0.8	0.0	0.3** (74.0)
Number of SNF days per 1,000 beneficiaries	464	863	−399***	−150 (−24.4)
Percent with one or more home health visit, past three months	2.2	3.8	−1.6***	−0.3 (−11.8)
Total number of home health visits per 1,000 beneficiaries, past three months	408	1,324	−916***	−471*** (−53.6)
Percent with one or more home visit by a nurse or therapist, past three months	2.0	3.2	−1.2***	−0.2 (−7.2)
Total number of home visits, by nurse or therapist per 1,000 beneficiaries, past three months	209	626	−417***	−209** (−50.0)
Percent with one or more home visit by an aide, past three months	0.8	1.9	−1.1***	−0.4* (−30.5)
Number of home visits by aide, per 1,000 beneficiaries, past three months	209	767	−558***	−276*** (−56.9)

*Significant at the .10 level, two-tailed test.
**Significant at the .05 level, two-tailed test.
***Significant at the .01 level, two-tailed test.
†The numbers in parentheses are HMO impacts expressed as a percent of the expected service use for enrollees had they remained in the FFS sector, which we estimate here by the enrollee mean for service use in the HMO sector minus the HMO impact. Sample sizes range from 6,350 to 6,408 for enrollees and from 5,727 to 5,848 for nonenrollees.

Impacts of the Risk Program on Costs to HCFA

Two models were estimated to assess the effects of the risk program on costs to HCFA—one to project what FFS reimbursements would have been for enrollees and one to predict the AAPCC capitation payment for enrollees. Separate reimbursement and capitation equations were estimated for Part A and Part B using the nonenrollee sample, then used to project values for the enrollee sample. Impacts were then disaggregated to determine the sources of the costs or savings.

Projecting FFS reimbursements for enrollees

The estimated reimbursement equations for Part A and B explained only a small fraction of the variance in the Medicare reimbursements of nonenrollees ($R^2 = .06$ for Part A, .11 for Part B), as is typical for models of Medicare reimbursement (Thomas and Lichtenstein 1986a,b; Whitmore et al. 1989; Ellis and Ash 1988), but a number of variables were found to have large and statistically significant effects in the expected direction (see Appendix 1A for coefficient estimates). The coefficients on all five of the health status measures from the survey were statistically significant for Part B reimbursements, and four of the five were significant for Part A reimbursements. Coefficients on whether the individual died in the nine months following the interview and whether there was a history of serious illness (cancer, heart disease, or stroke) were especially large. Measures of attitudes toward health and health care also had significant effects on reimbursements: those who worried about their health problems more than most people had much higher reimbursements than the overall average (by about 50 percent), whereas those who said they avoided doctors whenever possible had reimbursements that were 20 percent lower than average. Beneficiaries with a usual place of care also had much higher than average Part A and Part B reimbursements.

Medigap coverage led to higher than average Part B reimbursements but did not affect Part A reimbursements. Socioeconomic variables (income, education, race) had little effect, as expected. Reimbursements tended to increase with certain AAPCC factors (age, Medicaid eligibility, nursing home residence), as expected, but the patterns were somewhat erratic due to the availability of detailed data on health status and modest sample sizes for some cells.

To predict FFS reimbursements for enrollees from these estimated equations it was necessary first to predict whether they would have had Medigap coverage and a usual source of care, as noted earlier. Using the models for these characteristics estimated on nonenrollees, we predicted that 76 percent of enrollees would have purchased Medigap coverage, slightly higher than the 72 percent of nonenrollees with such coverage, and that 92 percent of enrollees (versus 91 percent of nonenrollees) would have had a usual source of care. The higher predicted proportion of enrollees that would have purchased Medigap coverage is due to the much lower proportions of enrollees who had Medicaid coverage or who were disabled, both characteristics associated with a low probability of having Medigap coverage. The proportion of enrollees predicted to have had a usual place of care is higher than the 85 percent who said they had a usual place before enrolling, but lower than the 100 percent who have a usual place as a member of an HMO. Thus, the estimates seem reasonable for these characteristics.

Inserting enrollee mean values for the explanatory variables into the estimated FFS reimbursement equations yielded an estimated average reimbursement of $2,344 for enrollees had they remained in FFS, about 17 percent less than the actual mean reimbursements for the nonenrollees ($2,811). Predicted reimbursements were $1,213 for Part A and $1,131 for Part B.

Estimated capitation payments for enrollees and effects on HCFA costs

The capitation equation was obtained by regressing Part A and Part B Medicare reimbursements for nonenrollees on the AAPCC risk factors only (including site dummies), a subset of the regressors used in the reimbursement equation. Without the more detailed survey characteristics, the percent of variance explained dropped to about 2 percent for Part A and 4 percent for Part B, about one-third of the value of the R^2 statistics obtained for the full cost model. These low estimates of the percent of variance explained by the AAPCC risk factors are comparable to (or slightly higher than) estimates obtained by other authors (Hornbrook 1984; Anderson et al. 1986; Thomas and Lichtenstein 1986a,b). The coefficients in general follow the expected pattern, increasing with age, Medicaid coverage, and nursing home residence.

Inserting mean values on these explanatory variables for enrollees into the estimated equations, we project that the average AAPCC rate for the enrolled individuals would have been $2,608. Multiplying by .95 to reflect the payment rate formula, we estimate that capitation payments would have been $2,478.

Comparing these estimates to the projected FFS costs (Table 1.6) shows that HCFA paid HMOs about 5.7 percent more per beneficiary per year than would have been paid in reimbursements for these individuals had they received their Medicare-covered care on a FFS basis. Over three-fourths of the $134 overpayment is for Part A services, for which payments exceeded projected FFS costs by 8.5 percent. Capitation payments for Part B services exceeded projected FFS costs by only 2.7 percent. Thus, rather than saving 5 percent on the risk program, HCFA is losing over 5 percent.

Table 1.6   Comparison of Average Annual Predicted Capitation
Payments (AAPCC) and Predicted FFS Reimbursements per
Enrollee, 1989

	Time Period		
	Part A	*Part B*	*Total*
Predicted* AAPCC, AAPCC model†	$1,385	$1,223	$2,608
Predicted capitation payments, 95 percent of predicted AAPCC	$1,316	$1,162	$2,478
Predicted FFS reimbursements‡	$1,213	$1,131	$2,344
Difference between predicted capitation and predicted FFS reimbursement	$103	$31	$134
Percent difference between predicted capitation and predicted FFS reimbursement	8.5%	2.7%	5.7%

*Predicted reimbursements and capitation payments were obtained for the sample of
6,475 enrollees.

†Capitation payments were imputed for enrollees from a regression model estimated on
nonenrollees, with Medicare reimbursements (plus pass-through and administrative costs)
as the dependent variable and AAPCC risk classifications and binary site variables as the
independent variables. Capitation was computed for each enrollee as 95 percent of the
predicted AAPCC from this model.

‡FFS reimbursements were imputed for enrollees from a regression model estimated on
nonenrollees with Medicare reimbursement (plus pass-through and administrative costs)
as the dependent variable and the full list of independent variables in Table 1.2, plus site
characteristics. FFS reimbursements were predicted for each enrollee in the sample, based
on the enrollee's predicted probabilities of having Medigap coverage and having a usual
source of care, and the enrollee's actual values for all other variables.

Sources of overpayment

The overpayment by HCFA is due to favorable selection—beneficiaries
who enroll in HMOs need and desire less care on average than beneficiaries who do not enroll—and these differences are only partially captured
by the factors included in the AAPCC payment formula (average reimbursements for nonenrollees are $467 greater than the projected FFS
reimbursements for enrollees; the AAPCC adjustments explain only $203,
or 43 percent of this difference). If we can determine which differences
between enrollees and nonenrollees account for the failure to correctly
predict reimbursements, it may be possible to identify feasible ways to
reduce or eliminate the overpayment.

Our straightforward regression models for FFS reimbursements
and AAPCC capitation payments provide a simple and intuitive way

to identify these differences. Recall from our discussion of the methodology for predicting payments that the capitation equation is a restricted version of the FFS cost equation. The difference between the average projected AAPCC payment for enrollees (from Equation 2) and the average projected FFS reimbursement that HCFA would have paid out for them (from Equation 1) can be written as:

$$\hat{Y}^e_{AAPCC} - \hat{Y}^e_{FFS} = \bar{X}^e_A \hat{c}_a - (\bar{X}^e_a \hat{b}_a + \bar{X}^e_o \hat{b}_o) \tag{3}$$
$$= \bar{X}^e_a (\hat{c}_a - \hat{b}_a) - \bar{X}^e_o \hat{b}_o$$

A convenient property of regression analysis enables us to convert this expression into one that is solely a function of the more detailed survey characteristics (X_o) that are not part of the AAPCC formula. Because the capitation equation is a "shortened" version of the "full" FFS reimbursement model, the coefficients $\hat{c}_a$ from the short regression can be shown to be exactly equal to the coefficients on these same variables in the full regression plus an additional term that is a function of the coefficients on the X_o variables that appear only in the full regression:

$$c_a = (X'_a X_a)^{-1} X'_a Y \tag{4}$$
$$= (X'_a X_a)^{-1} X'_a (X_a \hat{b}_a + X_o \hat{b}_o + \hat{u})$$
$$= \hat{b}_a + (X'_a X_a)^{-1} X'_a X_o \hat{b}_o$$
$$= \hat{b}_a + P_{ao} \hat{b}_o$$

Each column of matrix P_{ao} is a vector of regression coefficients from the "auxiliary" regression of the corresponding new survey variables (X_o) on the set of characteristics incorporated in the AAPCC risk adjustment (X_a).

If we insert the expression for $\hat{c}_a$ from Equation 4 into Equation 3 we find:

$$\hat{Y}^e_{AAPCC} - \hat{Y}^e_{FFS} = \bar{X}^e_a (\hat{c}_a - \hat{b}_a) - \bar{X}^e_o \hat{b}_o \tag{5}$$
$$= \bar{X}^e_a (\hat{b}_a + P_{ao} \hat{b}_o - \hat{b}_a) - \bar{X}^e_o \hat{b}_o$$
$$= \bar{X}^e_a P_{ao} \hat{b}_o - \bar{X}^e_o \hat{b}_o$$
$$= (\hat{X}^e_o - \bar{X}^e_o) \hat{b}_o$$

where $\hat{X}^e_o = \bar{X}^e_a P_{ao}$, the average predicted value of the detailed survey characteristics for enrollees, obtained from a regression of these characteristics on the AAPCC risk factors $(X_a X_a)$ for nonenrollees. That is, the difference between the average AAPCC capitation and the average projected FFS reimbursement that would have been incurred for enrollees is equal to the product of the error in predicting the mean of the X_o variables from the X_a variables (using the auxiliary regressions) and the coefficients on these X_o's from the full FFS reimbursement regression (Equation 1). The predicted values of the X_o variables for enrollees are obtained by inserting mean values for X_a for enrollees into the auxiliary regressions, which were estimated on the nonenrollees.

The interpretation of these results is straightforward and appealing; it enables us to identify exactly which characteristics of enrollees account for the cost increases to HCFA. If $\hat{b}_o$ for some characteristic (income, etc.) is zero—that is, the characteristic has no effect on FFS reimbursements—then enrollee values on this characteristic, which is not included in the AAPCC formula, have no effect on costs to HCFA. Conversely, even if the characteristic does affect FFS reimbursements, if the AAPCC factors are able to predict this excluded characteristic reasonably well on average, having excluded it from the capitation formula will not result in AAPCC rates that are too high or too low. This feature of our estimates is consistent with the concept behind the AAPCC. If the characteristics included in the AAPCC rate structure are good proxies on average for other characteristics that are difficult to measure, the AAPCC will be an accurate projection of the costs that would have been incurred for enrollees under FFS care, and HCFA will save the intended 5 percent. The poorer the ability of AAPCC risk indicators to capture the effects of excluded characteristics, and the more important these characteristics are for determining Medicare reimbursements, the larger the gap is likely to be between the AAPCC and the costs that would have been incurred under FFS coverage.

There are actually two other ways that the impact of risk contracting on costs to HCFA would be equal to zero. If enrollees had the same unadjusted mean values for X_a and X_o as nonenrollees, or if the *auxiliary relationships* (the P_{ao}) between X_a and X_o were identical for enrollees and nonenrollees, we would observe no effect on costs to HCFA for enrollees. These conditions are also appealing: if enrollees looked like nonenrollees on average, there would be no biased selection and we would expect HCFA to save 5 percent as intended (assuming the AAPCC accurately projects cost for *nonenrollees*). Alternatively, if the relationship between AAPCC characteristics and other personal characteristics were identical for enrollees and nonenrollees, the AAPCC characteristics would fully account for the observed differences in means in these other characteristics (see Hill et al. 1992, for details).

None of the four conditions that would lead to no effect on costs to HCFA are satisfied:

- Many of the coefficients (b_o) on survey variables that are not used in AAPCC rate determination are large and significantly different from zero (see Appendix 1A).

- The AAPCC factors fail to predict accurately the values of the other survey variables.
- The unadjusted means for enrollees on X_o and X_a are quite different from the unadjusted means for nonenrollees (see Table 1.2).
- The relationship of AAPCC factors to beneficiary characteristics from the survey is quite different for enrollees and nonenrollees (see Hill and Brown 1992).

Therefore, it is not surprising to find that the AAPCC rate for enrollees exceeds what their FFS reimbursements would have been, by 11 percent.

The estimates we obtain from the decomposition given in Equation 5 show that 83 percent of the observed difference between the average AAPCC rate projected for enrollees ($2,608) and the average FFS reimbursement that would have been incurred for them ($2,344) is due to the effects of health status variables that are not captured by the AAPCC risk indicators. As Table 1.7 shows, the number of ADL impairments; numbers of IADL impairments; a history of heart disease, cancer, or stroke; and a self-rating of health as "poor" all contributed substantially to the increase in costs to HCFA. Having a history of serious illness is the most important single factor, accounting for about 38 percent of the cost increase, nearly half of the effect of the set of health measures. The importance of this measure is due to the large effect it has on Medicare reimbursements and to the inability of the auxiliary regression to explain the large difference between enrollees and nonenrollees on this measure. Interestingly, the variable indicating death within the nine-month period following the interview had no effect on the cost increase to HCFA. Although those who died had much higher Medicare reimbursements (the coefficients in the FFS reimbursement model are very large for both Part A and Part B), the mortality rate for enrollees (4.6 percent) was predicted very accurately by the auxiliary regression on AAPCC factors (the predicted mean was 4.7 percent).

Attitudes toward health care also contributed somewhat to the increased costs to HCFA, but socioeconomic characteristics had little effect. Beneficiaries who worry less about their health than others and those who avoid going to the physician generate significantly lower Medicare reimbursements than other beneficiaries and there are higher proportions of enrollees than nonenrollees with these characteristics. The auxiliary regression underpredicts slightly the proportions of enrollees who would have these characteristics, leading to AAPCC rates that are too high. These differences account for 14 percent of the cost increase to HCFA. Differences on socioeconomic factors (education, race, income, Medigap

Table 1.7   Effects of Enrollee Characteristics on Difference between AAPCC Rate and Projected FFS Reimbursements for Enrollees

	Effect on AAPCC Rate–FFS Reimbursement	*Percent of Total Difference*
Health Status Indicators		
ADL impairments	$ 40.29	15.3%
IADL impairments	$ 31.66	12.0%
History of cancer, heart disease, stroke	$ 100.61	38.2%
Poor health	$ 44.08	16.7%
Died during nine-month postinterview period	$ 2.47	0.9%
Total effect of health status measures	**$ 219.11**	**83.1%**
Attitudes toward Health Care		
Worries about health more	$ 19.20	7.3%
Avoids seeing physicians	$ 15.15	5.7%
Has usual source of care	$ 2.23	0.9%
Total effect of attitudinal variables	**$ 36.58**	**13.9%**
Socioeconomic/Ethnic Characteristics		
Income	$−17.58	−6.7%
Whether nonwhite	$ 13.23	5.0
Education	$ 6.16	2.3
Has Medigap coverage	$ 6.19	2.3
Total effect of socioeconomic variables	**$ 8.00**	**2.9%**
Difference between AAPCC and Projected FFS Reimbursement	**$ 263.70**	**100.0%**

coverage) account for only 3 percent of the difference, since none of these factors has much effect on Medicare reimbursements. Beneficiary income is estimated to have a *negative* effect on both Part A and Part B reimbursements, although the coefficients are very small and not significantly different from zero (a $10,000 increase in income decreases predicted total reimbursements by about $26, or about 1 percent). Medigap coverage has a modest effect on reimbursements ($292 higher for those with Medigap), but the predicted proportion of enrollees with Medigap coverage is overestimated only slightly by the auxiliary regressions.

Conclusion

Our estimates indicate that although the Medicare risk program succeeds in providing health care more efficiently than FFS, it increases costs to HCFA rather than saving the intended 5 percent. HMOs effectively reduce the use of hospital days and other Medicare covered services to rates below those that they would have used under FFS care. They do so not by reducing the number of individuals who receive care of a given type, but by reducing the *amount* of such care received. HMOs discharge patients from the hospital quicker, shorten SNF stays, reduce the number of home health visits per recipient, and reduce the number of beneficiaries who visit physicians frequently (once a month or more on average). But they do not affect the rate of admissions to hospitals, the likelihood of receiving home health care, or the average number of physician visits. Furthermore, HMOs *increase* the likelihood that the enrollee will have at least one visit to a physician, a physical exam, and even (slightly) a SNF stay. However, due to the favorable selection experienced by the HMOs and the insensitivity of the AAPCC to measurable differences between enrollees and nonenrollees, Medicare pays out 5.7 percent more for enrollees in capitation payments than the costs it would have incurred in FFS reimbursements for these individuals. While HMOs are paid 12 percent less than the average FFS reimbursement for nonenrollees—since enrollees are younger and less likely to be in nursing homes or on Medicaid, and because payments are set at 95 percent of the AAPCC—the FFS reimbursements for enrollees had they not joined an HMO would have been about 17 percent below the nonenrollee average.

Qualifications

Although our estimates appear to be plausible and most of our findings are consistent with estimates from other studies, there are four concerns about our estimates that should be raised. The sample appears to be representative of the Medicare population on a number of dimensions, and our estimated models have sensible and highly significant coefficient estimates. But there are two potential problems with the models we use, and two concerns about the data should be acknowledged.

First, it is possible that the models fail to account for selection bias. That is, the insignificant test for biases from our use of econometric techniques for dealing with unobserved differences between enrollees and nonenrollees may simply reflect an inadequate model of enrollment behavior rather than absence of selection. While this criticism is always applicable to studies without random assignment, we believe that the detailed survey data on health status as well as on attitudes toward health care and financial access to care enable us to control for virtually all of the major sources of correlation between health care use (or costs) and the probability of joining a Medicare risk plan. (Our impact estimates are much different when we control only for the characteristics usually available.) Other circumstantial evidence is provided by the absence of an estimated HMO effect on hospital admissions. It is implausible that HMOs *increase* hospital use, but that is what would be implied if there are unobserved factors (such as strong physician ties) that both decrease the likelihood of joining an HMO and increase expected utilization. Arguing that HMOs actually do reduce hospital admissions, given our estimates to the contrary, would require arguing that there are unmeasured characteristics that would increase both utilization and the likelihood of enrollment. Given that all of the *observed* differences between enrollees and nonenrollees are in the opposite direction, this seems highly unlikely.

The second potential modeling problem is that some control variables in our models, especially the health status and attitudinal variables, may have been influenced by the HMO and, therefore, including them in the model may mask some program effects. This argument has some merit, because half of the enrollees had belonged to the HMO for three years or more at the time of interview. However, Brown et al. (1986) found enrollee-nonenrollee differences of similar magnitude on such characteristics at the time of enrollment, using data from the Medicare Competition Demonstrations. Furthermore, Retchin et al. (1992) find no HMO effects on the change in measures of functioning using those earlier data. Also, using data from the current study, Hill and Brown (1992) find a significantly higher rate of serious illness history among those who had been enrolled for at least two years than among those who had enrolled more recently, after controlling for age and other AAPCC risk factors. Thus, we feel reasonably confident that HMO effects on these health status variables (if any) have been minimal, and that omitting the variables from the models would be more likely to create bias in our impact estimates than to lessen it.

The third concern is a data issue: our Medicare reimbursement and use measures were for the year prior to interview, when all individuals were alive, but program effects on both costs to HCFA and service use for the terminally ill may be quite different. We have some evidence that HMO effects on utilization are greatest for those who need the most care, so our estimates of impacts on service use may indeed be understated. However, we do not think that the estimated effects on costs to HCFA are likely to be affected much, given the apparent ability of the AAPCC factors to account for the moderate difference between the two groups in mortality rates.

Finally, another data concern is that we do not compare projected FFS reimbursements to actual AAPCC capitation payments but rather to *predicted* payments, based on a model to simulate the AAPCC for survivors. While explanations for why we take this approach are provided, the results do not reflect any over- or under-payments due to errors in AAPCC predictions of costs for those who remain in the FFS sector. Other studies suggest that the AAPCC predicts average cost per beneficiary for the United States reasonably well, so our estimates of average overpayments should not be far off. In any case, assessing errors in the AAPCC for nonenrollees is beyond the scope of this chapter. The approach we take yields estimates of costs or savings to HCFA even if the AAPCC *perfectly* predicted average FFS reimbursements for nonenrollees in each area, as it is intended to.

Implications

Our findings suggest that although the program currently increases costs to HCFA, the addition of a single variable to the AAPCC payment formula could essentially eliminate the overpayment. The capitation equation was reestimated to include a binary variable indicating whether the beneficiary had a history of cancer, heart disease, or stroke, and the projected capitation payments for enrollees under this new AAPCC formula were compared to their projected FFS reimbursements. The estimates showed that average payments under this formula (assuming HCFA continued to pay 95 percent of the AAPCC) would be about 1.1 percent *lower* than average projected FFS reimbursements would have been for enrollees. (Although the added variable accounts for only 38 percent of the overpayment according to Table 1.7, its coefficient in the revised capitation equations also reflects the influence of the other excluded health status measures on costs.)

Clearly this approach would require further investigation concerning an appropriate definition for the variable, the feasibility of collecting the necessary information, and the manner in which to incorporate it into the payment formula. However, such a variable has several features that make it much more attractive than other proposed changes to the AAPCC: (1) it is readily verifiable and thus cannot be easily manipulated by HMOs, unlike measures such as functional abilities; (2) it would need to be updated only for the relatively small proportion of patients in a given year that develop one of these conditions for the first time; (3) it would encourage HMOs to seek a more neutral selection of patients and to retain patients who develop such problems; and (4) it encompasses a sizable fraction of all Medicare beneficiaries (about one-third, according to our survey).

The reduction in average payment to HMOs that would result from incorporating this factor into the payment mechanism could force some HMOs out of the risk program. However, our estimates of the reductions in service use that HMOs are able to achieve, especially for expensive hospital services, together with any price breaks that HMOs are able to negotiate, suggest that most HMOs should be able to prosper. It remains to be seen whether the higher beneficiary premiums that would probably result from such a change would drive enrollees out of HMOs and HMOs out of the risk program.

Notes

1. This decline in risk plans is due almost entirely to HMOs discontinuing their risk plans. Consolidation or mergers of plans accounted for a very small portion of the decline in the number of risk contracts. See McGee and Brown (1992) for further information on HMOs that discontinue their risk contracts.
2. Measures based on pre-enrollment use patterns will also overstate enrollee-nonenrollee differences in health status if enrollees postpone needed, schedulable procedures in anticipation of enrolling in the HMO, with its more comprehensive coverage. However, Brown et al. (1986) found Medicare enrollees at the time of enrollment to be *less* likely than nonenrollees to claim that they were aware of a health problem that might require a hospital stay.
3. These enrollee-nonenrollee differences shrink somewhat when age and other AAPCC risk factors are controlled for, but they remain statistically significant (see Hill and Brown 1992).
4. The coefficient on λ in the modified utilization equation provides an estimate of S_{eu}/S_e, where S_{eu} is the covariance between the disturbance terms in the enrollment and utilization equations and S_e is the standard error of the enrollment equation.
5. The projected average reimbursement for enrollees was negative due to the large but statistically insignificant coefficient on the selection bias term. The size of the coefficient may be due in part to the small variation in values for λ for nonenrollees.
6. Our Medicare reimbursements measure includes the administrative cost allowance incorporated into the AAPCC, which HCFA sets at 0.5178 percent of direct Part A reimbursements and 2.6494 percent of Part B reimbursements.
7. The AAPCC payment to an HMO for a particular enrolled beneficiary is equal to the AAPCC rate for the enrollee's county of residence multiplied by the demographic risk factor for the enrollee (with separtate rates and risk factors for Part A and Part B). The risk factor depends on the rate cell into which the beneficiary falls. The 60 rate cells are defined by the interaction of the following factors: age (five categories), sex (two categories), disability status (two categories), and Medicaid/institutional status (three categories). In our models we have used metropolitan areas rather than counties as the geographic unit and have treated the site effect as additive rather than multiplicative, thereby ensuring that the mean predicted value for nonenrollees is equal to the mean actual value in eact site. To eliminate very small cell sizes, we have also collapsed the 60 cells into 25 cells by including all of the institutionalized beneficiaries in a single rate cell, and by classifying all disabled beneficiaries as members of a new single age category (under 65). Thus, we have 12 age/sex cells for those not in institutions or on Medicaid, 12 age/sex cells for those in institutions (see Appendix 1A).
8. We present only the extimated impacts here. Coefficients on control variables, standard errors, and R^2 statistics are presented in Hill et al. (1992).

References

Anderson, G., J. Cantor, E. Steinberg, and J. Holloway. "Capitation Pricing: Adjusting for Prior Utilization and Physician Discretion." *Health Care Financing Review* 8, no. 2 (Winter 1986): 27–34.

Bradbury, R. C., J. H. Golec, and F. E. Stearns. "Comparing Hospital Length of Stay in Independent Practice Association HMOs and Traditional Insurance Programs." *Inquiry* 28 (Spring 1991): 87–93.

Brown, R. "Biased Selection in the Medicare Competition Demonstrations." Princeton, NJ: Mathematica Policy Research, Inc., 1988.

Brown, R., J. Bergeron, D. Clement, J. Hill, and S. Retchin. "The Medicare Risk Program for HMOs—Final Summary Report on Findings from the Evaluation." Princeton, NJ: Mathematica Policy Research, Inc., August 1992.

Brown, R., K. Langwell, K. Berman, A. Ciemnecki, L. Nelson, A. Schreir, and A. Tucker. "Enrollment and Disenrollment in Medicare Competition Demonstration Plans: A Descriptive Analysis." Princeton, NJ: Mathematica Policy Research, Inc., 1986.

Dowd, B., R. Feldman, S. Cassou, and M. Finch. "Health Plan Choice and the Utilization of Health Care Services." *The Review of Economics and Statistics* 73, no. 1 (February 1991): 85–93.

Dowd, B. E., A. N. Johnson, and R. A. Madson. "Inpatient Length of Stay in Twin Cities Health Plans." *Medical Care* 24, no. 4 (April 1986): 294–310.

Duan, N., W. G. Manning, Jr., C. N. Morris, and J. P. Newhouse. "A Comparison of Alternative Models for the Demand of Medical Care." *Journal of Business and Economic Statistics* 1, no. 2 (April 1983): 115–26.

Eggers, P. "Risk Differential between Medicare Beneficiaries Enrolled and Not Enrolled in an HMO." *Health Care Financing Review* 1, no. 3 (1980): 91–99.

Eggers, P., and R. Prihoda. "Pre-Enrollment Reimbursement Patterns of Medicare Beneficiaries Enrolled in 'At Risk' HMOs." *Health Care Financing Review* 4, no. 1 (September 1982): 55–73.

Ellis, R. P., and A. Ash. "Refining the Diagnostic Cost Group Model: A Proposed Modification to the AAPCC for HMO Reimbursement." Boston: Boston University, February 1988.

Gruenber, L., D. Pomeranz, and F. Porrell. "Evaluation of the Accurary of the AAPCC." Boston: Bigel Institute for Health Policy, Heller Graduate School, Brandeis University, August 1988.

Heckman, J. J. "Dummy Endogenous Variables in Simultaneous Equation System." *Econometrica* 46, no. 6 (July 1978): 931–59.

———. "Sample Selection Bias as a Specification Error." *Econometrica* 47, no. 1 (January 1979): 153–61.

Hill, J., and R. Brown. "Health Status, Financial Barriers, and the Decision to Enroll in Medicare Risk Plans." Princeton, NJ· Mathematica Policy Research, Inc., June 1992.

Hill, J., and R. Brown. "Biased Selection in the TEFRA HMO/CMP Program." Princeton, NJ: Mathematica Policy Research, Inc., 1990.

Hill, J., R. Brown, D. Chu, and J. Bergeron. "The Impact of the Medicare Risk Program on the Use of Services and Costs to Medicare." Princeton, NJ: Mathematica Policy Research, Inc., June 1992.

Hornbrook, M. C. "Examination of the AAPCC Methodology in an HMO Prospective Payment Demographic Project." *Group Health Journal* 5, no. 1 (Spring 1984): 13–21.

Johnson, A. N., B. Dowd, N. E. Morris, and N. Lurie. "Difference in Inpatient Resource Use by Type of Health Plan." *Inquiry* 26, no. 3 (Fall 1989): 388–98.

Lichtenstein, R., J. Thomas, B. Watkins, J. Lepkowski, C. Pinto, J. Adams-Watson, B. Simone, and D. Vest. "The Relationship between Marketing Strategies and Risk Selection in Medicare At-Risk HMOs." Ann Arbor, MI: Department of Health Services Management and Policy, School of Public Health, University of Michigan, December 1989.

Luft, H. S. *Health Maintenance Organizations: Dimensions of Performance.* New Brunswick, NJ: Transaction Books, 1987.

Maddala, G. S. *Limited-Dependent and Qualitative Variables in Econometrics.* New York: Cambridge University Press, 1983.

Manning, W. G., A. Leibowitz, G. Goldberg, W. Rogers, and J. Newhouse. "A Controlled Trial of the Effect of a Prepaid Group Practice on Use of Services." *New England Journal of Medicine* 310, no. 23 (7 June 1984): 1505–11.

McCombs, J. S., J. D. Kasper, and G. F. Riley. "Do HMOs Reduce Health Care Costs? A Multivariate Analysis of Two Medicare HMO Demostration Projects." *Health Services Research* 25, no. 4 (October 1990): 593–613.

McGee, J., and R. Brown. "What Makes HMOs Drop Their Medicare Risk Contracts?" Princeton, NJ: Mathematica Policy Research, Inc., May 1992.

Nelson, L., and R. Brown. "The Impact of the Medicare Competition Demonstrations of the Use and Cost of Services." Washington, DC: Mathematica Policy Research, Inc., January 1989.

Palsbo, S. J. "The AAPCC Explained." Research Brief No. 8. Washington, DC: The Group Health Assocation of America, Inc., February 1989.

Prospective Payment Assessment Commission. "Medicare and the American Health Care System. Report to Congress." Washington, DC: ProPAC, June 1991.

Retchin, S., R. Brown, R. Cohen, D. Gurnick, M. Stegall, and B. Abujaber. "The Quality of Care in TEFRA HMOs/CMPs." Richmond, VA: Medical College of Virginia, June 1992.

Riley, G., J. Lubitz, and E. Rabey. "Enrollee Health Status Under Medicare Risk Contracts: An Analysis of Mortality Rates." *Health Services Research* 26, no. 2 (June 1991): 137–65.

Stern, R. S., P. I. Juhn, P. J. Gertler, and A. M. Epstein. "A Comparison of Length of Stay and Costs for Health Maintenance Organizations and Fee-for-Service Patients." *Archives of Internal Medicine* 149 (May 1989): 1185–88.

Thomas, J. W., and L. Lichtenstein. "Functional Health Measures for Adjusting Health Maintenance Organization Capitation Rates." *Health Care Financing Review* 7, no. 3 (Spring 1986): 85–95.

Thomas, J. W., and R. Lichtenstein. "Including Health Status in Medicare's Adjusted Average per Capita Cost Capitation Formula." *Medical Care* 26, no. 3 (March 1986): 259–75.

Whitmore, R. W., J. E. Paul, D. A. Gibbs, and J. C. Beebe. "Using Health Status Indicators in Calculating the AAPCC." In *Advances in Health Economics and Health Services Research. Vol. 10,* edited by R. M. Scheffler and L. F. Rossiter. Greenwich, CT: JAI Press, Inc., 1989.

Yelin, E. H., M. A. Shearn, and W. V. Epstein. "Health Outcomes for a Chronic Disease in Prepaid Group Practice and Fee-for-Service Settings—The Case of Rheumatoid Arthritis." *Medical Care* 24, no. 3 (March 1986): 234–47.

Appendix 1A   Regression Models for 1989 Medicare Costs and
                   Payment Rates

	FFS Reimbursement Equations		Capitation Rate Equations	
	Part A	*Part B*	*Part A*	*Part B*
Intercept	−242	−280	979	760***
	(.762)†	(.289)	(.169)	(.002)
AAPCC Risk Indicators‡				
Noninstitutionalized, Non-Medicaid	−347	−568***	132	−348*
Male, disabled (under 65)	(.564)	(.004)	(.824)	(.081)
Male 65–69	§	§	§	§
Male 70–74	221	−45	234	−22
	(.575)	(.727)	(.558)	(.873)
Male 75–79	258	320**	488	396***
	(.562)	(.029)	(.280)	(.009)
Male 80–84	930*	654***	1,315***	789***
	(.066)	(.000)	(.010)	(.000)
Male ≥ 85	685	4	1,592**	383*
	(.283)	(.984)	(.012)	(.072)
Female, disabled (under 65)	8	−15	841	371
	(.990)	(.946)	(.224)	(.110)
Female 65–69	−104	−8	−310	−122
	(.793)	(.951)	(.439)	(.365)
Female 70–74	163	227*	79	196
	(.663)	(.067)	(.834)	(.123)
Female 75–79	−46	157	−85	158
	(.909)	(.239)	(.834)	(.248)
Female 80–84	879*	239	1,038**	349**
	(.051)	(.107)	(.021)	(.021)
Female ≥ 85	285	−6	1,033**	325**
	(.569)	(.971)	(.035)	(.048)
Noninstitutionalized, Medicaid	1,689*	29	1,927	98
Male, disabled (under 65)	(.063)	(.923)	(.032)**	(.746)
Male 65–69	1,444	2,390***	2,344	2,557***
	(.446)	(.000)	(.221)	(.000)
Male 70–74	658	336	1,115	295
	(.602)	(.420)	(.382)	(.491)

Continued

Appendix 1A Continued

	FFS Reimbursement Equations		Capitation Rate Equations	
	Part A	Part B	Part A	Part B
Male 75–79	−2,123	406	99	1,174*
	(.261)	(.514)	(.959)	(.067)
Male 80–84	4,534**	1,161	5,761**	1,478*
	(.048)	(.123)	(.013)	(.058)
Male ≥ 85	−2,112	−225	170	352
	(.278)	(.726)	(.931)	(.591)
Female, disabled (under 65)	607	206	1,240	551
	(.568)	(.555)	(.242)	(.121)
Female 65–69	853	37	1,248	141
	(.423)	(.917)	(.243)	(.695)
Female 70–74	406	678**	640	743**
	(.668)	(.030)	(.500)	(.020)
Female 75–79	87	57	451	180
	(.934)	(.868)	(.667)	(.609)
Female 80–84	−237	196	574	442
	(.830)	(.589)	(.604)	(.234)
Female ≥ 85	71	113	1,336	547
	(.949)	(.759)	(.229)	(.143)
Nursing home resident	1,168**	−156	3,407***	861***
	(.043)	(.412)	(.000)	(.000)
Socioeconomic/Demographic Variable				
Minority race (not white)	223	−114		
	(.557)	(.359)		
Race information missing	1,830*	149		
	(.070)	(.653)		
Education				
College	−84	153		
	(.783)	(.128)		
High school graduate, no college degree	−76	75		
	(.731)	(.299)		
Education data missing	504	−216		
	(.390)	(.263)		

Continued

Appendix 1A   Continued

	FFS Reimbursement Equations		Capitation Rate Equations	
	Part A	Part B	Part A	Part B
Access to Care				
Income ($1,000)	−1	−1		
	(.659)	(.214)		
Income data missing	−120	−34		
	(.658)	(.705)		
Medigap coverage	123	169**		
	(.594)	(.027)		
Health Status				
Number of ADL impairments	430***	253***		
	(.002)	(.000)		
Number of IADL impairments	105	96***		
	(.187)	(.000)		
Poor health	774**	351***		
	(.024)	(.002)		
Ever had cancer, heart disease, or stroke	1,183***	527***		
	(.000)	(.000)		
Died during nine months following interview	1,532***	648***		
	(.001)	(.000)		
Missing data, poor health	1,376	1,704***		
	(.122)	(.000)		
Missing data, cancer, heart disease, stroke	2,216*	−338		
	(.051)	(.364)		
Preferences for seeking care				
Avoid doctors	−300	−295***		
	(.158)	(.000)		
Missing data, avoid doctors	146	−87		
	(.825)	(.687)		
Worry about health	840***	561***		
	(.000)	(.000)		
Missing data, worry about health	365	−224		
	(.465)	(.174)		
Usual place of care	621*	591***		
	(.062)	(.000)		

Continued

Appendix 1A Continued

	FFS Reimbursement Equations		Capitation Rate Equations	
	Part A	Part B	Part A	Part B
Mean of Dependent Variable	$1,558	$1,254	$1,558	$1,234
R^2	0.058	0.110	0.020	0.037
N	6,107	6,107	6,107	6,107

*Significantly different from zero at the .10 level, two-tailed test.

**Significantly different from zero at the .05 level, two-tailed test.

***Significantly different from zero at the .01 level, two-tailed test.

†Numbers in parentheses are p-values for 2-tailed tests of the hypothesis that the coefficient is zero for the population.

‡Each model also included a set of 43 binary site variables. See Hill et al. (1992) for these estimates.

§The reference category for the set of binary variables indicating the AAPCC risk classification categories in males age 65–69. Thus, all of the coefficients on AAPCC risk indicators are expected costs relative to this reference group.

Chapter 2

The Twin Cities Medicare Health Plans Market: Choice, Cost, and Health Status

Catherine Wisner, Roger Feldman, and Bryan Dowd

The Twin Cities of Minneapolis and St. Paul have provided a natural experiment for capitated delivery systems and, recently, a limited test of managed competition. HMOs have been offered in the Twin Cities for over 30 years and have participated in the Medicare program since the Medicare capitation demonstration project in the early 1980s. In this paper, we summarize the results of several studies that focused on the Twin Cities Medicare health plans market. The first study provided information on the characteristics of Medicare beneficiaries who choose different types of health plans. The second study investigated bias in HCFA payments to Medicare HMOs. The third examined the effect of health plan membership on the health status of enrollees. Finally, we discuss how the results from these studies bear on our proposal for a competitive pricing system in the Medicare program.

Background

In 1970, the metropolitan area of Minneapolis and St. Paul had one HMO. By 1978, seven HMOs were operating in the Twin Cities. HMO enrollment reached 240,854 members, or 12 percent of the area's population (Minnesota Department of Health 1979). Thus, when HCFA released a Request for Proposals (RFP) in 1978 to solicit demonstrations of prospective risk contracts for Medicare, the Twin Cities was a logical area in which to test this new program. HCFA signed a contract with InterStudy, a Minneapolis-based HMO "think tank," to act as a broker in recruiting several of the area's HMOs into the risk contracting demonstration.

Originally, six Twin Cities HMOs agreed to participate in the demonstration. Group Health Plan, the largest HMO, chose not to participate from the beginning. During negotiations among the HMOs, InterStudy, and HCFA, two other HMOs dropped out because they objected to establishing a fixed premium, wanting instead to collect coinsurance and deductibles as beneficiaries incurred them (Galblum and Trieger 1982). The remaining four plans would not have participated in the demonstration had HCFA not permitted them to subject potential enrollees to health screening outside a 30-day annual open enrollment period. However, health screening was permitted, and the four HMOs signed on. The participating plans and their startup dates were: SHARE Health Plan (December 1980); MedCenters Health Plan (July 1981); Nicollet-Eitel Health Plan (July 1981); and HMO Minnesota (July 1981).

Initial enrollment in the demonstration was slow to occur. Only 1,000 beneficiaries signed up in three plans during their first open enrollment. These three HMOs offered marginal additional benefits. Only SHARE Health Plan, by using minimal health screening, achieved a substantial initial enrollment of 5,269 (Galblum and Trieger 1982). However, 2,000 of these members were converted from a previous Medicare cost contract.

One of the primary purposes of the Medicare capitation demonstration was to test the feasibility of developing prospective capitation methodologies and to determine whether the resulting payment systems were acceptable to HCFA and the HMOs. The critical reimbursement issue that surfaced was the accuracy of the AAPCC (adjusted average per capita cost) methodology. Early evidence (Eggers and Prihoda 1982) from three demonstration HMOs outside the Twin Cities showed that two of them (Fallon Community Health Plan and Kaiser, Portland) experienced favorable selection as evidenced by their enrollees' use of medical care prior to enrollment. Enrollees in the Marshfield, Wisconsin, Medical Foundation had significantly higher prior use of outpatient and physician services, although total Medicare reimbursements for enrollee and nonenrollee groups were not significantly different. As a result of the Eggers and Prihoda study, the Congressional Budget Office (1982) estimated that HMOs would increase Medicare's costs in the short run.

Despite these early findings, public interest in the HMO concept for Medicare developed rapidly, with activity on several fronts. The Tax Equity and Fiscal Responsibility Act of 1982 (TEFRA) contained provisions that would lead to a national program for Medicare HMOs. At the same time that regulations to implement TEFRA were being drafted,

27 HMOs and "Competitive Medical Plans" (CMPs) entered the Medicare market under a second demonstration program.[1] The key feature of this demonstration was the willingness of HMOs and CMPs to accept financial risk for providing Medicare benefits to enrolled beneficiaries (Langwell et al. 1987; Langwell and Hadley 1989).

Although Minneapolis was not a site for the Medicare competition demonstration, it experienced rapidly increasing Medicare HMO activity during the early 1980s. Physicians' Health Plan, a Minneapolis-based IPA, joined the program in 1981 and by the end of 1981, Medicare enrollment in the five HMOs increased to 8,534 (Minnesota Department of Health 1981).[2] In 1983 MedCenters and Nicollet-Eitel Health Plan merged. Medicare enrollment in the four remaining plans increased by 59 percent from 1982 to 1983, with 34,013 enrollees in 1983 (Minnesota Department of Health 1983). SHARE Health Plan still had the most enrollees (20,378) in 1983. In the following year, Group Health Plan began enrolling Medicare beneficiaries, as well as NWNL (Northwestern National Life) Health Network, a Competitive Medical Plan that became operational in March 1984. Regulations to implement TEFRA were published in January 1985, and the Twin Cities plans converted from demonstration status to TEFRA program status. Under TEFRA rules, they were required to give back to enrollees, in the form of reduced premiums and copayments or increased benefits, profits above a level negotiated by HCFA and the HMO.

Total Medicare HMO enrollment increased to 161,466 in 1986 (Minnesota Department of Health 1986). The following year, First Plan HMO, a prepaid group practice based in northeastern Minnesota, joined the program; but for the first time since 1981, total enrollment increased slowly, to 173,535 (Minnesota Department of Health 1987). As we get to more recent history, Table 2.1 shows the Medicare HMO enrollment by plan from 1987 to 1991.

The next critical year for Medicare HMO enrollment was 1988, when total enrollment dropped by over 25,000, largely due to sharp declines at Physicians' Health Plan and HMO Minnesota (renamed Blue Plus in 1988) and, to a lesser extent, at SHARE and MedCenters. To understand the cause of these declines, we need to look at where they occurred. Those enrollees were dropped by the HMOs, and they were all outside the Twin Cities (*Minneapolis Star Tribune*, 8 November 1987). The HMOs said they had no choice, blaming the federal government for paying less for rural patients than for urban ones, even though the cost of treating them might not differ.

There was no question that Medicare payment rates were lower in the affected rural areas. Physicians' Health Plan, for example, withdrew from six rural counties where the average AAPCC payment rate in 1987 was $159.57 (*St. Paul Pioneer Press*, 15 December 1987). This contrasts

Table 2.1   Total Minnesota Medicare HMO Enrollment*, 1987–1991

	Year				
Plan Name	1987	1988	1989	1990	1991
First Plan HMO	838	854	908	917	955
Group Health Plan	15,172	18,185	18,808	21,363	22,271
HMO Minnesota	18,785	9,471	14,540	16,543	14,665
MedCenters Health Plan	29,005	28,499	12,625	19,267	17,469
Physicians' Health Plan	58,786	41,138	40,759	39,877	40,883
NWNL Health Network	2,899	2,348	44	0	0
SHARE Health Plan	47,674	41,046	41,279	41,634	42,623
Minnesota Health Plans	0	4,554	4,287	0	0
Other HMOs	376	169	566	213	239
Total	173,535	146,264	133,816	139,814	139,105

Source: Minnesota Department of Health. 1987, 1988, 1989, 1990, 1991.
*Refers to all products for the elderly sold by HMOs, not just enrollment in TEFRA-risk plans.
†Name Changes: HMO Minnesota = Blue Plus (1988); SHARE Health Plan = Medica Primary (1990); Physicians' Health Plan = Medica Choice (1990).

with an AAPCC rate of $257.51 in Hennepin County (Minneapolis) and $252.86 in Ramsey County (St. Paul). A representative of one HMO, in a personal communication to the authors, alleged that the low AAPCC in rural areas is due to low utilization of health care services in these areas, which takes away the HMO's technological advantage over the fee-for-service delivery system. Another factor that the HMOs did not count on was that many rural patients, once in an HMO, would start going to the doctor for the first time in years. Newspaper accounts (*Minneapolis Star Tribune*, 8 November 1987) suggested that this occurred because the rural elderly had been avoiding medical care due to the expense, and now they did not need to worry about doctors' bills. The implication is that many rural elderly, in contrast to urban elderly, did not have Medicare supplementary insurance prior to joining the HMO. These policies increase the use of services in the FFS sector, which increases the urban AAPCC. Unfortunately, no rigorous study of this unique event—Medicare HMO withdrawal on a large scale from rural areas—was conducted.

Since 1989, Medicare HMO enrollment in Minnesota has stabilized at about 140,000 enrollees. However, this aggregate total hides a major shift in the type of contracts established between the HMOs and HCFA. Medica Choice (formerly Physicians' Health Plan) and Blue Plus converted from TEFRA risk-bearing contracts to "Health Care Prepayment

Plans" (HCPPs) in 1990. Under this type of contract, the HMO bears no risk for covered services. Benefits in an HCPP must match or exceed those of Medicare; enrollees can obtain care outside the plan, at standard Medicare cost-sharing rates. Most significantly, the HCPP can subject potential enrollees to health screening. This represents a significant advantage over TEFRA risk-bearing contracts and is one of the reasons why HCFA has supported legislation to eliminate this option (Wilensky and Rossiter 1991).

In the last five months of 1989, MedCenters began participating in the Diagnostic Cost Grouping (DCG) Demonstration Project, designed to test an alternative payment program for risk contractors using a form of health status adjustment. The DCG Demonstration enabled MedCenters to realize an additional 10 percent revenue over what they would have received under the AAPCC payment method (Riley, Walton, and Johnson 1992). When the demonstration ended in 1992, MedCenters also converted its Medicare contract to a HCPP. Among the factors cited by MedCenters (in addition to loss of the DCG revenue) were: aging of the population in the risk contract; flat AAPCC payment rates in the Twin Cities; and minimal new enrollment. In general, HMOs consider the Twin Cities Medicare market to be saturated. With about 60 percent of the elderly population enrolled, the HMOs believe that the remaining 40 percent will not switch from the fee-for-service sector—either because these persons do not want to be locked into an HMO or because they have well-established relationships with their current health care providers.

Our final point is that the HMO industry in the Twin Cities has been undergoing structural changes equally significant as those experienced in the Medicare market segment. In the last decade, the HMO industry in the Twin Cities has been marked by consolidation. The current Blue Plus HMO, which is affiliated with Blue Cross and Blue Shield of Minnesota, was created in 1988 from a merger between Coordinated Health Care and HMO Minnesota. This merger added about 20,000 enrollees to the 40,000 in HMO Minnesota.

A more significant consolidation occurred in 1987–1988 when Physicians Health Plan and SHARE Health Plan joined forces as Medica, the area's largest HMO. SHARE (now known as Medica Primary) and PHP (known as Medica Select) are both managed by United HealthCare Corporation.

The movement toward HMO consolidation took a huge leap early in 1992, when Group Health and MedCenters Health Plan announced a proposed "partnership" (*Minneapolis Star Tribune*, 6 March 1992). Details of the partnership, later published in the Twin Cities newspapers, indicate that it was in fact a merger. The merger partners announced that they would submit bids to provide coverage to two Minnesota employer coalitions. The HMOs also announced the creation of an institute with the Mayo Clinic and Park Nicollet Medical Center to measure and monitor quality of care in the consolidated organization. The merger of Med-Centers and Group Health surpasses any previous consolidation in this market. It brings together the number two and three HMOs to create the largest HMO in the state and in the Twin Cities.

Implications of these mergers for the Medicare market are unclear. They will, however, significantly reduce the number of independent sellers of Medicare HMO products in the Twin Cities. This may have an effect on the number of products offered and on premiums and enrollment in the remaining plans.

Health Plan Choice

One of the first questions that must be addressed in an analysis of a health plan market is choice of health plans by enrollees. Not only is the question of health plan choice of intrinsic interest, but health plan choice equations are an important component of the econometric correction for endogenous sample selection bias that arises in studies of utilization of services, expenditures, and health status, when enrollees are not assigned randomly to health plans. Previous studies by Eggers (1980), Luft (1981), Eggers and Prihoda (1982), Dowd and Feldman (1985), Wilensky and Rossiter (1986), Garfinkel et al. (1986), Hellinger (1987), Brown (1988), and Feldman et al. (1989) generally have found a pattern of selection that favors HMOs over the FFS sector. Several of these studies focused specifically on Medicare beneficiaries.

Our data were collected in the Twin Cities market area in 1988. At that time, the enrollment in Medicare HMOs was as shown in Table 2.2.

A survey questionnaire was administered, in person, to a random sample of Medicare beneficiaries who met five eligibility criteria: a resident of the seven-county Twin Cities metropolitan statistical area, over age 65, currently eligible for both Part A and Part B benefits, not Medicaid eligible (and thus not a Medicaid "buy-in" beneficiary), not a member of a social HMO, and not eligible for supplemental security income.[3] The survey instrument requested basic demographic data as well as self-reported information on physical functioning, chronic health conditions, and perceived health status.

The interviews took place between November 1987 and April 1988. During the course of analyzing the data, we discovered that HCFA inadvertently had selected only beneficiaries younger than age 88. To correct the error, HCFA drew another sample of beneficiaries in January 1990 from the population meeting the eligibility criteria as of November 1,

Table 2.2   1988 Distribution of Medicare Enrollees across Health Plans

Plan	TEFRA-Risk Enrollees*	% of TEFRA-Risk Enrollees	% of All Beneficiaries
HMO Minnesota	3,480	4.2	2.1
Physicians Health Plan	28,200	30.8	15.5
MedCenters	9,780	10.7	5.4
Group Health	12,060	13.2	6.6
Share	37,800	41.2	20.8
Total HMO Sector (TEFRA-risk)	91,680	100.0	50.4
FFS Sector	90,325		49.6
Total Eligible Beneficiaries	182,005		

*These numbers do not match the earlier enrollment data because these data refer only to TEFRA-risk enrollees.

1987, and survey data were collected for individuals in this sample who were 88 years and older as of that date.[4] If the beneficiary had died or was otherwise incapable of responding, the survey was completed by a proxy. Fifty-six percent of the interviews for beneficiaries over age 88 were administered to proxies, compared to 3 percent proxies for beneficiaries under age 88. There were 2,375 completed interviews. The response rates were 90 percent in the FFS sector, 71 percent in the HMO sector, and 82 percent overall.

Respondents and nonrespondents were compared in a variety of ways. Fifty-seven percent of the eligible sample was in the FFS sector, but 63 percent of respondents were in the FFS sector.[5] Despite the lower response rate in the HMO sector, there were no significant differences in age, sex, or county of residence between respondents and nonrespondents in the HMO sample. Respondents were found to be younger than nonrespondents, on average, although the difference in mean age was not large (75.89 years for the entire sample, versus 75.48 for respondents). The discrepancy in age is due to underrepresentation of the oldest age cohort among respondents. The proportions of males and females over age 85 in the full sample were .06 and .11, respectively, but only .05 and .10 among respondents. The age discrepancy arises primarily in the FFS sector. The difference in age between respondents and nonrespondents was significant in the FFS sector, but not in the HMO sector.

Response bias does not pose a problem for our statistical models if it is limited to differences in the means of reported variables between respondents and nonrespondents. It becomes a problem only if the underlying models, for example, the model of health plan choice, differ significantly between respondents and nonrespondents. In this case, models estimated from the sample of respondents cannot be generalized to the whole Medicare HMO population. The hypothesis that underlying models differ for respondents and nonrespondents can be tested for variables that are available for both groups. The results of that test are presented in the next section.

Means and standard deviations of variables used in the analysis of health plan choice are shown in Table 2.3.

Analysis of variance comparisons of the variables in Table 2.3 for individual health plans and the aggregate HMO and FFS sectors were performed, followed by estimation of multinomial logit models of health plan choice. In the multinomial logit analysis the health plans were grouped into four categories: (1) basic FFS (no supplement), (2) FFS with a supplement, (3) IPA (PHP and HMOM), and (4) network plans (MedCenters, Group Health, and SHARE).

Both the ANOVA and multinomial logit analyses showed that the youngest enrollees are found in network HMOs. Except for hearing problems, the chronic illness variables are negatively associated with choice of all sectors relative to basic FFS, although the effect is significant at the .05 level only for skin problems in network HMOs. Network HMO enrollees are significantly more likely to be married than beneficiaries in the basic FFS sector. This may be due, in part, to the mobility required to reach the clinics of network HMOs. That hypothesis is supported by the positive coefficient of HOURDR, to the extent that having more children within an hour drive improves the beneficiary's access to more distant HMO clinics.

Income has the strongest and most consistent effect on health plan choice. Beneficiaries whose annual income is greater than $10,000 (HI-INC) are significantly more likely to be found in all sectors other than basic FFS Medicare. The strongest effect is for IPAs, where moving from the "under $10,000" range to the "over $10,000" range of income is associated with a nearly fourfold increase in the probability of choosing an IPA over basic FFS Medicare. Beneficiaries who do not live in the Twin Cities all year are significantly more likely to choose the FFS sector with a supplement. Completion of high school (HS) increases the probability of choosing both the IPA or FFS sector with a supplement, relative to basic FFS Medicare. College graduates (COLLEGE) are significantly less likely to choose network HMOs over basic FFS Medicare. The way in which coverage is purchased strongly affects choice. Beneficiaries who purchase any of their coverage through a group (GRPPOL) or receive a subsidy (OTRPAY) for any coverage are significantly more likely to choose the FFS sector with a supplement, relative to basic FFS Medicare.[6] Beneficiaries

Table 2.3 Variable Definitions and Descriptive Statistics: Health Plan Choice Model

Variable	Mean	s.d.	Description
Dummy Variables for Presence of Medical Conditions*			
DIAB	0.090	0.287	Respondent reports presence of diabetes
ASTHMA	0.094	0.291	Emphysema or chronic bronchitis
NERVE	0.041	0.198	Nerve or muscle problems
SKIN	0.083	0.276	Chronic skin problems
SPEECH	0.036	0.186	Speech problems
HEAR	0.327	0.469	Hearing problems
Continuous Demographic Variables			
AGE	75.234	76.445	Age, from HCFA records
KIDS	2.440	1.933	Number of living children
HOURDR	1.701	1.594	Number of children living < 1-hour drive
LIVETC	53.612	21.209	Number of years respondent has lived in the Twin Cities
Dummy Demographic Variables*			
HIINC	0.655	0.475	Income > $10,000
INCMIS	0.075	0.264	Income data missing
TECH	0.038	0.191	Technical or vocational school without high school diploma
HS	0.513	0.500	High school diploma
COLLEGE	0.126	0.332	College degree
EDMIS	0.006	0.078	Education data missing
MALE	0.410	0.492	Respondent is male
ALONE	0.330	0.294	Respondent lives alone
ALLYEAR	0.904	0.294	Respondent lives in the Twin Cities all year
MARRIED	0.341	0.474	Respondent is married
OTRPAY	0.187	0.390	Someone besides the beneficiary contributes to the premium
OTRMIS	0.015	0.122	Data on OTRPAY missing
GRPPOL	0.381	0.486	Respondent has any health insurance purchased through a group policy
GRPMIS	0.016	0.124	Data on GRPPOL missing

Sample Size = 2,326 (275 in basic FFS, 1,191 in FFS with a supplement, 308 in IPAs and 552 in network HMOs)

*Dummy variables are equal to 1 if the condition or criterion is present and 0 if it is not. The omitted education category is no high school diploma/no technical school.

with group policies are significantly less likely to choose IPAs, relative to the basic FFS sector.

When we compared the predicted (most likely) health plan choice from the model with the actual choice, we found that the model predicted quite well for basic FFS Medicare and FFS with a supplement. Seventy percent and 79 percent of the actual choices were predicted by the model for these sectors. However, the model predicted less well for network HMOs (57 percent), and it performed poorly for IPA plans (4 percent). Since random guessing would have predicted some choices correctly, we also calculated a statistic for the reduction in predictive errors afforded by knowledge of the model (Hildebrand, Laing, and Rosenthal 1977). Overall, the multinomial logit choice model reduced the predictive errors by 32 percent, compared with simple guesswork.

We examined response bias by comparing the means of variables for respondents and nonrespondents, as discussed earlier. As a further test of response bias, we reestimated the multinomial logit model of health plan choice as a function of data available for respondents and nonrespondents (age, sex, and county of residence of the enrollee). Health plans were classified as FFS, IPA, and network HMO, since data on FFS supplements were available only for respondents. We combined age and sex into dummy variables corresponding to the AAPCC rate cells, and predicted health plan choice by the age/sex dummy variables and the beneficiary's county of residence. Each age/sex and county variable also was interacted with another dummy variable that equaled one if the beneficiary responded to the survey, and zero otherwise. Coefficients of the interaction variables test whether the effect of the variable on health plan choice is significantly different between respondents and nonrespondents.

Among the response interaction terms, the intercept (representing respondent versus nonrespondent) was significant and negative for both IPAs and network HMOs, indicating that respondents were less likely than nonrespondents to choose those two sectors, relative to the FFS sector. The interaction coefficient for females over age 85 was significant and positive in both the IPA and network HMO equations, and the interaction coefficient for males over age 85 was significant and positive in the network HMO equation. These results indicate that respondents in the oldest age category were more likely than nonrespondents to choose those sectors over FFS Medicare. A possible explanation for this finding is that, although the oldest beneficiaries were least likely to be in HMOs, those who were in HMOs may have found them especially attractive, and thus they may have been more willing to answer the survey. Overall, the tests for nonresponse bias indicate that the multinomial logit results may overstate slightly the negative effect of age on choice of the IPA and network HMO sectors. The effect of nonresponse bias should not be large, however, because it appears only in the oldest age category, which contains only 17 percent of beneficiaries in the total sample.

The multinomial logit model assumes that the error terms in the beneficiary's utility function for each choice are uncorrelated. Feldman et al. (1989) found that that assumption did not apply to health plan choice in the Twin Cities *employed population*, where the plans could be grouped into "nests," depending on the number of participating providers in the plan. To test the nesting hypothesis in our data, we dropped the network HMO observations (and thus the people who chose them) from the data and reestimated the multinomial logit model. Dropping the network HMOs did not alter the "FFS with a supplement" and IPA coefficient vectors, using the Hausman-McFadden (1984) test.

Expenditure Analysis

The second area of analysis concerned expenditure on health care services. The scope of this research was limited to examination of potential bias in the adjusted average per capita cost (AAPCC) payment system for Medicare HMOs in the Twin Cities during the period of observation (roughly calendar year 1988). Bias in the AAPCC–based payment formula is an important policy topic. Currently, payment to Medicare HMOs is based on the predicted cost of a person in the same county with similar values of age, sex, institutional, and welfare status. If there are additional, unobserved variables that influence both choice of the HMO versus FFS sector *and* subsequent expenditures, HMO payments will be biased. The fact that a number of studies have documented favorable selection into HMOs on the basis of *observed* variables leads one to suspect the presence of favorable selection attributable to unobserved variables, as well. The association of unobserved variables both with choice of the HMO versus FFS sector and with subsequent values of a variable of interest, such as expenditures, is referred to as selectivity bias or endogenous sample selection bias. Our objective in this analysis was to determine whether significant selectivity bias remained after including the AAPCC variables in the health plan choice (sample selection) and expenditure equations.

Our study collected prospective expenditure data from HCFA claims files on individuals in the sample of 1,446 beneficiaries who chose basic FFS Medicare or FFS with a supplementary insurance policy. Each individual was followed for one year, beginning at the time of the in-person interview. Claims were allowed to accrue for a minimum nine-month "lag" period following the close of the observation period. HCFA estimates that a nine-month lag will result in expenditure data that are 95 percent complete. Among the 1,446 FFS beneficiaries, 686 had positive HCFA reimbursements and approximately 80 percent had supplementary insurance.

One of the first, and perhaps most important, findings of our analysis was that the average annual reimbursement for FFS beneficiaries in our sample was $1,434.76, compared to the average AAPCC payment, weighted by the percentage of the sample in each of the seven Twin Cities counties, of $3,220.96. This discrepancy is much greater than the 10 to 20 percent underrepresentation that one can expect due to hospital cost pass-throughs and periodic reconciliations of HCFA claims data (Langwell and Hadley 1990). The discrepancy is also larger than that found by Nelson and Brown (1989) and reported by Langwell and Hadley (1989). We did not correct the latter figure for the AAPCC variables, however. This difference is not caused by "short years" due to death of some beneficiaries in our sample. These beneficiaries were included in both the numerator and denominator of our calculated average FFS expenditures. This is exactly how HCFA calculates the AAPCC. Also, the difference is not due to response bias, because we calculated average expenditures for all FFS beneficiaries in the sample (both respondents and nonrespondents). Consequently, the difference between $1,434.76 and $3,220.96 remains a major unresolved problem—either in our data or in the AAPCC.[7]

There are three estimation problems in the expenditure analysis: (1) sample selection bias arises from endogenous health plan choice; (2) zeros are concentrated in the expenditure data; and (3) errors in the expenditure equation, even conditional on health plan choice and some positive expenditures, are not normally distributed. To address problems of endogenous health plan choice and concentration of zeros in the expenditure data, we estimated both a selectivity-corrected Tobit model (Dowd et al. 1991) and a selectivity-corrected two-part model. The two-part model utilizes separate equations for the probability of some Medicare expenditures and the value of positive expenditures. The non-normality problem was addressed by taking the natural log of positive expenditures.

The expenditure equation included *only* explanatory variables from the AAPCC: age/sex cells and dummy variables for county of residence. Males between the ages of 65 and 69 and Hennepin County served as the reference categories. The health plan choice equation, which serves as the sample selection equation, must begin with the same specification as the expenditure equation, because to include other variables that might be related to expenditures would bias the findings towards "no selectivity bias."[8] However, the robustness of the selectivity test depends importantly on including variables in the health plan choice equation that do not appear in the expenditure equation (Manning, Duan, and Rogers 1987). We included two such variables (and their missing data counterparts): GRPNEW (and GRPMIS) and OTRNEW (and OTRMIS), which indicate whether the beneficiary obtains any health insurance through a group policy and whether anyone outside the family contributes to health plan premiums, respectively. Analysis showed that these variables are significant predictors of health plan choice, but there is no theoretical reason why they should affect expenditures, except through choice of health plan.

Three specifications of the choice equation were tested: (1) a dichotomous logit equation for the choice of the FFS versus HMO sector; (2) a trichotomous logit equation where the choices were FFS coverage, IPAs, and network HMOs; and (3) a polychotomous logit equation in which the choices were basic FFS coverage, FFS with supplementary coverage, IPAs, and network HMOs. In the final, four-choice model, the number of estimated coefficients became intractably large, and we were forced to limit the AAPCC variables in the choice equation to dummy variables representing the oldest age categories for males and females.

Table 2.4 summarizes the selectivity correlations in the expenditure equations.

The selectivity correlation measures the relationship between the error terms in the health plan choice and FFS expenditure equations due to common omitted variables. Based on the results of our analysis, shown in Table 2.4, we must reject the hypothesis of significant selectivity. So, the bottom line with respect to selectivity bias is that the current

Table 2.4 Estimates of Selectivity Correlations (Asymptotic t-Statistic in Parentheses)

		Two-Part Model	
Choice Model	*Tobit Model*	*Some vs. No Expenditure*	*Positive Expenditure*
FFS/HMO	0.0586	0.1079	−0.1232
	(0.580)	(0.952)	(−0.931)
FFS/IPA/Network HMO	0.0580	0.1060	−0.1206
	(0.575)	(0.935)	(−0.910)
Basic FFS/FFS + supp/IPA/ Network HMO	−0.0048	0.0292	−0.1242
	(−0.087)	(0.460)	(−1.673)

AAPCC formula is an accurate predictor of FFS Medicare expenditures for beneficiaries who join HMOs.

This conclusion must be offered with the following qualifications, however. First, the selectivity coefficient almost attained statistical significance at the .10 level in the four-way choice model. At this point, we cannot be sure if this result is due to separating basic FFS Medicare from FFS with a supplementary policy, or to the combination of age and sex categories in the four-way choice equation. As we noted previously, this model was estimated with a reduced number of choice variables to make it tractable. Exclusion of other variables related to choice and expenditures may be the cause of selectivity bias in this model.

Second, the selectivity correlation measures only the linear relationship among omitted variables (Dowd et al. 1991). We cannot rule out the possibility of more complex, nonlinear relationships between omitted variables that affect Medicare health plan choice and expenditures. Finally, this may not be a fair test of the allegation of selectivity bias, since HMOs are facing payments based on national AAPCC weights, not locally adjusted weights.

Health Status

The few studies that have assessed the effects of HMOs on the health of their enrollees have either demonstrated an advantage in health status for HMO enrollees or no significant differences between FFS and HMOs in their effect on health status. Ware et al. (1986) used RAND Health Insurance Experiment data to compare health outcomes of individuals between 14 and 62 years of age in prepaid and FFS systems. They found that "for most people, and particularly for those with higher incomes, GHC care (the HMO) saved money and, if anything, may have been better for health." For low-income people who began the experiment with health problems, however, "health status was in some respects worse at GHC than in the Seattle FFS system." Wagner and Bledsoe's (1990) findings were similar to those of Ware et al. for the general population, but they did not find that HMO care had adverse effects on health for the low-income, sick individuals. Sloss et al. (1987) also evaluated the RAND Health Insurance Experiment data and found no differences in the health status measures between the FFS and HMO samples.

HMO versus FFS sectors

Physical functioning. Wisner (1992) analyzed two different measures of health status: physical functioning and general perceived health status. The first dependent variable was a ten-item physical functioning scale with a range of scores from 10 to 40, where a score of 10 indicates no limitations in physical functioning, and a score of 40 indicates severe limitations on all ten measures. This information was collected only for beneficiaries younger than age 88.

When physical functioning was regressed on the explanatory variables in Table 2.3, the distribution of residuals was severely non-normal. The Jarque-Bera test statistic (Jarque and Bera 1981)[9] had a value of 135.6 with two degrees of freedom for the HMO sector, and 223.3 for the FFS sector. A log transformation of the dependent variable reduced the Jarque-Bera statistic to 15.4 in the HMO sector and 26.5 in the FFS sector, still outside the critical range. The reciprocal and square-root transformations of the dependent variable produced similar results. Estimates from the untransformed, log, and reciprocal transformations were compared for statistical significance, and the results were virtually identical. The log transformation was chosen for its relatively close approximation to normally distributed errors and the ease of retransforming the log scale to obtain predictions.

In the log scale estimates, no selectivity bias was found for either the HMO ($\rho = -0.097$; $p = .36$)[10] or FFS ($\rho = 0.098$; $p = .31$) sector, supporting the hypothesis that no unobserved variables affect both choice of the health plan and health status of Medicare beneficiaries, after controlling for variables included in the AAPCC. Having rejected the hypothesis of sample selection bias, the model was reestimated without the sample selection term to simplify computation of the standard error of the contrast ($Y_{FFS} - \hat{Y}_{HMO}$). The smearing estimator (Duan 1983) was used to retransform the predictions back to the original functional status scale.

Health status was predicted separately in each sector. The regression model is:

$$\log(Y) = X\beta + u$$

and the predicted Y in the original scale is:

$$predicted\ Y = \hat{Y} = \exp(X\beta) * S$$

where

$S = \sum_i (\exp e_i)/n;$

e_i = the observed residuals from the log-transformed regression; and

n = the number of observations.

The variance of the difference in the prediction of Y in the FFS versus HMO sectors is computed by the delta method (Sobel 1982). The test statistic for comparing mean scores in the original scale is:

$$t\text{-statistic} = \frac{\sum_i (\hat{Y}_{FFS} - \hat{Y}_{HMO})}{SQRT\ (Variance[\hat{Y}_{FFS} + \hat{Y}_{HMO}])}$$

The mean physical functioning scores predicted for all beneficiaries if they had enrolled in the FFS and HMO sectors were 5.39 and 5.15, respectively. The t-statistic for the difference in predicted physical functioning was 1.015. Thus, the model predicts that had everyone in the sample joined an HMO, their physical functioning score would not have been significantly different than if they had chosen the FFS sector.

Two analyses were performed to answer the question: Does the HMO or the FFS sector produce better health in low-income individuals? First, the impact of plan membership on low-income people was evaluated using a single regression equation with interactions among plan membership, income level, and health status. A second analysis was performed using only the low-income (less than $20,000 per year) beneficiaries.[11]

Neither method indicated the presence of selectivity bias in the data. The first analysis of physical functioning replicated Ware et al.'s (1986) result: low-income people fared worse in the HMO. That model is restricted, however, in its assumption that the other coefficients are identical for high- and low-income people. In the second analysis, predicted health status was not significantly different between HMO and FFS enrollees ($\hat{Y}_{FFS} = 1.547$; $\hat{Y}_{HMO} = 1.542$; t-statistic = 0.009), thus failing to reject the hypothesis that the FFS and HMO sectors are associated with equal levels of physical functioning for low-income beneficiaries.

General perceived health status. Health status was also modeled using the general health perceptions scale of Davies and Ware (1981): "Do you rate your health as excellent, good, fair, or poor?" The theoretical model underlying the analysis assumes the existence of an underlying continuous index of perceived health status, denoted HS^*, which equals $X\beta + \sigma u$, with u distributed $N(0,1)$. The *observed* values of perceived health status (denoted HS), however, take on one of four ordered values: 0 = excellent health, 1 = good health, 2 = fair health, and 3 = poor health. Both ordered probit and ordered logit models were estimated for the ordered dependent variable. In this analysis, we used all beneficiaries who could answer the survey for themselves, including those age 88 and over.

In addition to the ordered values of the dependent variable, the estimation method also must account for potential bias arising from endogenous selection of the HMO versus FFS sector. Again, the approach to this problem is to estimate a health plan choice equation and to allow the error terms in the choice equation and the perceived health status equation to be correlated. The selectivity correlations were insignificant in both the FFS sector ($\rho = -0.1135$; $p = .244$) and the HMO sector ($\rho = 0.0051$; $p = .962$).

Perceived health status equations were estimated separately for the HMO and FFS sectors, but predictions were made using all beneficiaries in both sectors, as before. The mean perceived health status scores in the FFS and HMO sectors were 0.6774 and 0.6059, respectively. The resulting t-statistic was 2.998, indicating that perceived health status for all beneficiaries in this sample would have been higher in the HMO sector than in the FFS sector.

As in the case of physical functioning, the model also was estimated using only the low-income (less than \$20,000 per year) beneficiaries. Again, there was no indication of selectivity bias, and the difference in predicted perceived health status between the FFS and HMO sectors for low-income beneficiaries was not significant ($\hat{Y}_{FFS} = 0.7498$, $\hat{Y}_{HMO} = 0.7199$, t-statistic = 0.7814).

Basic FFS coverage versus FFS with a supplementary policy

Physical functioning. We also estimated differences in predicted health status for beneficiaries in the basic FFS sector (no supplementary policy) and beneficiaries with a supplementary policy (denoted "FFS-Plus"). This analysis addresses the question concerning whether beneficiaries with supplementary policies have better health than those with basic FFS Medicare.

Selectivity-corrected regressions were estimated for predicted health status, measured by the log of the physical functioning scale, for both sectors. The estimated selection terms were insignificant for both FFS ($\rho = 0.0197$; $p = .901$) and FFS-Plus ($\rho = 0.0502$, $p = .818$). Regressions then were estimated without the selection correction, and the predictions were transformed back to the original scale. We found no significant differences in predicted physical functioning between the FFS and FFS-Plus sectors ($\hat{Y}_{FFS+} = 1.305$; $\hat{Y}_{FFS} = 1.573$; t-statistic = -1.27).

General perceived health status. The same analysis was repeated using perceived health status as the dependent variable. In this case, the sample selection correlation coefficient was significant in the basic FFS sector ($\rho = 0.590$; $p = .001$), but not in the FFS-Plus sector ($\rho = 0.151$; $p = .345$). The difference in predicted health status between FFS and FFS-Plus also was significant ($\hat{Y}_{FFS+} = 0.901$; $\hat{Y}_{FFS} = 1.640$; t-statistic = -18.53), indicating that supplementary insurance is associated with higher perceived health status than the basic FFS sector.

Discussion

The most striking result from the analysis of health plan choice was that the oldest, poorest, and to some extent, the sickest Medicare beneficiaries in the Twin Cities have basic FFS Medicare. The effects of age and illness on choice of basic FFS Medicare versus FFS with a supplementary policy probably are due to a combination of medical underwriting by FFS supplementary insurers and other factors, such as physician loyalty and access, which influence the choice between the FFS sector and network HMOs or IPAs. Since our data were collected, three of the TEFRA risk plans (including both IPAs) have converted to HCPPs, which can practice medical underwriting. Thus, elderly beneficiaries with health problems may find their choices much more restricted today than in 1987–1988.

In the under-65 population, several states, including Minnesota, are experimenting with underwriting reform that limits insurers' ability to base premiums on risk. Pauly (1984) has pointed out that prohibiting insurers from varying premiums with the individual's risk may create, rather than alleviate, incentives for discrimination against high-risk individuals. The practice of individual risk rating appears to be confined primarily to the individual and small-group insurance market, although some large firms and insurers have expressed interest in the idea.

Another approach to insurance rating reform is to reorganize the individual and small-group market so that it more closely resembles the large employer market, where medical underwriting is much less prevalent and high-risk employees are pooled with low-risk employees. We have proposed that approach to reforming the Medicare market, which currently resembles the individual health insurance market (Dowd et al. 1992). Annual open enrollment periods with limited plan switching between open enrollment periods, and uniform premiums charged by participating insurers, could improve dramatically the access of the oldest and sickest Medicare beneficiaries to all health plans in the market. Open enrollment also would improve the information of the health plans on their enrolled populations. When beneficiaries enroll in groups of 20,000, the insurer needs to know only the sample mean expenditure for the group, rather than the estimated mean and variance for each beneficiary, as in the individual market, where beneficiaries enroll one at a time. Because medical underwriting would be greatly reduced or eliminated under this proposal, administrative cost savings also could be substantial.

Another important factor limiting the growth of Medicare HMOs appears to be the subsidy of supplementary FFS insurance by Medicare and employers. The current subsidy of supplementary FFS insurance by Medicare reduces employers' and employees' incentives to shop carefully for supplementary coverage (Dowd 1991). If this subsidy were eliminated, employers and employees might be more likely to turn to TEFRA-risk HMOs for their supplementary Medicare coverage. Many employers also subsidize the choice of supplementary FFS policies, thereby limiting the growth of Medicare HMOs. It is important for HCFA to continue its examination of the relationship between employment-based retiree plans and Medicare HMOs (Health Care Financing Administration 1991). Finally, the fact that beneficiaries who do not live in the Twin Cities all year are more likely to choose the FFS sector might be of interest to HMOs considering open-ended options (Christianson, Dowd, and Feldman 1992).

The finding of insignificant selectivity bias in the expenditure equations was surprising in light of earlier studies of HMO selection and our own health plan choice equations. It is clear that there are important differences in enrollee characteristics *within* and between the HMO and FFS sectors. The poorest, oldest beneficiaries in the Twin Cities tend to be found in basic FFS Medicare, but basic FFS Medicare comprises only 20 percent of the FFS Medicare sector in the Twin Cities. Network HMOs enjoy limited favorable selection, but there do not appear to be important differences between IPA-model HMOs and the "FFS plus supplement" sector. Thus, in the Twin Cities, the difference between the aggregate HMO and FFS sectors is diminished by within-sector variation in selection.

Insignificant selectivity bias in the Twin Cities during a period when five TEFRA-risk HMOs were operational has important implications for HCFA policy. First, *if average cost in the Twin Cities' FFS sector was computed correctly by HCFA during the study period*, HMO payments based on 95 percent of FFS costs yielded a 5 percent savings to HCFA. In addition, Nelson and Brown (1989) find "average reimbursements computed from HCFA claims data are considerably lower than the values implied by the county AAPCC values," and our data also show average FFS reimbursements to be considerably below AAPCC payment rates in the Twin Cities. Thus, even in the absence of selectivity bias, HCFA may have overpaid HMOs simply because the computation of average FFS expenditures in the AAPCC cells was incorrect.

The finding of no selectivity implies that it is unnecessary for HCFA to add further variables to the AAPCC in order to correct a payment bias. In fact, adding further variables actually might *create* selectivity bias. The finding of no selectivity could be due to variables with opposite effects (some favorable to HMOs and some favorable to FFS) offsetting each other. Adding one set of variables to the payment formula without adding the offsetting variables could create selectivity bias.

The overall conclusion from the analysis of health status in the Twin Cities is that the HMO and FFS Medicare sectors are associated with similar levels of physical functioning in beneficiaries younger than age 88. The same result holds for low-income beneficiaries. HMOs were associated with better perceived health status when beneficiaries older than age 88 were included in the sample and health status was measured as general health perceptions.

When the analysis of health status was limited to the FFS sector, no significant differences in physical functioning were found between the basic FFS sector and "FFS plus a supplementary policy." However, the difference in perceived health status was statistically significant, indicating better perceived health status associated with the "FFS plus a supplementary policy" sector.

The health status results also have important implications for the competitive pricing proposal for Medicare. A potential criticism of a system in which the federal government's contribution to Medicare premiums is limited to the lowest price submitted by a health plan in a market area is the likelihood that many low-income beneficiaries would choose the cheapest plan. Critics fear that the cheapest plan will skimp on quality of care.

In fact, the poorest beneficiaries in the Twin Cities are now choosing the cheapest plan: basic FFS Medicare, which costs $31.90 per month (the 1992 Part B premium). This is no bargain, in terms of the effect on health status. Wisner's (1992) results indicate that health outcomes would be better for all beneficiaries in the "FFS with a supplementary policy" sector versus basic FFS. She found no difference between the FFS sector as a whole, which is dominated by the "FFS plus a supplementary policy" sector, and the HMO sector, for low-income beneficiaries. Thus, based on these preliminary analyses, the indication is that low-income beneficiaries would have no worse, and perhaps better health, in an HMO than in the basic FFS sector.

Acknowledgments

This research was supported, in part, by the Health Care Financing Administration under cooperative agreements 17-C-99040/5-01 and 99-C-99169/5-04. The views expressed herein are solely those of the authors.

The authors wish to thank their project officers, Gerald Riley and Jim Beebe, as well as Jim Lubitz and Janet O'Leary for their helpful advice and comments during the course of the projects.

Notes

1. Competitive Medical Plans (CMPs) are HMOs that were not federally qualified, or other organizations such as preferred provider organizations.
2. All Medicare HMO data attributed to the Minnesota Department of Health (MDH) are reported for the state of Minnesota. MDH does not present

breakdowns of Medicare enrollment for the Twin Cities versus the rest of the state. This is most problematic for HMOs with service areas that include both the Twin Cities and other parts of the state (e.g., HMO Minnesota and Physicians' Health Plan).

3. A Social/HMO (S/HMO) is a health care financing and delivery system designed to transfer some money spent on acute care for the elderly to long-term care and, especially, to noninstitutional long-term care. Group Health Plan offers a S/HMO in the Twin Cities through a TEFRA risk contract. We excluded S/HMO enrollees from the survey because the S/HMO benefit package differs significantly from other Medicare HMOs. Medicaid "buy-in" beneficiaries were excluded because they supposedly were ineligible for Medicare HMO coverage. Elderly Supplemental Security Income (SSI) recipients are likely to be in an institution. We excluded this group because their choice of health plans and the effect of HMOs on their use of services might differ systematically from those of other elderly Medicare beneficiaries.

4. Information on physical functioning was not collected for the oldest beneficiaries.

5. The lower HMO response rate may have been due to the "bad press" that Medicare HMOs were getting at that time for withdrawing from rural areas (see pages 57 and 58 for a discussion of this problem). In the Twin Cities, Medicare HMOs were posting higher premiums for the supplementary benefits they offered under TEFRA risk contracts. This may have contributed to a bias among HMO enrollees against responding to our survey.

6. Many employers contribute to Medicare supplemental policies on behalf of their employees. Such contributions should increase the likelihood of choosing FFS with a supplement, both because they reduce the price of supplementary coverage of any kind, and because they are often limited to Medicare supplements offered by the employer's FFS health plan.

7. A significant number of claims in the HCFA MADRS data had no date of service. These claims were omitted from this study, but are being analyzed in another current study. Preliminary results indicate an increase in mean expenditures to $2,100, still far short of the average AAPCC payment of $3,220.96, and no substantial changes in the results regarding selectivity.

8. We wanted to determine if there is selectivity bias in the current AAPCC payment formula. Had we wanted to test for selectivity bias in *any* possible payment formula, we would have included additional explanatory variables in both the expenditure equation and the health plan choice equation.

9. The Jarque-Bera test statistic has a critical value of 5.991 with two degrees of freedom for normally distributed errors (Jarque and Bera 1981).

10. r is the correlation of the error terms in the health plan choice equation and the physical functioning equation.

11. Wisner's (1992) definition of low income (below $20,000) differed from that used in the analysis of health plan choice and expenditures (below $10,000). She chose this cutoff point because the median income in our sample is approximately $20,000.

References

Brown, R. S. "Biased Selection in Medicare HMOs." Paper presented at the Fifth Annual Meeting of the Association for Health Services Research, San Francisco, CA, June 26–28, 1988.

Christianson, J., B. Dowd, and R. Feldman. "Open-Ended Options in TEFRA-Risk Contracts with HMOs." Minneapolis: Division of Health Services Research and Policy, University of Minnesota, 4 May 1992.

Congressional Budget Office. *Cost Estimate for H.R. 3399*. Washington, DC: Government Printing Office, 26 May 1982.

Davies, A., and J. Ware. *Measuring Health Perception in the Health Insurance Experiment*. Santa Monica, CA: RAND Publication, R-2711-HHS, October 1981.

Dowd, B., and R. Feldman. "Biased Selection in Twin Cities Health Plans." In *Advances in Health Economics and Health Services Research, Vol. 6*, edited by R. M. Scheffler and L. F. Rossiter. Greenwich, CT: JAI Press, 1985.

Dowd, B., R. Feldman, S. Cassou, and M. Finch. "Health Plan Choice and the Utilization of Health Care Services." *Review of Economics and Statistics* 73, no. 1 (February 1991): 85–93.

Dowd, B., I. Moscovice, R. Feldman, M. Finch, C. Wisner, and S. Hillson. "Health Plan Choice in the Twin Cities Medicare Market." *University of Minnesota: Institute for Health Services Research*, 1992.

Duan, N. "Smearing Estimate: A Nonparametric Retransformation Method." *Journal of the American Statistical Association*, 78, no. 383 (September 1983): 605–10.

Eggers, P. "Risk Differential Between Medicare Beneficiaries Enrolled and Not Enrolled in an HMO." *Health Care Financing Review* 1, no. 3 (Winter 1980): 91–99.

Eggers, P. W., and R. Prihoda, "Pre-Enrollment Reimbursement Patterns of Medicare Beneficiaries Enrolled in 'At-Risk' HMOs." *Health Care Financing Review* 4, no. 1 (September 1982): 55–73.

Feldman, R. D., M. Finch, B. Dowd, and S. Cassou, "The Demand for Employment-Based Health Insurance Plans." *Journal of Human Resources* 24, no. 1 (Winter 1989): 115–42.

Galblum, T. W., and S. Trieger, "Demonstrations of Alternative Delivery Systems Under Medicare and Medicaid." *Health Care Financing Review* 3, no. 3 (March 1982); 1–11.

Garfinkel, S., W. E. Schlenger, K. R. McLeroy, F. A. Bryan, J. G. York, G. H. Dunteman, and A. S. Friedlob. "Choice of Payment Plan in the Medicare Capitation Demonstration." *Medical Care* 24, no. 7 (July 1986): 628–40.

Hausman, J., and D. McFadden. "Specification Tests for the Multinomial Logit Model." *Econometrica* 52, no. 5 (September 1984): 1219–39.

Health Care Financing Administration. "Expanding Medicare Coordinated Care Choices for Employer Group Retirees: The Report of the Health Care Financing Administration's Employer Group Task Force." U.S. Department of Health and Human Services, Washington, DC, June 1991.

Hellinger, F. J. "Selection Bias in Health Maintenance Organizations: Analysis of Recent Evidence." *Health Care Financing Review* 9, no. 2 (Winter 1987): 55–64.

Hildebrand, D. K., J. D. Laing, and H. Rosenthal. *Prediction Analysis of Cross Classification*. New York: John Wiley and Sons 1977.

Jarque, C., and A. Bera. "An Efficient Large-Sample Test for Normality of Observations and Regression Residuals." Manuscript, Australian National University, Canberra, 1981.

Langwell, K., L. Rossiter, R. Brown, L. Nelson, S. Nelson, and K. Berman. "Early Experience of Health Maintenance Organizations Under Medicare Competition Demonstrations." *Health Care Financing Review* 8, no. 3 (Spring 1987): 37–55.

Langwell, K. M., and J. P. Hadley. "Evaluation of the Medicare Competition Demonstrations." *Health Care Financing Review* 11, no. 2 (Winter 1989): 65–80.

Luft, H. S. *Health Maintenance Organizations: Dimensions of Performance*. New York: Wiley, 1981.

Manning, W. G., N. Duan, and W. H. Rogers. "Monte Carlo Evidence on the Choice Between Sample Selection and Two-Part Models." *Journal of Econometrics* 35 (1987): 59–82.

Minneapolis Star Tribune. "HMOs Rushing to Discontinue Coverage for the Elderly." 8 November 1987.

———. "2 HMOs, Clinic May Become Partners." 6 March 1992.

Minnesota Department of Health. *Statistical Report on Health Maintenance Operations in Minnesota*. Minneapolis: MDH, 1979–1991.

Nelson, L., and R. S. Brown. *National Medicare Competition Evaluation: Impact of Medicare HMOs on the Use and Cost of Services*. Final report to HCHA. Washington, DC: Mathematica Policy Research, Inc., January 1989.

Pauly, M. V. "Is Cream-Skimming a Problem for the Competitive Medical Market?" *Journal of Health Economics* 3, no. 1 (1984): 87–95.

Riley, P. A., B. Walton, and N. Johnson, "Risky Business—Shifting from a TEFRA-Risk Contract to a Health Care Prepayment Plan: MedCenters Health Plan's Experience." Paper presented at 1992 Aetna Health Plans Government Programs Workshop, Tucson, AZ, March 26–28, 1992.

St. Paul Pioneer Press. "PHP Defends Rural Pullout, Cites Losses." 15 December 1987.

Sloss, E., E. Keeler, R. Brook, B. Operskalski, G. Goldberg, and J. Newhouse. "Effect of a Health Maintenance Organization on Physiologic Health." *Annals of Internal Medicine*, 106, no. 1 (1987): 130–38.

Sobel, M. "Asymptotic Confidence Intervals for Indirect Effects in Structural Equation Models." In *Sociological Methodology*, edited by S. Leinhardt. San Francisco: Jossey-Bass, 1982.

Wagner, E., and T. Bledsoe. "The Rand Health Insurance Experiment and HMOs." *Medical Care* 28, no. 3 (1990): 191–200.

Ware, J. E., R. H. Brook, W. H. Rogers, E. B. Keeler, A. R. Davies, C. D. Sherbourne, G. A. Goldberg, P. Camp, and J. P. Newhouse. "Comparison of Health Outcomes at a Health Maintenance Organization with Those of FFS care." *The Lancet* (3 May 1986): 1017–22.

Wilensky, G., and L. Rossiter. "Patient Self-Selection in HMOs." *Health Affairs* 5, no. 1 (Spring 1986): 66–80.

Wilensky, G. R. and L. F. Rossiter. "Coordinated Care and Public Programs." *Health Affairs* 10 no. 4 (Winter, 1991): 62–77.

Wisner, C. "Health Plan Effects on the Health Status of Medicare Beneficiaries." *University of Minnesota: Institute for Health Services Research,* 1992.

Chapter 3

Responses and Discussion

Thomas Rice

Both papers—by Brown and Hill, and by Wisner, Feldman, and Dowd—provide excellent and timely analyses of the Medicare risk contracting program. This commentary briefly goes over some of the authors' central findings and then draws some more general policy implications about the way in which Medicare pays HMOs.

Brown and Hill use recent data—from 1990—to compare two groups of Medicare beneficiaries: those in HMOs that have Medicare risk contracts, and those in the fee-for-service component of Medicare. A remarkable thing about the study is the number of telephone interviews they conducted (almost 13,000) to obtain detailed and current information on the health status of these individuals. This aspect of the study is extremely useful because Medicare data on prior utilization alone may not capture differences in the health status of beneficiaries, and therefore in how many services they are likely to use in the future.

The first finding by Brown and Hill was that Medicare HMOs did have the *potential* to provide savings. But the way in which these savings were garnered was a surprise. The authors found that Medicare HMO admission rates were no lower than those in the fee-for-service sector, but that hospital lengths of stay were about 17 percent lower. The finding that HMO admission rates are no different than those in FFS comes as something of a surprise because it is generally believed that HMOs achieve their savings through lower admission rates. The authors suggest that the reason these savings may not have occurred in their sample is because FFS admissions had already dropped dramatically.

The finding that length of stay is lower in HMOs than in fee-for-service, although not in line with most previous research, is consistent with two recent studies that showed 15 percent shorter lengths of stay in the HMO setting (Bradbury, Golec, and Stearns 1991; Stern et al. 1989). The finding also makes a certain amount of sense. If, as the authors found, Medicare HMO admission rates are no lower than FFS, then these HMOs must find new ways to compete to keep their premiums down. Apparently they are beginning to do this by reducing length of stay to levels even lower than are being accomplished through the Medicare prospective payment system.

In summary, Brown and Hill found that, controlling for selection effects, people in Medicare HMOs spend 17 percent less than they would spend in the fee-for-service setting. Despite this, the authors conclude that Medicare risk contracts actually cost the program 6 percent more than if enrollees had remained in FFS. This is because the AAPCC is unable to control for the substantial amount of favorable selection into HMOs. Nevertheless, these new estimates are lower than the 15–33 percent losses the authors found in previous research from the Medicare Competition Demonstrations in the mid-1980s (Langwell and Hadley 1989).

Wisner, Feldman, and Dowd focused on Medicare HMOs in the Twin Cities as they looked not only at selection bias but, to the degree possible, at the impact on health status of enrollment in an HMO. Like the Brown and Hill study, this one relied, in part, on a large survey—over 2,000 in-person interviews with Medicare beneficiaries in 1987 and 1988.

Like previous studies, this one found that beneficiaries who remained in the fee-for-service setting tended to be older, poorer, and perhaps a little sicker. Where their findings differ from those of Brown and Hill is in a lack of evidence that selection bias, per se, is costing Medicare money, at least in the Twin Cities. What seems to be costing the Medicare program is rather its inability to calculate the costs of treating a person in the fee-for-service sector.

Their findings on this issue are startling. Wisner, Feldman, and Dowd calculate that fee-for-service beneficiaries in their sample were responsible for less than $1,500 each in Medicare reimbursements. AAPCC payments to HMO beneficiaries, however, were more than twice as high, averaging over $3,200.

The health status findings are encouraging; there is little evidence to suggest that the savings experienced by Medicare HMOs resulted in poorer quality care although, clearly, much more research is still necessary. Nor was there much evidence to indicate (as Ware et al. [1986] did from the RAND Health Insurance Experiment) that HMOs were differentially harmful to the poor.

Although methodology in both studies appears to be sound, it is difficult to reconcile the different findings regarding whether or not selection bias is responsible for program losses. While Brown and Hill calculated

Medicare losses on the order of 6 percent, Wisner, Feldman, and Dowd found no losses. Although the implications of these differences for reform of the AAPCC is important, the actual size of the difference is small, and may simply be due to the differences in the mix of patients in the Twin Cities compared to those in the nation as a whole.

The continued use of the AAPCC by Medicare

After over ten years during which Medicare has paid HMOs on a risk rather than cost basis, researchers continue to complain that the AAPCC is simply not up to the task. Estimates of its low predictive power are by now legendary, and investigators report that its use is costing Medicare money.

One problem with the AAPCC's low predictive power is that HMOs may perceive their participation in Medicare risk contracts as a crap shoot. Because the formula does not explain expenditures, HMOs may view the payment mechanism as almost random, and there is concern that they could very well lose money. This is surely partly responsible for the low levels of Medicare HMO enrollment—only 4 percent of beneficiaries are in HMOs, compared to 20 percent of people with employer-sponsored health insurance (Sullivan and Rice 1991). There appears to be a severe shortage of HMOs that are willing to take these risks.

The other central problem with the low predictive power of the AAPCC is that—as Brown and Hill show—Medicare may lose money. This finding has been known for over four years, however. Although Wisner, Feldman, and Dowd are among the first researchers *not* to detect a problem with regard to the AAPCC, they do detect a potentially greater one—that the program severely overestimates the cost of the fee-for-service sector, which in turn grossly inflates Medicare payments to HMOs through the AAPCC.

For whatever reasons—its low explanatory power, its sensitivity to selection bias, or the difficulty it has in calculating Medicare fee-for-service costs—the continued use of the AAPCC does not seem justifiable. This seems especially true since alternative payment mechanisms have been available for years.

Numerous researchers have shown that the formula could be made more effective by including measures of previous utilization, objective or perceived measures of health status, or even the presence of particular diagnoses. Brown and Hill claim that simply including a variable for whether the beneficiary has a history of cancer, heart disease, or stroke would effectively solve the problem. In another in this group of papers [chapter 11], Rossiter argues that a new risk adjustment formula, developed by Robinson et al. (1991), shows a great deal of promise and could be implemented in a short period of time.

Although these modifications are, in my opinion, long overdue, they miss the crux of the problem, which is that *HMO payments should not be based on fee-for-service costs*. This is true for two primary reasons. First, fee-for-service costs are a poor barometer of what it costs to provide care efficiently because they give providers a financial incentive to overprovide services. Even though Medicare has recently revamped its physician payment system through the adoption of the resource-based relative value payment system, physicians still earn more by doing more.

Second, unless the AAPCC is perfectly specified, linking HMO payments to fee-for-service costs is inherently unstable. As more relatively healthy people enroll in HMOs, a sicker cohort remains in FFS, which in turn increases HMO payments when, in fact, the opposite should be occurring. This problem will become greater over time as FFS gets smaller, since the AAPCC payments will be based on a smaller, and perhaps less representative cohort.

Exactly what should be done in place of even a modified AAPCC is not obvious. One possibility would be to conduct time-and-motion studies to determine the true costs involved for HMOs in treating Medicare patients. Unfortunately, such studies are riddled with problems, and they leave unsolved how payments vary according to selection bias in each particular case.

In other research, Dowd et al. (1992) suggest a competitive bidding approach. Although their particular proposal may have difficulties overcoming political barriers, the idea is appealing. Not only would HMOs be paid on the basis of treating patients in the HMO rather than the fee-for-service sector, but selection bias problems would be obviated to the extent that the HMOs could predict their own enrollment patterns.

I believe that HCFA and the Congress have had enough information to address this problem for some time; the findings by Brown and Hill underscore the cost of waiting longer. HMOs have repeatedly been shown to save money and many people want to join them; however, Medicare's use of the AAPCC has the remarkable effect of dissuading HMOs from taking Medicare patients, while allowing HMOs that do take this risk to experience windfall profits.

The new administration in Washington should take as one of its main priorities correcting this problem, either by modifying the AAPCC or, better yet, by replacing it with something better. This may be easier to talk about than to accomplish, however. Most of the numerous health care reform proposals before Congress focus on everything *except* Medicare. For example, the HealthAmerica bill (S. 1227) sponsored by many prominent congressional Democrats aims to provide universal health care coverage through a "play or pay" approach and by reforming the private health insurance market, but it makes almost no changes to Medicare. Similarly, a very different bill that calls for managed competition (HR 5936), sponsored by the Conservative Democratic Forum, revamps nearly everything in the health care sector, but leaves Medicare almost untouched.

Congress seems frightened to make substantial changes to Medicare, probably because of its not-too-distant memory of the passage and then ultimate repeal of the Medicare catastrophic legislation. But changes are long overdue; an excellent beginning—and one that would stimulate real competition—would be major reforms in the way Medicare pays HMOs.

References

Bradbury, R. C., J. H. Golec, and F. E. Stearns. "Comparing Hospital Length of Stay in Independent Practice Association HMOs and Traditional Insurance Programs." *Inquiry* 28, no. 2 (Spring 1991): 87–93.

Dowd, B. E., J. Christianson, R. D. Feldman, C. Wisner, and J. Klein. "Issues Regarding Health Plan Payments Under Medicare and Recommendations for Reform." *Milbank Quarterly* 70, no. 3 (1992): 423–53.

Langwell, K. M., and J. P. Hadley. "Evaluation of the Medicare Competition Demonstrations." *Health Care Financing Review* 11, no. 2 (Winter 1989): 65–80.

Robinson, J. C., H. S. Luft, L. B. Gardner, and E. M. Morrison. "A Method for Risk-Adjusting Employer Contributions to Competing Health Insurance Plans." *Inquiry* 28, no. 2 (Summer 1991): 107–16.

Stern, R. S., P. I. Juhn, P. J. Gertler, and A. M. Epstein. "A Comparison of Length of Stay and Costs for Health Maintenance Organizations and Fee-for-Service Patients." *Archives of Internal Medicine* 149 (May 1989): 1185–88.

Sullivan, C., and T. Rice. "The Health Insurance Picture, 1990." *Health Affairs* 10, no. 2 (Summer 1991): 104–15.

Ware, J. E., R. H. Brook, W. H. Rogers, E. B. Keeler, A. R. Davies, C. D. Sherbourne, G. A. Goldberg, P. Camp, and J. P. Newhouse. "Comparison of Health Outcomes at a Health Maintenance Organization with Those of FFS Care." *The Lancet*, (3 May 1986): 1017–22.

Jan Malcolm

The two papers, by Brown and Hill and Wisner, Feldman, and Dowd, appear well documented and analytically credible. While they clearly contribute to understanding the specific questions examined by the authors, the significance of Medicare's experience with risk contracting plans to the current health care reform debate calls for a broader perspective on the questions.

The TEFRA program contains within it many elements thought to be desirable for health care reform. The central concept is that risk-assuming plans take responsibility to organize and guarantee access to the full range of needed services for a defined population of enrollees. The budget discipline created by prospective per capita reimbursement should drive such systems to organize resources more rationally and to emphasize primary and preventive care. This is striking by contrast to the predominant (at least in the Medicare market) fragmented fee-for-service nonsystem, where the incentives to increase unit costs and generate volume are powerful. A TEFRA plan can be held "accountable" in ways unattainable in FFS. The potential—if not demonstrated—effects of TEFRA plans on the cost, quality, and outcomes measured at the population level rather than at the level of the individual patient are important to test.

For the TEFRA program not to be a clear success on a national scale over time, therefore, causes some serious depression among true believers in organized care systems. To the extent that analyses in these two papers tend to portray the TEFRA program as unsuccessful, either by their direct conclusions or by inference, it is important to revisit how success is being measured.

These comments address each of the two papers separately and then conclude with some general observations.

Brown and Hill

The effects of Medicare risk HMOs on Medicare costs and service utilization. The increased sophistication and timeliness of this analysis over prior studies is notable. In particular, quantification of the degree to which health status variables account for differences between average projected AAPCCs and average projected FFS costs may be useful in the ongoing search for health status adjustments to the reimbursement formula. The suggestion that the formula specifically account for cancer, heart disease, and stroke deserves exploration.

It is apparent that great care was taken in the methods by which the authors estimated the differences between HMO enrollees and fee-for-service users and predicted what the enrollees' fee-for-service costs would have been. However, given the realities of enrollment distribution, it was not possible for the analysis to avoid significantly overrepresenting Los Angeles and Dade counties. Therefore, if the AAPCCs in those two counties are of questionable accuracy, which seems possible, if not likely, the validity of the overall findings is open to question.

In some respects, the estimated effects of the risk program on service use do not square with Group Health Inc.'s/MedCenters' own experience. We believe we are reducing hospital admission rates as well as length of stay, partially through more extensive use of home health and skilled nursing facility services than this paper suggests is true on the average. For instance, we believe we admit patients of higher acuity to SNFs than is typically true in FFS, and that we provide more services in that setting as well as in home health than would be reimbursable under FFS rules.

With respect to HMO impact on use of physician services, it would be interesting to evaluate the appropriateness of the more frequent ambulatory visits of the FFS population. This could be one area where the incentives inherent in FFS reimbursement are operating to generate more frequent "call-backs" than might be medically necessary. It would also be interesting to see whether observed differences in ambulatory use rates would hold true for selected conditions, including chronic conditions, or whether HMO substitution of ambulatory for inpatient care would be more evident there.

To put the central finding in perspective, the result of an extra 5 percent cost to HCFA holds only if the AAPCC is an accurate predictor of FFS costs. Since the USPCC is sometimes off by 2 or 3 percent, some inaccuracy at the county level is also to be expected.

It would be helpful to clarify what on the surface seem to be disparate results. For example, the authors state that HCFA is "losing" 5.7 percent on the TEFRA program rather than saving the intended 5 percent. They later report that the AAPCC for enrollees exceeds their fee-for-service costs by 11 percent. They again mention the 5.7 percent figure for capitation overpayment, but wind up saying that due to demographics, the actual FFS costs for enrollees would have been 17 percent below the nonenrollee average. A reconciliation of these numbers for nontechnicians would be useful.

While the authors express their belief that the "qualifications" noted to the conclusions are not likely to produce significantly different results, those issues go to the heart of much of the debate about payment accuracy and HMO effectiveness, and therefore deserve deeper analysis. Perhaps it is only intuitive rather than statistically significant, but the ability of HMOs to better manage complex, high-cost, and chronic cases seems important given the nature of the cost management challenges particular to the Medicare population.

Wisner, Feldman, and Dowd

The Twin Cities Medicare health plans market: choice, cost, and health status. As a possible window into future patterns in other markets, this paper's historical accounting of Medicare offerings in the Twin Cities over the last 12 years is useful. I share the authors' regret that the rural experience was not studied. And additional research into the impact on total Medicare expenditures over this period, especially given the shifts from risk-based back to cost-based contracting, would be enlightening.

This research, conducted in a sophisticated Medicare HMO market produced results significantly different from prior studies on selection bias. This seems especially impressive, given that the data were drawn from a period not long after the HMOs stopped health screening, which might have been expected to produce more selection bias in the results. That it did not seems important to the debate.

The paper briefly notes the MedCenters Health Plan experience with the DCG (diagnostic cost group) demonstration. It has always been striking that the DCG results, under a system that clearly has greater predictive power than the current AAPCC cells, were so strongly different from earlier findings, based on prior-use analyses, that MedCenters was favorably selected. Those contradictory results need to be carefully analyzed.

Most plans contend that adding a health status adjustment to the formula is important, to increase confidence that plans are being appropriately rewarded for managing rather than avoiding risk. Many plans as well have provider capacity constraints that tend to place them in a situation with a fairly stable and aging group of enrollees, so that health status changes within the group can become critical.

The paper's finding that the oldest, poorest, and sickest beneficiaries in the Twin Cities had unsupplemented FFS Medicare in 1988 is not surprising, given the prevalence of medical underwriting in the market (even among HMOs until 1985). It might be interesting to rerun this analysis on more recent data to see if the distribution has changed.

HMOs in Minnesota are interested in better understanding the authors' competitive pricing proposal. The HMOs would agree that pooled purchasing is an important ingredient for small-group and individual insurance market reform. It would be helpful for the Twin Cities group to explain more clearly how Medicare is subsidizing FFS supplementary insurance.

As a small footnote to explain the Group Health/MedCenters affiliation, it is indeed a merger of administrative capabilities, but both separate HMO licenses will continue to function with provider network and benefit differences between them.

General comments

Both of these papers are careful and sophisticated in their approaches. They add to our knowledge on important topics. To the extent that some holes are left in the picture of how the risk contracting program has performed for beneficiaries, the government, and the plans, perhaps we in the industry should be challenged to contribute our own analyses.

We should try to understand what drives the reality that the risk program is now successful in only a limited number of areas in the country, characterized by high fee-for-service expenditures. More plans have lost money, or have barely broken even than have profited significantly from risk contracting. For most plans, input prices are rising faster than their AAPCCs.

The enrollment experiences of HMOs often do not conform to what the studies show. Perhaps the hard-to-measure effects of pent-up demand or anticipatory switching are more significant than have been shown so far.

Few if any analyses mention Medicare's low reimbursement rates relative to those of other buyers. Either Medicare uniquely knows what services are worth, or it is cost-shifting to less powerful buyers. This may be relevant only to the discussion of whether risk contracting should truly be judged solely, or primarily, on whether Medicare shaves another 5 percent off its already deeply discounted rates.

The more relevant measure of HMO cost savings might be of total beneficiary expenditures, since Medicare fails to capture a large portion of the costs paid out-of-pocket for noncovered services or in cost sharing.

Other important measures of TEFRA's success might include increasing access to care, especially for the low-income beneficiaries, and increasing the percentage of eligibles who receive primary and preventive care like immunizations and various screenings. And to reiterate an earlier point, more emphasis should be placed on the ability of HMOs to better manage the costs, and quality, of complex cases.

Finally, to judge fairly whether the TEFRA program is a model for reform, its long-term versus short-term effects must be studied. It may be that HMO success in increasing access to preventive care produces greater cost savings long-term relative to those covered only by basic Medicare. At the overall community level, using again the experience of the Twin Cities, TEFRA plans have had important effects on the restructuring of the community's care delivery system and on significantly reducing the rate of growth in total Medicare expenditures.

General Discussion

A participant pointed out that the broader policy of real concern is how to provide health insurance to the elderly with acceptable coverage in a cost-effective manner. But its cost to HCFA is only a part of the question. If one were to factor in the amount that FFS people are paying for Medigap policies, the figure would be much larger; the total insurance cost for FFS would be larger than the total amount of money for health insurance for the elderly in the HMO sector. The authors were asked if that is a reasonable thing to conclude from their data.

Bryan Dowd said that the statement is probably accurate. Another way of asking the question is, Where does the money go? If HCFA does overpay, what happens to that extra money? HMOs are filling in a lot of the premiums and deductibles that are the reasons the FFS people are buying Medigap policies. So from society's point of view, the Medicare HMO program may be a cost-effective way to provide more comprehensive health insurance coverage to the elderly. One participant commented that this was not meant as a criticism of the Wisner, Feldman, and Dowd study, but from the point of view of the big policy picture, it would be useful to study these issues in more detail.

There was a question whether some of the difference between these two papers and some of the differences between the perception of traditional HMOs and these studies might relate to the readers' sense that everybody comes in through open enrollment. In the Brown and Hill study population, the median enrollment tenure is roughly three years. That simply bears no resemblance to the median enrollment tenure of the Twin Cities or of other traditional HMOs. So are these actually two very different populations—one of which comes in through open enrollment with all the selection pressures, while the other population has aged in without the benefits to the HMO of the open-enrollment filtration process?

Conferees agreed that a substantial difference does exist between people who have "aged in" and people who come in through open enrollment. In many HMOs, probably fewer than 10 percent would have been in the plan three years previously. Some people may have been in the HMO when they were employed and aged in. What was measured by the HCFA data was when they enrolled in the Medicare risk plan. But you can't necessarily infer from the Brown and Hill data how long these beneficiaries had been associated with the HMO. The subjects were not asked how long they had been in that HMO; they were asked whether they had to change physicians when they joined. This implies a negative response by people joining an IPA and continuing with the same physician they had under FFS. The question was designed to focus on the need for switching, not on longevity in the plan.

One participant mentioned that in his own study he compared people who come in during open enrollment with similar information on those who were aged in, and there is a substantial difference that is not reflected in a simple reading.

Randall Brown was asked about the survey response rate of enrollees. He answered that it was about 82 percent for enrollees and 74 percent for nonenrollees. He explained that they sent out a letter to enrollees selected at randon from HCFA's list of all people who were enrolled. For nonenrollees, the sample was drawn from the beneficiary files. HCFA did not have phone numbers for either group, and many of the addresses were bad, so finding them required a fair amount of work. Letters were sent on HCFA stationery to inform beneficiaries that they would be contacted. Then these beneficiaries were called and an interview was requested. If they had an unlisted number, which was frequently the case, beneficiaries received a second letter asking them to call in. The response rate was based on the original pool. Dr. Brown said that they got very few refusals, less than 5 percent, once they were able to reach the people by telephone. The trick was to get a decent phone number.

It was pointed out that the data in the Brown and Hill paper were self-reported services data, while the Wisner, Feldman, and Dowd data were claims data. Dr. Dowd reported that he had no self-reported utilization data.

A further comment concerning the Brown and Hill study stated that a fairly good-sized proportion of Medicare risk plan enrollees were covered completely, with no supplemental premiums, and many were covered for prescription drugs as well. So they paid absolutely nothing except a small surcharge for each visit. Comparing this model with FFS, HCFA does not know how much these people paid for prescription drugs, mental health and preventive services, deductibles, copayments, and/or premiums. It is possible to draw a superficial conclusion that HCFA overpays for Medicare in HMOs, when in fact Medicare covers only about 50 or 60 percent of the total cost for nonenrollees, whereas HMOs cover almost 100 percent of the cost.

Randall Brown responded that his study examines whether the program accomplished what he interpreted HCFA's intent to be, that is, cost savings to Medicare for Medicare-covered services. Is Medicare paying more now than it would have if the person had stayed in FFS? This is a different issue than whether total expenses (including both Medicare payments and beneficiaries' out-of-pocket payments) would have been higher under FFS. Then HCFA can decide whether it wants to provide a subsidy from taxpayers to *some* Medicare beneficiaries, as it is now doing. They probably wouldn't choose to distribute it primarily to beneficiaries in Miami and Los Angeles, which is basically what is happening because of the geographic concentration of Medicare HMO enrollment.

Another participant commented that the Brown and Hill findings were not anti-HMO at all. Their research actually found some savings.

So in some ways, whether HCFA is saving money or not is not the big issue. The important point is, if HMOs are more efficient and can save money, we need to find a way to pay them in a way that makes HMOs want to participate. An important point to consider is how to encourage beneficiaries to join Medicare HMOs. It does not appear that Medicare is doing very well in setting an appropriate payment, whether or not HCFA is losing money in the experiment.

Another aspect of this issue is related to the fact that the whole Medicare program for HMOs is different from the regular HMO, non-Medicare enrollee program. Typically HMOs are dealing with large groups that have an open enrollment season once a year. The marketing costs are relatively small until there is a major advertising campaign. Medicare enrollment typically requires marketing to individuals, and people can come and go each month. On the Medicare side this imposes substantial costs that do not appear as services or utilization. They do not show up in the studies here, and they are not explicitly incorporated in the AAPCC in terms of Medicare costs. So Medicare can say they want to knock 5 percent off what it costs them for services, while the HMOs are saying that those costs have to cover both services and marketing.

Dr. Brown was asked if his figures include ambulatory care. He responded that beneficiaries were asked how many ambulatory care visits they had in the last 30 days as well as interval questions about how many they had had in the past year (any, fewer than three, three to eleven, twelve or more). They found that HMO members were more likely to have seen a physician at least once in the past year and more likely to have had a physical examination, but they were less likely to have had *many* visits (more than 12) last year.

A follow-up question was, What is the ambulatory care visit rate per thousand members per year in FFS and in the HMO? The investigators did not have the data to address this question, but they did learn that HMO enrollees report less use of specialists and less follow-up and monitoring for some conditions. This finding was challenged by one of the participants.

Dr. Dowd voiced concern that discrepancy in the findings on over-payment might be taken away from the discussion. He wanted to em-phasize that the 5 percent overpayment versus no overpayment is well within the range of error of the different methodological approaches used in his study. If the Wisner, Feldman, and Dowd study had started with a similarly specified cost equation and then had compared the predicted level of cost for HMO versus FFS enrollees, the investigators might have replicated the Brown and Hill result. It is possible that if Brown and Hill had started with a bare-bones AAPCC equation and a bare-bones choice equation, with just enough variables in the latter to identify the cost equation, they might not have found selectivity there and thus might have replicated the Wisner, Feldman, and Dowd results. So Dowd cautioned against making too much of the apparent differences. It should be emphasized that the authors have reported their findings but that no attempt has been made to reconcile the differences in the two studies. That includes taking into consideration all of the other obvious differences such as location.

Randall Brown commented that while it is true that his study might have found a result similar to Bryan Dowd's, it is unlikely and would actually only show misspecification of that model. His study, he said, had *real* data on beneficiaries' health status; he found that enrollees *are* healthier, and that the AAPCC does not control fully for this. That is favorable selection. There might be little or none of it in the Minneapolis plans, but nationwide it exists.

Part **II**

Enrollee Satisfaction

Chapter 4

Satisfaction with Access and Quality of Care in Medicare Risk Contract HMOs

Dolores Gurnick Clement, Sheldon M. Retchin, and Randall S. Brown

Overview: Satisfaction with Care

Beneficiary satisfaction with a health maintenance organization is an important concern for the Medicare risk contract program. HMOs with risk contracts are compensated to ensure access and coverage of the enrolled beneficiaries while managing utilization and costs. Enrollment in an HMO offers a Medicare beneficiary wider coverage of benefits for some services. Yet a persistent concern has been that financial incentives for HMOs to control utilization and costs can affect the quality of care. Measures of beneficiary satisfaction serve as indicators of the perceived quality of care delivered by HMOs and can be used to assess various aspects of the structure, process, and outcome of care. Satisfaction with medical care and the system through which it is delivered is influenced by the characteristics of patients, characteristics of providers, and factors related to the delivery and use of health care services. Medicare beneficiaries' satisfaction with their access to care and the quality of care they receive is measured and analyzed in this paper.

Maintaining a high level of satisfaction with HMO care is critical both to an HMO's financial performance and to achievement of the Health Care Financing Administration's goal of expanding beneficiaries' choices of health care delivery systems. HMOs that participate in risk-based contracts cannot expect enrollment to grow if their enrollees are not at least as satisfied as fee-for-service (FFS) beneficiaries. Furthermore, enrollment and disenrollment are costly, so avoiding turnover is desirable. The fact that Medicare beneficiaries are permitted to disenroll with a month or less notice means that participating risk contract HMOs must be consistent in maintaining high-quality services and amenities in order to maintain beneficiary satisfaction and thus avoid high disenrollment rates. From a medical perspective, satisfaction with care is important, too, because it affects patient compliance to prescribed therapy as well as subsequent care-seeking behavior.

Background: Satisfaction Measurement

Patient satisfaction is a measure of the patient's perception of the match between desires, expectations, and needs, and the care that is received. Specific dimensions of patient satisfaction that address the patient/ system relationship have been investigated over a broad range of settings and conceptualizations. Ware et al. (1978) identify eight dimensions that contribute to a patient's satisfaction or dissatisfaction with care: the art of care, technical quality, accessibility, convenience, finances, physical environment, availability, continuity, and efficacy/outcomes. The multidimensionality of the concept of patient satisfaction is reflected in its assessment over time.

Thomas and Penchansky (1984) and Aday, Andersen, and Fleming (1980) explored the access dimension—the fit between the patient and the system—by measuring several variables: availability, acceptability, accommodation, affordability, and accessibility. They found that differences in utilization were associated with various levels of satisfaction with access in different populations.

Other distinctions, such as having a regular source of care and knowledge about the system, enhance the understanding of satisfaction with access to care. Doyle and Ware (1977) demonstrated that the relationship between overall satisfaction and the continuity of care (having a regular source of care) was stronger for those patients who were better educated. Newhouse, Ware, and Donald (1981) measured knowledge about the medical delivery system and how it pertained to the consumer's ability to make a good choice. They hypothesized that a weak correlation exists between consumer sophistication and satisfaction with medical care. The results indicated that more informed persons tend to be more critical in evaluating providers and services, and that dissatisfaction triggers the search for alternatives.

Ware and Davies (1983) found that differences in satisfaction influence subsequent patient behavior, as measured by intentions to maintain provider continuity. Greater satisfaction with care was associated with the intention to continue with a specific provider, while dissatisfaction was associated with the intention to try different doctors or change the delivery system. The results of a different, longitudinal study of actual behavior indicated that consumer satisfaction with medical care predicts changes in medical care providers (Marquis, Davies, and Ware 1983). The study concludes that the probability of changing provider increases as satisfaction with care decreases.

Dimensions of satisfaction also influence the decision to enroll in prepaid health plans. Medicare demonstration studies indicate that elderly beneficiaries respond to HMO marketing to the extent that they are dissatisfied with coverage, costs, and the perceived quality of care received from their existing FFS providers. Friedlob and Hadley (1985), Garfinkel et al. (1986), and Brown et al. (1986) all reported that, as dissatisfaction with prior usual source of care increases, Medicare beneficiaries are more likely to switch to an HMO. In addition, the burden of paperwork was found to be an even more important aspect of satisfaction than fees, travel, and waiting time.

The only randomized, controlled trial comparing satisfaction with care between HMO enrollees and FFS beneficiaries was done as part of the RAND Health Insurance Experiment, and studied a nonelderly (age 17 to 61) population. In this study, the typical person assigned to an HMO was found to be significantly less satisfied overall than the typical fee-for-service respondent, although those who chose the HMO alternative were equally as satisfied overall with their care (Davies et al. 1986).

Assessment of Satisfaction in Geriatric Populations

Although it has been found that both young and old persons are satisfied with the overall quality of the care they receive, differences exist in the relative influence of indicators on patient satisfaction (Linn, Linn, and Stein 1982). Satisfaction for the elderly is associated with the expectation of physical improvement, and their compliance is associated more with the personal qualities of the provider and with the cost and convenience of care. The elderly also are less likely to complain about long clinic waits.

Although the determinants of patient satisfaction have been studied extensively, there is less empirical knowledge of older adults' satisfaction with care in a prepaid setting. Medicare beneficiary satisfaction in HMOs has been examined for the Medicare Capitation Demonstrations and in the National Medicare Competition Evaluation (NMCE). The first analysis focused on beneficiaries enrolled in HMOs in Minneapolis in 1982, and found very high levels of overall enrollee satisfaction, ranging from 85.9 percent to 91.5 percent, across the four plans studied (Friedlob and Hadley 1985). The NMCE found somewhat lower levels of overall satisfaction (80.8 percent). Although the differences in these results could represent a decline in satisfaction as risk-based contracting under Medicare expanded during the period, it is more likely that they simply reflect differences in the HMOs studied, the ability of the particular HMOs to influence enrollee satisfaction, the market environment and understanding of the HMO concept, survey research methods, or the characteristics of enrollees in the two demonstrations.

The results of the NMCE study on patient satisfaction suggest that continuing HMO enrollees are as satisfied overall with their health care arrangements as are fee-for-service Medicare beneficiaries, although they are somewhat less satisfied with the quality of the care available to them (Rossiter et al. 1988). However, the high disenrollment rates in some HMOs and the relationship between satisfaction and disenrollment documented in the Rossiter et al. report suggest that the effects of HMO membership on beneficiary satisfaction in the Medicare risk program should continue to be monitored.

The flexibility of the disenrollment option of risk contract HMOs allows beneficiaries to examine coverage under an HMO that they might be reluctant to join if they have to commit to a longer enrollment period. Langwell et al. (1989) analyzed the disenrollment experience of the risk contract program. Their report showed that a high proportion of Medicare beneficiaries continue to disenroll from TEFRA HMO/CMP risk contracts over time. They found that approximately 7 percent of Medicare beneficiaries disenroll within the first three months of enrollment. This pattern was the same during the demonstration period and throughout their study period of 1985–1988. However, their findings also indicated that in areas with multiple risk plans some competition among plans existed for Medicare enrollments. This accounted for some of the disenrollment. They also found higher disenrollment from HMOs and CMPs in areas where enrollees reported below average satisfaction with selected dimensions of quality in the demonstration analysis.

Purpose of the Analysis

The purpose of the analysis is to determine whether enrollees in the Medicare risk-based plans have different levels of patient satisfaction than fee-for-service Medicare beneficiaries (nonenrollees). Differences are identified between enrollees and nonenrollees on the personal characteristics of beneficiaries that seem to be most associated with the highest level of satisfaction (reported as excellent). A logistic model is developed to estimate the differences between enrolled and nonenrolled respondents' satisfaction with various aspects of care and care delivery, controlling for differences between the groups on key characteristics, including age, income, race, gender, health status, activities of daily living (ADL) characteristics, and behavioral characteristics. Probabilities of being satisfied, holding these characteristics constant, are calculated from the model estimates and are tested to determine the magnitude of the effects; they are presented for enrollees and nonenrollees. The effect HMO membership has on various dimensions of satisfaction with access and quality of care is examined to determine current beneficiaries' perceptions of managed care and implications of these perceptions for the risk contract program.

Data: Beneficiary Survey

The study is based on the analysis of a 1990 survey of a stratified random sample of Medicare beneficiaries who were enrolled in one of the 75 HMOs with established risk contracts, and a comparable stratified random sample of Medicare beneficiaries who continued to receive their care in fee-for-service (FFS) settings. The nonenrollees who were selected resided in one of the 44 market areas in which risk contract HMOs were operating on April 1, 1990. The survey is described in more detail in the final report of the evaluation of access and satisfaction with care in the TEFRA evaluation (Clement et al. 1992).

This analysis is focused on Medicare beneficiaries who are over the age of 64. It is limited to this group because of concerns that beneficiaries under age 65 who are entitled to Medicare for disability or end-stage renal disease may exhibit very different care-seeking behavior. Fewer than 3 percent of the enrollees are under 65.

Other data sources

The beneficiary survey is the main source of data for our analyses, although several data sources maintained by HCFA (Bureau of Data Management and Strategy 1989a,b) were also used. For enrollees, data on age, sex, race, welfare status, disability status, and dates of entitlement and enrollment were obtained from the Group Health Plan Operations (GHPO) file. For nonenrollees, these data were obtained from the Medicare master beneficiary file (URHIMRS). Plan characteristics (premiums, benefits, and model type) were obtained from the monthly Office of Coordinated Care, Policy, and Planning (OCCPP) reports.

Logistic regression model methods

In addition to descriptive bivariate comparisons of enrollees and nonenrollees for satisfaction with care, the difference is estimated between the two groups using statistical methods to control for the effects other characteristics might have on satisfaction and access. Since most of the dependent variables that are examined are binary, logit models are used to estimate the relationship between the probability that an individual is satisfied and the beneficiary's characteristics, including enrollment status. The logit model for the probability of being satisfied ($Y = 1$) is represented by:

$$\text{prob}(Y = 1) = 1/(1 + e^{-aE - bX})$$

where

E = 1 for enrollees and 0 for nonenrollees;
X = the set of control variables; and
a and b = parameters to be estimated with the logistic model.

The odds that $Y = 1$ for enrollees is $p(Y = 1)/p(Y = 0) = e^{a + bX}$; the odds that $Y = 1$ for nonenrollees is e^{bX}; and the enrollee-to-nonenrollee ratio of these odds is e^a. The statistical significance of the effect of HMO enrollment is determined by the t-statistic for the coefficient a.

The results are presented in the form of HMO effects on the *probabilities* of a beneficiary's satisfaction with care. These estimates are obtained by using the estimated logit model to compute the predicted probability for each individual in the sample that $Y = 1$, first assuming that the individual is an enrollee and then assuming that the individual is a nonenrollee (regardless of his or her actual status). The difference between these two estimates is the predicted effect of HMO enrollment on this individual's probability of being $Y = 1$. These predicted effects are then averaged across all sample members to obtain the overall effect. The predicted probabilities displayed in the results tables are the raw mean for the nonenrollees (to provide a reference point); for enrollees, the displayed probability is the nonenrollee mean plus the estimated effect.

Dependent variables

The survey questions on dimensions of satisfaction with personal attention, access, cost, and quality of care are the base of our dependent variables. Interviewers required beneficiaries to rate their satisfaction with various aspects of care on a four-point scale (excellent, good, fair, poor). The responses were recoded to make each of these variables into a binary indicator (excellent versus good, fair, or poor) in order to assess estimated differences between enrollees and nonenrollees who reported their satisfaction as excellent. The dependent variables are listed with the results of the effects of enrollment status in Tables 4.3, 4.4, and 4.5 further on.

Independent variables

The control variables used in the logit model included the following types of variables:

- Demographic characteristics (age, gender, race, married status, education, whether live alone)
- Economic variables (income, employment status, whether own home)
- Behavioral variables (whether avoid physician visits, concern about health, whether smoke)
- Health and functioning indicators (ability to hear, ability to do activities of daily living, self-rating of health, history of serious illness).

Descriptive statistics of these variables are appended.

Since relatively unimpaired beneficiaries comprised the study sample, use of the individual indicators of impairment in the basic activities of daily living proved problematic. Many were not significant in the majority of models tested. In the interest of economy and following the lead of previous studies, we collapsed the ADL and instrumental activities of daily living (IADL) variables into a single dichotomous variable indicating whether or not an individual had any ADL or IADL impairment. The instrumental activities of daily living variables had been previously collapsed into a summative scale. The final specification for all of the independent variables included in the logistic regressions are listed in Table 4.1.

Results of Enrollee-Nonenrollee Comparisons

Medicare beneficiaries who remained in the fee-for-service sector were more likely to respond that satisfaction with various dimensions of care was excellent than those enrolled in risk contract HMOs. Although the statistically significant differences may show a lower proportion of enrollees who rated their satisfaction as excellent, the differences concern the degree of satisfaction rather than indicating dissatisfaction among enrollees. For example, responses to the question about how the respondent would rate the overall quality of care and services are presented in Table

Table 4.1   Independent Variable Definitions for Logit Model

Enrollment Status	Dichotomous variable indicating whether or not an individual was enrolled in an HMO
Demographic Variables	
Age	Continuous variable for age of sample person
Male	Dichotomous variable for gender: 1 = male, 0 = female
Caucasian	Dichotomous variable for race: 1 = Caucasian, 0 = other
Married, with spouse	Dichotomous variable indicating whether or not the sample person was married and living with spouse
Lives alone	Dichotomous variable indicating whether or not an individual lived alone or with others (not spouse)
Education	Continuous variable representing highest grade completed
Economic Variables	
Income	Continuous variable for annual income of beneficiary and spouse
Homeowner	Dichotomous variable indicating whether or not an individual owned own home
Working	Dichotomous variable indicating whether or not an individual is employed
Behavioral Variables	
Avoids doctor	Dichotomous variable indicating whether or not the sample person "will do just about anything to avoid going to the doctor"
Visit timing	Dichotomous variable indicating whether or not the sample person "usually goes to the doctor as soon as he/she starts to feel bad"
Health worries	Dichotomous variable indicating whether or not the sample person "worries about his/her health more than other people his/her age"
Tobacco use	Dichotomous variable indicating whether or not the sample person smokes or chews tobacco
Health and Functioning Variables	
Hearing	Dichotomous variable indicating whether or not the sample person has difficulty hearing
ADLs	Dichotomous variable indicating whether or not an individual needs assistance to perform any ADL task (i.e., eating, bathing, dressing, grooming, moving about)
IADLs	Number of instrumental activities of daily living needs help with (e.g., shopping, paying bills, etc.)
Self-rated health	Categorical variable for self-rated health condition (1 = excellent, 2 = good, 3 = fair, 4 = poor)
Serious illness	Dichotomous variable indicating self-reported history of cancer, heart disease, or stroke

4.2. Enrollees are significantly less likely than nonenrollees to rate overall quality as excellent. However, they are more likely to rate overall quality of care and services as good, fair, or poor.

For this analysis the "excellent" category is used only to differenti-ate the degree of satisfaction. Thus, the satisfaction rates and probabilities are lower, but the differences are greater in magnitude to have policy relevance. It should be noted that the analysis reported here was also replicated combining the excellent and good categories, as well as the fair and poor categories. Combining the excellent and good responses dilutes the effect that is being examined. Again referring to Table 4.2, it can be seen that 92.1 percent of enrollees respond excellent and good for satis-faction with overall quality of care versus 94.9 percent of nonenrollees, and the difference is reduced to 2.8 percentage points. Fewer than 10 percent of the sample responses were fair and poor, which considerably reduces the sample on which to determine an effect. Nonetheless, the results were similar but statistically significant differences were smaller in magnitude.

Satisfaction with personal attention

Logit estimates of the effects of enrollment status on the probability of Medicare beneficiaries rating their satisfaction with aspects of personal attention are presented in Table 4.3. Differences between enrollees and nonenrollees rating as excellent their satisfaction with the personal at-tention they received while under care range from 11 to 15 percentage points. Enrollees are consistently less satisfied than nonenrollees with explanations of care, attention they received as a patient, personal interest taken in their care, and their perception of respect and privacy. Enrollees

Table 4.2   Patient Satisfaction with Overall Quality of Care: Comparison of Survey Responses of Enrollees and Nonenrollees

Variable/Response	Enrollees	Nonenrollees	Difference†
Overall Quality of Care			
Excellent	44.9	51.7	−6.8*
Good	47.2	43.2	4.0*
Fair	6.5	4.3	2.2*
Poor	1.4	0.8	0.6*
	100.0	100.0	

*Significant at the .01 or 1% level, two-tailed test.
†Statistical significance tested using Mantel Haenszel Chi-square.

are also less likely than nonenrollees to rate as excellent the advice they receive on preventing health problems.

Satisfaction with access to care

Table 4.4 contains estimates of the effects of enrollment status on the probability of Medicare beneficiaries giving an excellent rating to their satisfaction with dimensions of access to care. HMO enrollees are less likely to be highly satisfied with the ease of seeing a physician of their choice, availability of emergency care, specialty care, and hospital care they receive, the ease with which they receive information or make an appointment over the phone, and the ease of getting a prescription filled. The probability that enrollees are satisfied with the convenience of office hours and waiting times (from appointment to visit and while at the office) is lower than that of nonenrollees. Thus, although it was found that access is similar for both groups (Clement et al. 1992), enrollees are less likely to express high satisfaction with the availability, convenience, and ease with which they can obtain care. Only the location of the office is considered equally convenient by enrollees and nonenrollees. For a number of measures (e.g., telephone appointments, ease of seeing a physician of choice, waiting time until an appointment can be scheduled), the differences are over 15 percentage points. For critical measures such as satisfaction with the availability of hospital care and the ease of filling prescriptions, the differences are smaller, although they remain statistically significant.

Table 4.3   Satisfaction with Personal Attention: Logit Estimates of Effects of Enrollment Status on Probability of Medicare Beneficiaries Satisfaction with Care (% Responses Excellent)

Dependent Variable	Enrollees	Nonenrollees	Difference
Explanations	.426	.539	−.113*
Attention to patient	.425	.560	−.135*
Preventive advice	.392	.501	−.109*
Personal interest	.404	.559	−.155*
Respect and privacy	.474	.591	−.117*
Sample Size†	5992	5158	

*Significant at the .01 level or higher, two-tailed test.
†Numbers refer to maximum sample size available for the satisfaction variables by enrollment status.

Table 4.4   Satisfaction with Access to Care: Logit Estimates of Effects of Enrollment Status on Probability of Medicare Beneficiaries Satisfaction with Care (% Responses Excellent)

Dependent Variable	Enrollees	Nonenrollees	Difference
Ease of seeing MD of choice	.429	.613	−.184*
Availability of emergency care	.488	.578	−.090*
Ease of making telephone appointments	.392	.566	−.174*
Convenience of office location	.493	.504	−.011
Convenience of office hours	.407	.483	−.076*
Availability of specialty care	.464	.556	−.092*
Availability of hospital care	.510	.562	−.052*
Wait from appointment to visit	.317	.472	−.155*
Wait at office	.317	.378	−.061*
Ease of obtaining information over the phone	.345	.473	−.128*
Ease of getting prescription filled	.526	.575	−.049*
Sample Size†	5992	5158	

*Significant at the .01 level or higher, two-tailed test.
†Numbers refer to maximum sample size available for the satisfaction variables by enrollment status.

Satisfaction with costs

The area in which HMO enrollees were more satisfied than nonenrollees was in the amount of out-of-pocket costs incurred with the care they received (Table 4.5). HMOs have succeeded in reducing the economic burden on the elderly by significantly lowering what the individual must pay for coverage. This is reflected in the difference (13 percentage points) in the degree of satisfaction with out-of-pocket costs for enrollees. This difference reflects the fact that about half of the enrollees belong to HMOs that do not charge a premium.

Satisfaction with the quality of care

Estimates of the effects of enrollment status on the probability of Medicare beneficiaries rating their satisfaction with dimensions of quality of care are presented in Table 4.5. Those enrolled in HMOs were significantly less likely than nonenrollees to rate as excellent the thoroughness of examinations, thoroughness of treatment, their perceived accuracy of

Table 4.5   Satisfaction with Costs and Quality of Care: Logit Estimates
of Effects of Enrollment Status on Probability of Medicare
Beneficiaries Satisfaction with Care (% Responses Excellent)

Dependent Variable	Enrollees	Nonenrollees	Difference
Satisfaction with Cost			
Amount of out-of-pocket costs	.534	.403	.131*
Satisfaction with Quality of Care			
Perceived quality of office/facilities	.498	.550	−.052*
Thoroughness of exams	.427	.521	−.094*
Perceived accuracy of diagnosis	.405	.508	−.103*
Thoroughness of treatment	.399	.497	−.098*
Perceived results of care	.405	.489	−.084*
Recommends provider to others	.935	.961	−.026*
Overall quality of care	.452	.529	−.077*
Sample Size†	5992	5158	

*Significant at the .01 level or higher, two-tailed test.
†Numbers refer to maximum sample size available for the satisfaction variables by
enrollment status.

the diagnosis, and the results of care. Enrollees were also less likely
than nonenrollees to recommend their provider to friends or relatives
needing medical care. Nonetheless, 93.5 percent of enrollees said they
would recommend their HMO to friends in need of health care.

Discussion of Results

Medicare beneficiaries who remained in the fee-for-service sector to obtain their medical care were more likely to respond that the overall
quality of their care and the services they received was excellent than
those enrolled in risk contract HMOs. In the design of the risk contract
evaluation it was thought that by 1990, with a quantity of beneficiaries who had considerable experience in managed care arrangements,
enrollees and nonenrollees would be equally satisfied with the overall
quality of care. The results do not support this premise, perhaps because
the time frame has not been long enough.

The results indicate that Medicare beneficiaries who enroll in HMOs
are consistently less highly satisfied with aspects of gaining access to a
system of managed care. Controlling for demographic, functional, behavioral, and health status factors, enrollees are less likely than nonenrollees
to be highly satisfied with (to rate as excellent) the ease with which they

can make telephone appointments, the ease of seeing the physician of their choice, the availability of hospital care, the availability of specialty care, the convenience of office hours, waiting time from appointment to visit, and the ease with which information is obtained by telephone. The only area concerning access to the delivery of care where no significant difference in satisfaction between enrollees and nonenrollees is found is the location of offices where care is received.

Similarly, Medicare beneficiaries who chose to enroll in risk contract HMOs are less satisfied with the personal attention they receive as patients than are those who did not enroll. Nonenrollees are more likely to rate as excellent their satisfaction with explanations of the care they receive, attention paid to them as patients, preventive advice, personal interest taken in their care, respect and privacy considerations, thoroughness of examinations, thoroughness of treatment, and the ease with which they are able to get prescriptions.

The enrollment of Medicare beneficiaries in HMOs with risk contract arrangements presents operational challenges that may strain the plans' capability to fully satisfy an older population. Indeed, obtaining care from a closed system of providers on a prepaid basis is still a relatively new concept for many people over 65 enrolling in these systems when all they have experienced up to this point in their lives may have been fee-for-service coverage. Although those who have enrolled in HMOs are able to access the systems, their expectations of service are not being met as well as the expectations of their counterparts who have remained in the fee-for-service area where they are perhaps more familiar with how delivery occurs. However, one could view this lower degree of satisfaction for enrollees as the trade-off that they make for the lower premiums and more extensive benefits they enjoy relative to nonenrollees with private Medicare supplementary insurance (Medigap) coverage or with no supplemental coverage.

This trade-off is evidenced in the higher satisfaction of HMO beneficiaries with the out-of-pocket costs required that are lower than fee-for-service costs for beneficiaries. It is interesting that only 40.3 percent of nonenrollees responded that they are satisfied with the amount of out-of-pocket cost incurred as opposed to 53.4 percent of enrollees. Nearly three-fifths of those who choose to remain with fee-for-service are somewhat less satisfied with the amount they are required to pay for medical care while fewer than half of those who join HMOs express the level of satisfaction with their payments as less than excellent.

It was thought that the satisfaction expressed by HMO enrollees with the perceived quality and outcomes of care they received would be at least equal to that expressed by their fee-for-service counterparts. The results indicate that enrollees are slightly less likely than nonenrolled beneficiaries to be satisfied with the perceived level of accuracy of the diagnosis and with the overall care received. The proportion of individuals highly satisfied on the perceived accuracy of diagnosis and on results of care is moderate for both enrollees and nonenrollees. The differences are statistically significant when controlling for demographic characteristics, functional status, behavioral characteristics, and health status; they warrant attention, since such perceptions may erode confidence in the provider of care and may be related to the differences detected in satisfaction with overall quality.

An interesting point is that, despite their somewhat lower satisfaction, 93.5 percent of enrollees would recommend their HMO to friends and relatives. While this rate is slightly below the 96 percent rate of provider recommendation found for nonenrollees, it is an overwhelmingly positive reaction to the trade-offs that accompany HMO coverage.

Conclusions and Suggestions for Further Research and Policy

Although overall satisfaction with services provided through the HMOs was high, enrollees were significantly less satisfied than nonenrollees with many aspects of the quality of care and medical services they received. The one exception was for out-of-pocket costs, where enrollees were substantially more likely to express satisfaction with their coverage. This latter finding, which duplicates the findings from the National Medicare Competition Evaluation, is not surprising, since it is due largely to the lower premium cost for HMO membership than for Medicare supplementary insurance, and to the more extensive coverage of benefits in HMOs (e.g., for prescription drugs, dental care). Indeed, about half of all enrollees belong to HMOs with risk contracts that do not charge a premium.

HMOs clearly offer wider benefits for some services that satisfy unmet needs for Medicare beneficiaries who choose to enroll. Benefits such as preventive health maintenance, vision care, and dental care are unique for the Medicare program; are heavily focused in ambulatory settings; concentrate largely on services aimed at maintaining functional status; and contrast sharply with the emphasis on specialized, high-intensity medical services provided in traditional fee-for-service settings. The low, or zero, premiums charged by HMOs for these benefits, as well as for coverage of Medicare's deductibles and coinsurance, allow individuals who otherwise could not afford such coverage to obtain it. For these individuals, the financial access to care is markedly increased.

Although enrollee satisfaction levels are high, they lag behind those of nonenrollees in part because beneficiaries have become accustomed to the unrestricted access to expensive resources provided by fee-for-service coverage. The findings that enrollees are less satisfied with components of care that involve uninhibited and speedy access (e.g., availability, convenience, and thoroughness) are derived in part from FFS expectations, and are not entirely surprising.

It is anticipated that, as the risk program becomes better established across the country and more widely understood, Medicare beneficiaries will be more knowledgeable about the HMO delivery system and thus will be more predisposed to join the type of managed care offered through an HMO. If so, satisfaction with care must be maintained and improved. To know if this is occurring, it must be monitored on an ongoing basis. Surveys should be done on a regular basis to evaluate trends in satisfaction and to monitor the progress of the program.

The promise of managed care for the aging Medicare population, both for constraining costs and providing new benefits, may not be realized without a price. Currently that price is a sacrifice in the degree of satisfaction of Medicare beneficiaries enrolled in risk contract plans. Policies aimed at ratcheting back the cost of acute care using capitated payments, in favor of providing benefits relevant to a geriatric population often afflicted with chronic illnesses, will have to address the trade-offs in perceived value.

References

Aday, L. A., R. A. Andersen and G. V. Fleming. *Health Care in the U.S.: Equitable for Whom?* Beverly Hills: Sage Publications, 1980.

Brown, R. A., K. Langwell, K. Berman, A. Ciemnecki, L. Nelson, A. Schreier, and A. Tucker. "Report on Enrollments and Disenrollments from Medicare HMOs." Report prepared under contract no. 500-83-0047 for Health Care Financing Administration, DHHS. Princeton, NJ: Mathematica Policy Research, Inc., June 1986.

Bureau of Data Management and Strategy. "1989 HCFA Statistics." Publication no. 03294. Baltimore, MD: Health Care Financing Administration, 1989a.

Bureau of Data Management and Strategy. "Data from the Medicare Statistical System." Baltimore, MD: Health Care Financing Administration, 1989b.

Clement, D. G., S. M. Retchin, M. H. Stegall, and R. S. Brown. "Evaluation of Access and Satisfaction with Care in the TEFRA Program." Draft report submitted to Health Care Financing Administration, Richmond, VA: Williamson Institute for Health Studies, 1992.

Davies, A. R., J. E. Ware, R. H. Brook, J. R. Peterson, and J. P. Newhouse. "Consumer Acceptance of Prepaid Medical Care: Results from a Randomized Controlled Trial." *Health Services Research* 21, no. 3 (1986): 429–52.

Doyle, B. J., and J. E. Ware. "Physician Conduct and Other Factors That Affect Consumer Satisfaction with Medical Care." *Journal of Medical Education* 52 (1977): 793–801.

Friedlob, A. S., and J. P. Hadley. "Marketing Medicare in a Competitive Environment." Baltimore, MD: Health Care Financing Administration Special Report, 1985.

Garfinkel, S. A., W. E. Schlenger, K. R. McLeroy, F. A. Bryan, B. J. G. York, G. H. Dunteman, and A. S. Friedlob. "Choice of Payment Plan in the Medicare Capitation Demonstration." *Medical Care* 24, no. 7 (July 1986): 628–40.

Langwell, K., S. Stearns, S. Nelson, J. Bergeron, L. Schopler, and R. Donahey. "Disenrollment Experience in the TEFRA HMO/CMP Program." Washington, DC: Mathematica Policy Research, Inc., 1989.

Linn, M. W., B. S. Linn, and S. R. Stein. "Satisfaction with Ambulatory Care and Compliance in Older Patients." *Medical Care* 20, no. 6 (1982): 606–14.

Manning, W. G., A. Leibowitz, G. A. Goldberg, W. H. Rogers, and J. P. Newhouse. "A Controlled Trial of the Effect of a Prepaid Group Practice on Use of Services." *New England Journal of Medicine* 310, no. 23 (1984): 1505–10.

Marquis, S. M., A. R. Davies, and J. E. Ware. "Patient Satisfaction and Change in Medical Care Provider: A Longitudinal Study." *Medical Care* 21 (1983): 821–29.

Newhouse, J. P., J. E. Ware, and C. A. Donald. "How Sophisticated Are Consumers about the Medical Care Delivery System?" *Medical Care* 19, no. 2 (1981): 316–28.

Rossiter, L. F., T. Wan, K. Langwell, J. Hadley, A. Tucker, M. Rivnyak, K. Sullivan, and J. Norcross. "An Analysis of Patient Satisfaction for Enrollees and Disenrollees in Medicare Risk-Based Plans." Report submitted to Health Care Financing Administration, DHHS, under contract No. 500-83-0047. Richmond: Medical College of Virginia, 1988.

Thomas, W., and R. Penchansky. "Relating Satisfaction with Access to Utilization of Services." *Medical Care* 22, no. 6 (1984): 553–68.

Ware, J. E., and A. R. Davies. "Behavioral Consequences of Consumer Dissatisfaction with Medical Care." *Evaluation and Program Planning* 6, no. 3 (1983): 291–97.

Ware, J. E., A. Davies-Avery, and A. L. Stewart. "Measurement and Meaning of Patient Satisfaction." *Health and Medical Care Service Review* 1, no. 1 (1978): 1–15.

Chapter 5

Satisfaction in the Social/Health Maintenance Organization:

A Comparison of Members, Disenrollees, and Those in Fee-for-Service

Robert Newcomer, Charlene Harrington, and Steven Preston

Patient satisfaction is important to any health plan. Low satisfaction may lead to disenrollment, or it may adversely affect the public image of the plan. If disenrollment occurs among the more healthy members, the plan may experience an unfavorable bias, leaving it with disproportionately more high-cost members. On the other hand, if dissatisfaction and any consequent disenrollment occurs among high users of service, the plan may gain a favorable bias in its members. Such concerns are common in studies of HMOs.

In 1985, the Health Care Financing Administration initiated a four-site demonstration program known as the Social/Health Maintenance Organization (S/HMO). These plans offer the health care benefits usually available through a Medicare risk contract HMO (e.g., hospital, physician, skilled nursing, home health, hospice, and durable medical equipment). They also offer expanded benefits in the form of outpatient prescription drugs, hearing aids, and eyeglasses. These expanded benefits help characterize S/HMOs as a "high-option" HMO. Both the basic and expanded benefits are available to all members.

A unique feature of S/HMOs is a chronic care benefit featuring homemaker, respite care, and custodial nursing home care. These benefits are limited to between $6,250 and $12,000 annually (depending on the plan), and they are available only to those who are functionally impaired or who have been certified as eligible for nursing home care. Medicare pays a capitation premium to finance the basic HMO component of the S/HMOs. This premium is adjusted based on the age, gender, and institutional status of the member. The plan receives 100 percent of the community's annual adjusted per capita cost for these subgroups. Private premiums help finance the expanded and chronic care component.[1]

Because of the range of benefits provided, S/HMOs are expected to be more successful than regular Medicare HMOs in retaining frail members—overcoming the propensity for sicker members to leave. To assess the effectiveness of S/HMOs in achieving member satisfaction we have compared disenrollment rates among members, controlling for health status; and we have examined reported satisfaction levels among both continuing members and those who have disenrolled. These results are also compared to a case-mix–matched sample of persons receiving fee-for-service (FFS) care within S/HMO service areas.

Satisfaction and Dissatisfaction with Health Care

A number of basic patterns or relationships have emerged from studies of individuals' perceptions of how well their needs and wants are met by their health plans:[2]

- Sociodemographic factors do not account for a large proportion of the variance in overall satisfaction, but poorer patients place more emphasis on cost and coverage factors than do those with higher income; female patients tend to be slightly more satisfied than males, and to place particular value on continuity of care.

- Satisfaction levels tend to be lower among those with poor health status or psychosocial disability. Medicare beneficiaries disenrolling from HMOs in their first year of membership are in poorer health (Tucker and Langwell 1989; Ward 1987). Patients in poor health are thought to be more likely to disenroll because they are more concerned about interpersonal relations and continuity of care (Davies and Ware 1988; Tucker and Langwell 1989).

- Medicare beneficiaries switching from one HMO to another have been found to be in better health than those going to fee-for-service. They were also less concerned with seeing the same physician and had less misunderstanding about the plan, but expressed more dissatisfaction with convenience factors (Tucker and Langwell 1989).

- The relationship between satisfaction and utilization has yielded mixed results. Recent studies generally have found no significant relationship; however, some have reported inverse relationships (Tucker and Langwell 1989; Pope, Freeborn, and Marks 1984). Individuals with more chronic illness and health problems may need more services than they are able to obtain in an HMO. Patients with higher use also tended to place more value on continuity in the patient-caregiver relationship, again possibly leading to dissatisfaction with an HMO.

- Surveys of HMOs have generally found disenrollees to be more dissatisfied than continuing members. Among Medicare beneficiaries, disenrollees have emphasized dissatisfaction with physicians, the failure to establish relationships with physicians, and a misunderstanding of plan procedures (particularly the need to switch physicians) at the time of joining (Rossiter et al. 1989; Tucker and Langwell 1989; Ward 1987).

- Among patients who are in better health, voluntary disenrollments seem to be primarily a response to cost/coverage factors and the relative cost of other plans (Sorenson and Wersinger 1981; Boxerman and Hennelly 1983). Cost/coverage concerns generally have lower salience in the disenrollment decisions of those in poorer health. These individuals tend to be more responsive to quality and continuity issues.

Dissatisfaction does not always lead to disenrollment, perhaps because of inertia, lack of satisfactory alternatives, lack of information about alternatives, or cost. These relationships are illustrated by a finding that substantial variation in Medicare HMO disenrollment occurred across market areas (Tucker and Langwell 1989). In areas with only one HMO, annual disenrollment rates (4.4 to 6.3 percent) were substantially lower than those within areas having multiple HMOs (6.6 to 27 percent). Luft's (1987) overview of disenrollment studies found that annual disenrollment rates were lower than 5 to 10 percent, except in years when premiums were raised.

The S/HMO evaluation of member satisfaction and disenrollment was guided by hypotheses derived from prior HMO studies and intended goals of the S/HMO model. In particular, we expected that functionally impaired members, those expressly targeted for the S/HMO chronic care benefits, would have lower disenrollment rates and satisfaction levels at least comparable to the more healthy members. Such findings would be counter to the experience of HMOs, where those with impairments have lower satisfaction rates and higher disenrollment.

We also expected differences in satisfaction levels and disenrollment rates across the S/HMOs. This could occur because of differences in the market areas and in the maturity among the four S/HMOs. Two of these plans (Seniors Plus serving the Minneapolis-St. Paul area of Minnesota, and Medicare Plus II serving Portland, Oregon) are essentially high-option plans that operate within the larger umbrella structure of preexisting HMOs. These are, respectively, Group Health Inc. and Kaiser Permanente Northwest. A further complicating factor is that approximately 40 percent of the Medicare Plus II enrollees were conversions from other Kaiser plans, while 60 percent of the Seniors Plus members were conversions from other Group Health plans. Such members presumably retained continuity in their care. Mature S/HMO plans can also be expected to have physicians experienced in HMO care, and to have a high proportion of members experienced with an HMO's methods for delivering care.

The remaining S/HMOs (Elderplan serving Brooklyn, New York, and SCAN Health Plan (SHP) serving Long Beach, California) were organizations that had their genesis as long-term care service providers and developed their HMO capacity while implementing this demonstration. These plans did not enjoy the advantage of a prior relationship with their enrollees. Most members had to change physicians when they enrolled. These plans had to establish operational relationships with medical groups and hospitals for the provision of health care. This affected continuity of care and interpersonal relationships with the physicians. Frequent turnover among the physicians further complicated these issues as well as the plan's relationship with its principal hospital at Elderplan. SHP's physician group was dissatisfied with their capitation contract. This is thought to have affected physician attitudes toward the plan and, through them, the attitudes of members (Harrington, Newcomer, and Friedlob 1989). Elderplan changed or added medical groups three times between 1985 and 1989. SHP terminated its contracts with both its original medical group and hospital in 1990.

Disenrollment from S/HMOs

During their first 36 months of operation, the S/HMOs experienced a composite disenrollment rate of 21.7 percent (with an additional 10.2 percent dying) from among those who initially joined these plans sometime between March 1985 and December 1986. Rates were lowest in the mature plans (i.e., 18.2 percent in Seniors Plus and 20.9 percent in Medicare Plus II), increasing with the newly formed plans (i.e., 26.0 percent in Elderplan and 33.8 percent in SHP).

The average annual S/HMO disenrollment rate (7.0 percent) is below the annual disenrollment rates of 10 to 30 percent found in other studies of general HMO members (Hennelly and Boxerman 1983; Luft 1987). It is also lower than the average rate of 15.5 percent found during the first year after enrollment in the 16 HMOs participating in the Medicare Competition Demonstration (Tucker and Langwell 1989).

Such comparisons show that the S/HMOs—even the newly formed plans—were at least as successful as typical Medicare risk contract HMOs in retaining members. Such comparisons need to be qualified, since these results are not adjusted for any differences in the membership and market area characteristics. To overcome this limitation we compiled the data shown in Table 5.1. These data compare S/HMO member disenrollment rates with those of Medicare beneficiaries selected from the same market areas.[3] These results again show that the S/HMOs, as a group, were

Table 5.1   S/HMO Disenrollment 1985–1989 by Site

Site	% Disenrolled To HMO	% Disenrolled To FFS	% Died
Brooklyn			
S/HMO	2.6	20.4	9.1
FFS†	8.6	NA	15.2
HMO*‡	NA§	NA	NA
Long Beach			
S/HMO	10.4	22.4	9.6
FFS	18.1	NA	13.7
HMO	30.9	10.5	7.9
Minneapolis			
S/HMO	11.0	5.5	9.5
FFS	15.2	NA	17.3
HMO	16.4	17.7	8.3
Portland			
S/HMO	10.2	8.2	11.3
FFS	24.4	NA	13.4
HMO	11.1	7.6	7.1
Total			
S/HMO	8.5	13.2	10.2
FFS	18.0	NA	14.6
HMO	20.6	10.7	7.1

*Brooklyn had no Medicare risk contract HMOs during the study period.

†FFS refers to fee-for-service, a probability sample of Medicare beneficiaries not enrolled in HMOs at the time the sample was drawn, March 1986.

‡HMO refers to a probability sample of persons who had enrolled in an HMO during the S/HMO's initial enrollment build-up period (i.e., between January 1985 and March 1986).

§Not applicable.

more successful than were other HMOs in retaining members who had enrolled during this same period. Newly formed S/HMOs had higher disenrollment than those based in established HMOs, but these differences were somewhat affected by the local context. Brooklyn had no Medicare risk contract HMOs during this period, so members were often unfamiliar with HMO lock-in features. The Long Beach area's experience with price competition among HMOs helped to produce volatile HMO disenrollment patterns among many plans.

More specific to the question of a S/HMO's relative success in retaining less healthy members are the results shown in Table 5.2. S/HMO disenrollment rates are compared with those of HMO members and FFS recipients from the same service area, time period, and health status. Rates are adjusted to exclude those who died during this period. The case-mix classes, briefly described in Figure 5.1, were derived using a grade of membership (GoM) procedure applied to the 31 health and functional characteristics contained within a baseline health status interview of study cases (Manton et al. 1992a,b).[4] GoM is a multivariate procedure that performs for discrete data the same type of analytic functions that factor analysis performs for continuous variables. GoM produces "pure type classifications" that are identical to factors except that they are constrained to be positive and to sum to one for a person. Based on their mix of attributes, each individual has a weighted probability of being in one or more of these "classes."

The classifications shown below were derived independently from prior service use and such demographic characteristics as age, gender, and marital status; and they were conducted with data for the FFS and S/HMO samples for all sites combined. Consequently, a person either in the FFS sample or a S/HMO, in any given site, with the same health and functional characteristics, has an identical classification.

When the total samples, and the "healthy," and the "older healthy" are considered, S/HMO members were only slightly more likely to leave their plans than FFS recipients were likely to join an HMO. This contrasts with those who began the period in HMOs, where substantially more changed health plans—many going to other HMOs.

Social/HMO and fee-for-service groups diverge more notably when other classes are considered. The acutely ill, those with chronic circulatory problems, and those with functional impairments are more likely to remain in FFS. This is consistent with the previously reported experience of other HMOs. S/HMO member disenrollment rates are not substantially higher in these classes than in the others, but higher proportions elect FFS than HMOs. A more favorable finding for the S/HMOs is that they are superior to their market area HMO group, in *all* classes, in retaining members.

Figure 5.1   Case-Mix Classes

1. **Healthy** is free of medical problems and impairment. This class is young (71 years), male, married, used few acute or long-term care services, and has low mortality.

2. **Acutely ill** has multiple medical problems (e.g., cancer and heart disease) but little impairment. It is similar in age to Class 1 (72.2 years) and is likely to be married and male. Class 2 used the most acute care in the prior year (e.g., hospitalization). Class 2 has mortality higher than Class 1 but lower than 3, 4, and 6. The phrase "acutely" ill is used to emphasize differences between case-mix classes. Some conditions associated with Class 2 persist and produce intermittent or terminal disability (e.g., cancer). However, "acute" seems appropriate given the seriousness of the illnesses and because they progress rapidly to death or recovery.

3. **IADL impaired** has impairments in instrumental activities of daily living, and mobility and neurological impairments. The IADLs (money management, telephoning, medications) suggest that this class is cognitively impaired. This class is older (78.8 years), dependent, uses long-term care, and has high mortality.

4. **Chronic circulatory** has diabetes, hypertension, atherosclerosis, and stroke. This class is old (81.1 years) and female with higher mortality than Class 2, the "acutely ill."

5. **Older healthy** is functional except for joint disorders. It is older than Class 1 (76.2 years) and more female. It has the second-highest marital rate. Service use, including long-term care, is low. Mortality is similar to Class 1.

6. **Frail** has multiple comorbidities and impairments. This class uses the most acute and long-term care services, and is old (89 years). It has the highest mortality.

Major reasons for S/HMO disenrollment

In spite of their favorable comparison to market area HMOs, an important pattern is present among S/HMO members: those with acute and chronic health conditions, as well as those with functional disability, are more inclined to leave a S/HMO than are the healthy members. To understand the dynamics affecting these patterns, we first examine the reported reasons for disenrollment. The major stated reasons are summarized in Table 5.3. These results compare functionally impaired persons with the unimpaired. Multiple reasons were sometimes given. Data were collected by telephone interview from those S/HMO members who were active at study baseline, but who disenrolled between June 1987 and September 1988.

Table 5.2   Case-Mix and Total Disenrollment Rates for S/HMO, HMO, and FFS Sample Service Episodes over Three Years, Mortality Eliminated

Case-Mix Class	Disenroll to:			Total Disenrollment Rate*	No Change
	S/HMO	HMO	FFS		
1. Healthy					
S/HMO	—	9.4%	13.0%	22.4%	77.6%
FFS†	1.5%	21.4	—	22.9	77.0
HMO‡	0.5	21.1	10.1	31.7	68.3
2. Acutely Ill					
S/HMO	—	8.3	16.4	24.7	75.2
FFS	1.6%	17.2	—	18.8	81.2
HMO	0.2	27.9	11.4	39.5	60.0
3. IADL Impaired					
S/HMO	—	7.1	23.3	30.4	69.3
FFS	1.8%	16.3	—	18.1	81.7
HMO	0.6	25.8	15.5	41.9	57.7
4. Chronic Circulatory					
S/HMO	—	7.8	16.0	23.8	75.0
FFS	0.8%	15.5	—	16.3	83.6
HMO	1.4	18.3	15.4	35.1	64.3
5. Older Healthy					
S/HMO	—	12.1	14.9	27.0	73.0
FFS	1.0%	23.0	—	24.0	76.0
HMO	1.0	19.5	10.8	31.3	68.8
6. Frail					
S/HMO	—	1.5	31.6	33.1	67.0
FFS	0.4%	10.7	—	11.1	89.2
HMO	1.3	19.2	31.8	52.3	47.4
Total Proportion					
S/HMO	—	9.4	14.7	24.1	75.4
FFS	1.3%	19.8	—	21.1	78.9
HMO	0.6	21.6	11.6	33.8	66.0

*Rows may not total to 100 percent due to rounding. Health status classes were derived from baseline health screening questionnaires using grade of membership procedures.

†FFS refers to fee for service, a probability sample of Medicare beneficiaries not enrolled in HMOs at the time the sample was drawn, March 1986.

‡HMO refers to a probability sample of persons who had enrolled in an HMO during the S/HMOs initial enrollment build-up period (i.e., between January 1985 and March 1986).

Dissatisfaction with physicians or medical care was a common reason for disenrollment among both functionally impaired and unimpaired groups. Chief among the factors comprising this were dissatisfaction with care by the physician or communications with the physician. Others disliked their choice of physicians or of having different physicians. Access to treatments, tests, or other care-related matters accounted for about one-quarter of the reported problems in this domain.

Other domains where the functionally impaired and unimpaired reported similar problems were referred to among those who either "moved from the area" or "spent time outside the area" (about 20 percent); and among those who were unhappy with access or "convenience" of the plan's hospital or clinic offices, e.g., location, appointment, waiting time (about 14 percent).

The samples diverged in the areas of "finances and benefits" and in "reputation." Unimpaired members (48.8 percent) were more than twice as likely to mention that premiums were too high, to complain about the dropping of dental coverage, or to state that they did not need the service or benefits, or that they had other problems related to cost and benefits. Impaired disenrollees, on the other hand, were more than twice as likely to express concern about the reputation of the plan.

These results all parallel findings from other HMOs. The major reasons for disenrolling varied by health plan (Table 5.4). Elderplan and SHP (the newly formed plans) had significantly higher proportions of their disenrollees (78 and 62 percent, respectively) reporting "physician or medical care" concerns. This is consistent with the problems these sites had in establishing and maintaining their acute and physician service network. Members in the more established plans (i.e., Medicare Plus II and Seniors Plus) had relatively less concern with physician and medical care. These plan members were more likely to express concern about total costs and benefits in return for the premiums being paid. Medicare Plus was the most expensive of the four S/HMOs, and Seniors Plus operated in a price-competitive market area. Members of the newly formed plan, particularly those at Elderplan, had comparatively more problems with hospital convenience factors. There were also differences among the plans with respect to members moving from the area, and understanding the plans. Neither of the latter differences was related to organizational maturity.

Health plan satisfaction in S/HMO and comparison populations

The third dimension of our analysis examines reported health plan satisfaction among plan members. Following the work of Rossiter and associates (1988), in their analysis of National Medicare Competition

Table 5.3   Major Reasons for Disenrolling from the S/HMOs

	Unimpaired (n = 392)	Impaired (n = 81)
All Physician/Medical Reasons†	44.0	46.7
Physician care unsatisfactory	11.2	16.0
Disliked choice of physicians	6.1	1.2
Difficult to get appropriate treatments/tests	4.1	6.2
Physicians not friendly or courteous	3.8	1.2
Disliked using different physicians	4.3	1.2
Physicians did not spend enough time	3.3	3.7
Poor communications	2.8	4.9
Wanted to keep former physician/hospital	6.4	0.0
Other care-related reason	6.1	12.3
All Cost/Benefit Reasons	48.8	20.8*
Cost of premiums too high	24.2	7.4
Dental coverage dropped	8.2	1.2
Did not need service or benefits	7.7	0.0
Premiums not covered by employer or union	2.6	1.2
Benefits exhausted	0.0	3.7
Too few chronic care benefits	1.3	2.5
Copayments and fees too high	1.3	1.2
Other	3.5	3.6
All Mobility Reasons	20.1	19.8
Moved out of service area	18.6	19.8
Spent time out of service area	1.5	0.0
Any Misunderstanding	10.7	8.6*
Service promised not offered	4.6	0.0
General misunderstanding/insufficient information	2.0	2.5
Medicare card could not be used elsewhere	2.0	2.5
Other	2.1	3.6
All Convenience Reasons	12.8	14.8
Did not get immediate care in emergency	1.5	0.0
Location of MDs or hospital not convenient	3.3	3.7
Hard to get appointments	2.0	2.5
Long wait for appointments	2.6	0.0
Other	3.4	8.6
Any Reputation or Other Reason	10.9	19.7*
Heard another HMO was better	2.3	0.0
Family recommended disenrollment	0.0	3.7
Other	8.3	16.0

*$p < .01$.

†Totals add up to greater than 100 percent as some respondents indicated more than one major reason for disenrollment.

Table 5.4   Major Reasons for Disenrolling from the S/HMOs, by Site

	Elderplan (n = 140)	Medicare Plus II (n = 109)	SCAN Health Plan (n = 118)	Seniors Plus (n = 106)
All Physician/Medical Reasons**†	78.4	17.4	61.9	6.5
Physician care unsatisfactory*	19.3	4.6	18.6	2.8
Disliked choice of physicians*	7.1	1.8	11.0	0.0
Difficult to get appropriate treatments/tests*	10.7	2.8	2.5	0.0
Physicians not friendly or courteous*	3.6	1.8	7.6	0.0
Disliked using different physicians*	10.0	2.8	0.0	0.9
Physicians did not spend enough time*	5.0	0.0	7.6	0.0
Wanted to keep former physician/hospital	2.1	0.0	4.2	0.9
Other care-related reason*	20.6	3.6	13.4	2.8
All Cost/Benefit Reasons**	17.8	55.0	37.0	89.3
Poor communications	6.4	0.9	2.5	1.9
Cost of premiums too high*	10.7	29.4	22.0	26.4
Dental coverage dropped*	0.0	0.0	0.8	30.2
Did not need service or benefits*	0.0	11.9	0.8	16.0
Premiums not covered by employer or union*	0.7	7.3	1.7	0.0
Benefits exhausted	0.0	0.9	0.8	0.9
Too few chronic care benefits	0.0	1.8	0.0	4.7
Copayments and fees too high*	2.1	2.8	0.0	0.0
Other*	4.3	0.9	10.9	11.1
All Mobility Reasons*	17.2	32.1	23.7	7.5
Moved out of service area*	14.3	31.2	23.7	6.6
Spent time out of service area	2.9	0.9	0.0	0.9
Any Misunderstanding**	10.7	0.9	8.5	10.4
Service promised not offered*	3.6	0.0	5.1	6.6
General misunderstanding/ insufficient information	7.1	0.9	3.4	3.8
All Convenience Reasons**	31.4	2.7	11.9	1.8
Did not get immediate care in emergency	7.9	0.0	0.0	0.0
Location of MDs or hospital not convenient	5.0	0.0	6.8	0.9
Hard to get appointments*	5.7	0.9	0.8	0.0

Continued

Table 5.4   Continued

	Elderplan (n = 140)	Medicare Plus II (n = 109)	SCAN Health Plan (n = 118)	Seniors Plus (n = 106)
Long wait for appointments*	10.0	0.0	1.7	0.0
Other	2.8	1.8	2.6	0.9
Any Reputation or Other Reason	9.9	14.6	16.8	8.3
Heard another HMO was better	1.4	2.8	3.4	0.0
Family recommended disenrollment	2.1	1.8	1.7	0.9
Other	6.4	10.0	11.7	7.4

*Significant at a probability level of less than .05 using a Chi-square test.
**Significant at a probability level of less than .01 using a Chi-square test.
†Totals add up to greater than 100 percent as some respondents indicated more than one major reason for disenrollment.

Evaluation (NMCE) risk contract HMOs, we adapted the Andersen behavioral model (1968) as our conceptual framework. This model, shown in Figure 5.2, postulates that continued plan membership is a joint function of predisposing, enabling, health status, utilization, and satisfaction factors. Predisposing factors refer to demographic characteristics (e.g., age, gender, education, marital status, living alone). The enabling factors may facilitate or impede beneficiary satisfaction. Included here are income, employment, and other public and private insurance. Adequate information is also a factor in making choices about health plan enrollment. The individual's health status is defined by level of physical and psychological functioning, perceived health, and reported health problems. Utilization includes physician visits, hospitalization, nursing home use, chronic care service use, and out-of-plan use. Patient satisfaction includes both specific dimensions (e.g., access, quality, interpersonal relations, costs and benefits) and overall indicators of satisfaction. Whether the plan is a mature HMO or a new one is used as a control for organizational characteristics.

Sample and data collection

The analysis of reported satisfaction is based on a two-staged sample drawn from three populations. The first stage consists of (a) S/HMO members (*n* = 7,136) who were active in these plans at study baseline (circa June 1986) and who continued to be enrolled through the summer of 1988; (b) a probability sample of Medicare beneficiaries (*n* = 8,170) from

Figure 5.2   Health Plan Satisfaction and Continuing Membership:
A Conceptual Framework

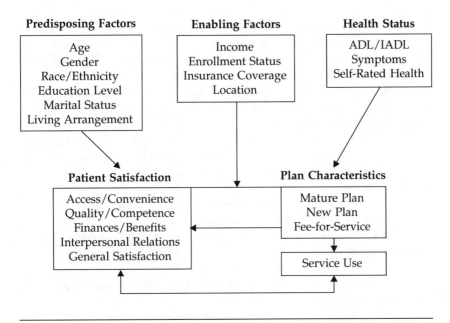

Predisposing Factors | Enabling Factors | Health Status
- Age, Gender, Race/Ethnicity, Education Level, Marital Status, Living Arrangement
- Income, Enrollment Status, Insurance Coverage, Location
- ADL/IADL, Symptoms, Self-Rated Health

Patient Satisfaction: Access/Convenience, Quality/Competence, Finances/Benefits, Interpersonal Relations, General Satisfaction

Plan Characteristics: Mature Plan, New Plan, Fee-for-Service

Service Use

Source: Adapted from L.F. Rossiter et al. (1988).

the S/HMO market areas who were receiving care in FFS (i.e., they were not enrolled as HMO members) at study baseline, and who continued to live in these market areas through the summer of 1988. Those who enrolled in HMOs or a S/HMO have been excluded from these analyses. (c) The third population includes those S/HMO members ($n = 473$) who were active at study baseline, but who disenrolled sometime between June 1987 and September 1988.

The sample frame assured that all S/HMO cases had a minimum of 12 months as members, and that these plans had been in operation more than two years. These constraints minimize two confounding factors common in Medicare HMO satisfaction studies: disenrollment being measured in a member's first year, when they are largely unfamiliar with the plan and its benefits; and the premature assessment of a plan's performance by reviewing it early in its development, before it reached a stable operation.

At stage two (June 1988), the S/HMO continuing members and comparison group samples were stratified into functionally unimpaired and impaired groupings. Health status, both at baseline and annually thereafter, was determined using a health status questionnaire (HSF). These instruments were generally administered by telephone among the comparison group and by mail among S/HMO members, but comparability in data quality was achieved through the efforts of S/HMO case managers. These individuals reviewed all member HSFs and made follow-up phone calls, if HSF items were incomplete or inconsistently answered.

HSFs contain commonly used measures of activities of daily living (ADLs) (e.g., toileting, dressing, bathing), instrumental activities of daily living (IADLs) (e.g., preparing meals, laundry, housework, managing money), and a variety of health conditions (e.g., diabetes, hypertension, neurological problems, lung and breathing problems). Persons reporting one or more ADL or two or more IADL limitations, whether at baseline or during an annual reassessment, were given a comprehensive assessment (CAF) to confirm this disability status. These were administered in the home by social worker or nurse assessors.[5]

Probability samples were selected from each impairment group.[6] The functionally impaired were defined as having one or more impairments in ADLs, or two or more impairments in IADLs. Persons without ADL impairments and with fewer than two IADL impairments were defined as unimpaired.[7]

The health plan satisfaction data were collected by telephone survey conducted between July 1988 and October 1988 among the second-stage samples. Almost 93 percent of the eligible continuing members completed interviews. This compares to just over 87 percent in the disenrollee group (a group much more difficult to locate). These rates are calculated on the basis of completions divided by the adjusted sample size within each original group.[8] No statistically significant differences in age, gender or living arrangement were found between those responding and not responding in these samples.[9] Just over 60 percent of the S/HMO disenrollees were in FFS care at the time of this survey.

Measuring patient satisfaction

A variation of the Patient Satisfaction Questionnaire (PSQ) was used in the S/HMO evaluation to measure member satisfaction. The PSQ is perhaps the most widely used instrument for surveys of health plan members' satisfaction. It was developed for the RAND Health Insurance Experiment (Ware et al. 1983). Among the other studies that have used variations of the PSQ are the National Medicare Competition Evaluation (NMCE) (Rossiter et al. 1989), and the Medicare Capitation Demonstration (MCD) (Friedlob and Hadley 1985). Both studies involved Medicare beneficiaries enrolled in HMOs.

Health plan satisfaction in the PSQ can be reported as a single cumulative score of a person's feelings about the care he or she is receiving (Figure 5.3), and by disaggregating the construct into subcomponents or domains of satisfaction.[10] Both Medicare HMO evaluations noted here used three of the PSQ domains (i.e., quality of care, interpersonal relations, and access/convenience) in addition to a global satisfaction measure. Our results are based on four satisfaction domains and a global measure of satisfaction:[11] These domains were compiled from 21 PSQ items.[12] The measure of overall satisfaction was developed using factor analysis, with 12 items loaded into this factor: general satisfaction, MD continuity, MD thorough, appointment wait, MD attends previous problems, convenience of the hospital, cost of premiums, MD knowledgeable, can get questions answered, copayments and deductibles, staff friendly and courteous, office waiting).

Satisfaction levels

Satisfaction levels were expected to be higher among members of the S/HMOs that were located in mature HMO organizations and among the functionally impaired. Tables 5.5 and 5.6 show the satisfaction rating for 21 specific items, and scale scores representing the dimensions of access, quality, interpersonal, finances/benefits, and a global satisfaction. The first table compares S/HMO members with beneficiaries receiving FFS care, the second, S/HMO members with disenrollees.

S/HMOs were generally able to satisfy their continuing members. The dimensional scores indicate that between 80 and 95 percent of S/HMO members were satisfied with access, quality of physician care, interpersonal relations and courtesy of staff, and finances and benefits associated with their health plan. Over 85 percent reported overall satisfaction with the plans. These levels of satisfaction are consistent with

Figure 5.3 Health Plan Satisfaction Domains

Access/Convenience (e.g., the time and effort required to get an appointment, waiting time at the office, convenience of hospital location)

Quality/Competence of Care (e.g., knowledge, competence and thoroughness of physicians, continuity and attentiveness to previous problems)

Finances and Benefits (e.g., comprehensiveness of benefits available, ability to save money, cost of premiums, copayments and deductibles)

Interpersonal Relations (e.g., courtesy, friendliness of physicians, can get questions answered, all needs met, doctor takes enough time, tests and treatments available, freedom to change physicians)

General Satisfaction (e.g., overall assessment of the care being received based on multiple dimensions of the satisfaction questionnaire)

---

the 80 to 91 percent rates of satisfaction reported from other studies of Medicare beneficiaries (Friedlob and Hadley 1985; Rossiter et al. 1988). Functionally unimpaired members tend to have slightly higher levels of satisfaction than those with functional impairments. This pattern is counter to our expectations, but consistent with HMO member satisfaction study results.

Comparisons between Social/HMO members and those receiving fee-for-service care show small but statistically significant differences. S/HMO *unimpaired* members tend to have higher levels of satisfaction than their counterparts in FFS. This occurs in all dimensions of care, except interpersonal relations, where there is no difference. Members with functional *impairments*, in contrast, generally have lower satisfaction scores than those in FFS. Such members are more satisfied only with "finances and benefits."

Disenrollees from the S/HMO were significantly more dissatisfied than continuing members in all dimensions of satisfaction: access, quality, interpersonal relations, finances/benefits, and global satisfaction. The difference between continuing members and disenrollees usually ranged between 5 and 15 points on individual items. The difference on scale scores was less than 10 percent. These differences were similar to those found in other studies that have compared disenrollees with continuing members (e.g., Mechanic, Weiss, and Cleary 1983; Boxerman and Hennelly 1983).

Disenrollees with functional limitations have the lowest reported satisfaction levels. These are usually about 10 percent lower than either unimpaired disenrollees or those with functional limitations in FFS. There is an even larger difference in the area of interpersonal relations.

Table 5.7 shows the satisfaction ratings by site for voluntary disenrollees and continuing members.[13] These calculations have been adjusted for the oversample of impaired individuals. Among continuing members of the four plans, there is little difference in any of the dimensions of satisfaction. There are, however, differences in the satisfaction levels of those who disenrolled. Disenrollees from Seniors Plus, located in Minneapolis, have satisfaction scores that are virtually equivalent to those of the plan's continuing members. This is true even for finances and benefits.

Medicare Plus II, the other S/HMO site with a mature HMO sponsor, reveals significant differences between members and disenrollees in access, quality, finances/benefits, and global satisfaction. Seniors Plus disenrollees show high satisfaction, and appear to be leaving for unmeasured reasons. In the case of Medicare Plus II, price is important, but not the single factor. These results suggest that in the relatively noncompetitive HMO environment of the study period, plan members had to be more dissatisfied before they disenrolled.

Table 5.5   Expressed Health Plan Satisfaction, S/HMO and
Fee-for-Service

Satisfaction Items, % Satisfied	S/HMO Sample		Fee-for-Service Sample	
	Impaired† (n = 488)	Unimpaired (n = 760)	Impaired† (n = 518)	Unimpaired (n = 568)
Access				
(Mean Scale Value)* abcd	8.0%	8.6%	8.7%	8.0%
Appointment wait‡	80.9	92.2	92.4	79.8
Office waiting	82.2	92.4	90.7	83.8
Convenience of hospital	80.7	90.9	94.4	80.1
Physician Quality				
(Mean Scale Value)* abcd	10.7	11.4	11.8	10.5
MD continuity	81.6	92.0	98.0	80.8
MD thorough	80.1	88.8	94.4	79.2
MD attends previous problems	78.1	83.6	93.3	73.4
MD knowledgeable	80.3	88.4	95.6	77.2
Interpersonal Relations/Courtesy				
(Mean Scale Value)a	17.2	17.2	17.4	17.3
MD spends enough time	85.0	87.4	87.0	88.6
All needs are met	94.1	93.9	93.7	93.3
Can get questions answered	86.9	82.8	92.4	86.4
Staff friendly and courteous	96.5	96.3	96.5	94.0
Freedom to change physician	89.5	91.4	95.0	94.2
Tests and treatment available	94.9	92.2	96.1	94.0
Finances and benefits				
(Mean Scale Value)* abcd	11.0	11.3	9.9	10.5
Happy with benefits	92.4	92.5	66.9	75.2
Saving money	82.2	80.5	37.4	62.9
Cost of premiums	75.4	89.2	48.0	74.5
Copays and deductibles	75.6	85.9	65.4	79.6
Global Satisfaction (Mean Value)abcd	32.4	34.2	34.5	32.3

*The Mean Scale Values shown for each group of scale items is the mean score summed across all items in that scale.

The maximum value for each scale is three times the number of items in that scale. Global Satisfaction represents the summed score of 12 items: appointment wait, office wait, convenience of hospital, MD continuity, MD thorough, MD attends previous problems, MD knowledgeable, can get questions answered, staff friendly and courteous, cost of premiums, copayments and deductibles, general satisfaction. Student-Neuman-Keuls tests were conducted on the scale scores to compare the differences between specific sites. aImpaired groups differ, bUnimpaired groups differ, cComparison groups differ, dS/HMO groups differ. All these results are at $p < .05$ (two-tailed).

†The classification of impairment used in this table is based solely on functional ability. Persons reporting two or more limitations in instrumental activities of daily living (IADL), or one or more limitations in activities of daily living (ADL), are defined as impaired.

‡The percentages shown for the individual items under each scale dimension were calculated based on the proportion reporting "satisfied."

Table 5.6   Expressed Health Plan Satisfaction, S/HMO Members and Disenrollees, by Impairment Level

	S/HMO Sample		Disenrollee Sample	
Satisfaction Items, % Satisfied	*Impaired (n = 488)*	*Unimpaired (n = 760)*	*Impaired (n = 81)*	*Unimpaired (n = 392)*
Access				
(Mean Scale Value)* bcd	8.0	8.6	7.6	8.4
Appointment wait	80.9	92.2	71.6	88.8
Office waiting	82.2	92.4	76.5	86.2
Convenience of hospital	80.7	90.9	77.8	81.4
Physician Quality				
(Mean Scale Value)* bcd	10.7	11.4	9.6	10.7
MD continuity	81.6	92.0	74.1	85.2
MD thorough	80.1	88.8	54.3	70.9
MD knowledgeable	80.3	88.4	70.4	79.6
Interpersonal Relations/Courtesy				
(Mean Scale Value)* abc	17.2	17.2	13.7	16.3
MD spends enough time	85.0	87.4	67.9	74.0
All needs are met	94.1	93.9	70.4	81.6
Can get questions answered	86.9	82.8	63.0	71.2
Staff friendly and courteous	96.5	96.3	84.0	89.0
Freedom to change physician	89.5	91.4	72.8	84.7
Tests and treatment available	94.9	92.2	79.0	87.8
Finances and Benefits				
(Mean Scale Value)* abd	11.0	11.3	10.4	10.7
Happy with benefits	92.4	92.5	72.8	79.8
Saving money	82.2	80.5	69.1	59.2
Cost of premiums	75.4	89.2	65.4	87.5
Copays and deductibles	75.6	85.9	59.3	80.1
Global Satisfaction (Mean Value)abcd	32.4	34.2	30.4	32.8

*The Mean Scale Values shown for each group of scale items is the mean score summed across all items in that scale.

The maximum value for each scale is three times the number of items in that scale. Global Satisfaction represents the summed score of 12 items: appointment wait, office wait, convenience of hospital, MD continuity, MD thorough, MD attends previous problems, MD knowledgeable, can get questions answered, staff friendly and courteous, cost of premiums, copayments and deductibles, general satisfaction. Student-Neuman-Keuls tests were conducted on the scale scores to compare the differences between specific sites. aImpaired groups differ, bUnimpaired groups differ, cDisenrollee groups differ, dS/HMO groups differ. All these results are at $p < .05$ (two-tailed).

†The classification of impairment used in this table is based solely on functional ability. Persons reporting two or more limitations in instrumental activities of daily living (IADL), or one or more limitations in activities of daily living (ADL) are defined as impaired.

‡The percentages shown for the individual items under each scale dimension were calculated based on the proportion reporting "satisfied."

Table 5.7 Health Plan Satisfaction among Members and Disenrollees in 1988 by Site

	Access	Quality	Interpersonal	Cost/Benefits	Global
Elderplan					
Member (n = 504)†	8.4	11.1	16.9	10.5	33.7
Disenrollee (n = 140)	8.3	11.0	14.5*	9.5	33.2
Medicare Plus II					
Member (n = 518)	8.4	11.2	17.4	10.7	32.4
Disenrollee (n = 109)	7.0**	9.1**	17.3	9.5*	29.4*
SHP					
Member (n = 505)	8.3	11.0	17.3	10.7	33.1
Disenrollee (n = 118)	8.2	10.8	15.3*	9.4*	32.1
Seniors Plus					
Member (n = 610)	8.4	11.2	17.4	10.9	34.2
Disenrollee (n = 106)	8.5	11.2	17.3	10.7	34.7

$*p < .05$, $**p < .01$, on comparisons between members and disenrollees.
†The number of member cases in each site has been weighted to proportionately adjust the original over sample of impaired cases.

Elderplan and SHP disenrollees vary from continuing members principally on the dimension of interpersonal relations and finances/benefits. The former aspect was expected to be the most sensitive to member satisfaction as these S/HMOs were enrolling new members, rather than switching old members into a high-option benefit. Access, quality, and general satisfaction showed no differences between those leaving and those remaining in the plans. SHP is located in an HMO market area of high price competition; Elderplan is in an area where the public has had little experience with HMOs.

Predicting disenrollment

The preceding results suggest at least five things: (1) new S/HMOs (from the perspective of their continuing members) have been competitive with the mature S/HMOs in satisfying access, quality, finances/benefits, and overall satisfaction; (2) the new S/HMOs have been less successful in establishing solid interpersonal relations between members and physicians; (3) members from the new S/HMOs have been more likely to disenroll than from the established S/HMOs if they are not relatively well satisfied with interpersonal relations and finances/benefits; (4) among all of the plans, satisfaction with quality, access, and even interpersonal relations is not sufficient to retain members if they are dissatisfied with the finances and benefits—particularly if the plan is in a highly price competitive market area such as Minneapolis and Long Beach; and (5) established plans in less competitive markets can retain members even when their satisfaction levels are relatively low.

A logit regression analysis was conducted to assess the validity of these assertions relative to the prediction of disenrollment from the S/HMOs. The equation takes the following form:

$$Y = f(HP, B, S)$$

where Y is a variable indicating whether one has disenrolled, HP is a vector of variables representing each S/HMOs (where SHP is used as the reference group); B is a vector of variables representing the predisposing, enabling, health status, and service use dimensions of our general behavioral mode; and S is a score representing the level of patient satisfaction.

Through these procedures, we have adjusted for the measured sociodemographic differences between the continuing members and the disenrollees. All items were binary variables coded as 1 for yes, except for age, frequency of physician visits, and satisfaction scores that were continuous variables. Positive coefficients indicate that attributes were associated with disenrollment. The analysis was conducted on 1,629 individuals, including the continuing S/HMO members and those who voluntarily disenrolled. Those who had moved were excluded.

Table 5.8 shows six different equations. Equation 1 is the basic model without satisfaction items. The remaining equations add a single satisfaction term. The exponential coefficient "EXP (B)," shown in parenthesis, indicates the factor by which the odds of disenrollment change when the coefficient increases by 1 unit. When the coefficient is 0, the factor equals 1, which leaves the odds unchanged. When the coefficient increases from 0 to 1, the odds are increased by the EXP (B) factor.

In the first equation, only one predisposing variable was significant—living alone, which was negatively associated with disenrollment. The enabling factor of having adequate information about the plan was negatively associated with disenrollment. Having an employer paying for the insurance, and having other insurance were both positively related to disenrollment. Those with employer-paid insurance had lower out-of-pocket expenses associated with the purchase of Medicare supplemental insurance. They may also have had more options for group membership enrollment.

Health status, in spite of the differentials in satisfaction levels between unimpaired and impaired persons shown previously, reveals generally negative associations with disenrollment. For the functionally

Table 5.8 Logit Regression of Factors Associated with S/HMO Disenrollment (Coefficient Shown with EXP B in Parentheses)

Equations (n = 1629)	1	2	3	4	5	6
Constant	0.993	2.044	1.209	1.600	6.321	5.304
Predisposing						
Age	−.020	−.020	−.02	−.020	−.030*	−.026*
	(0.98)	(0.98)	(0.98)	(0.98)	(0.97)	(0.97)
Female	−.084	−.071	−.081	−.075	−.039	−.030
	(1.09)	(1.07)	(1.09)	(1.07)	(1.04)	(1.03)
Education	−.062	−.072	−.064	−.070	−.047	−.079
	(1.06)	(1.07)	(1.07)	(1.08)	(1.04)	(1.08)
Married	−.145	−.121	−.139	−.130	−.090	−.073
	(1.16)	(1.13)	(1.15)	(1.14)	(1.09)	(1.08)
Alone	−.273**	−.256**	−.269**	−.262**	−.248**	−.233**
	(1.31)	(1.29)	(1.31)	(1.30)	(1.28)	(1.26)
Enabling						
Low income	.130	.120	.128	.120	.125	.120
	(0.88)	(0.89)	(0.88)	(0.89)	(0.88)	(0.89)
Employed	.081	.080	.082	.080	.112	.049
	(0.92)	(0.92)	(0.92)	(0.92)	(0.89)	(0.95)
Adequate information	−.310**	−.295**	−.309**	−.305**	−.065**	−.127**
	(1.36)	(1.34)	(1.36)	(1.36)	(1.07)	(1.14)
Other insurance	.647**	.640**	.646**	.643**	.568**	.652**
	(0.52)	(0.53)	(0.52)	(0.53)	(0.57)	(0.52)
Employer-paid insurance	.630**	.624**	.630**	.622**	.660**	.632**
	(0.53)	(0.54)	(0.53)	(0.54)	(0.52)	(0.53)
Health Status						
Impaired	−.249*	−.266*	−.253*	−.262*	−.217*	−.310*
	(1.28)	(1.31)	(1.29)	(1.30)	(1.24)	(1.36)
Excellent health	−.022	−.024	−.122	−.023	−.046	−.039
	(0.98)	(0.98)	(0.98)	(0.98)	(0.96)	(0.96)
Health problems	−.142*	−.132	−.139*	−.133	−.189*	−.122
	(1.15)	(1.14)	(1.15)	(1.14)	(1.21)	(1.13)
Health Service Use						
MD visits	.017	.020	.018	.017	.026	.032
	(1.02)	(1.02)	(1.02)	(1.02)	(1.03)	(1.03)
Hospital	−.203**	−.208**	−.205**	−.207**	−.211**	−.173*
	(1.23)	(1.23)	(1.23)	(1.23)	(1.23)	(1.19)
Nursing home	−.083	−.127	−.092	−.117	−.026	−.175
	(1.14)	(1.13)	(1.10)	(1.12)	(1.03)	(1.20)

Continued

Table 5.8 Continued

Equations (n = 1629)	1	2	3	4	5	6
Chronic care	−.376**	−.377**	−.376**	−.377**	−.392**	−.402**
	(1.46)	(1.46)	(1.46)	(1.46)	(1.48)	(1.50)
Out of plan	.170	.168	.170	.171	.059	.125
	(0.84)	(0.85)	(0.84)	(0.84)	(0.94)	(0.88)
S/HMO Site						
Brooklyn	−.031	−.021	−.026	−.021	−.107	−.002
	(1.03)	(1.02)	(1.03)	(1.02)	(1.11)	(1.00)
Minneapolis	−.152	−.135	−.103	−.102	−.057	−.127
	(1.17)	(1.14)	(1.49)	(1.39)	(1.06)	(1.13)
Portland	−.072	−.071	−.071	−.071	−.033	−.065
	(1.08)	(1.07)	(1.07)	(1.07)	(0.97)	(1.06)
Satisfaction						
Global	—	−.033*	—	—	—	—
	—	(0.97)	—	—	—	—
Access	—	—	−.20	—	—	—
	—	—	(0.98)	—	—	—
Quality	—	—	—	−.059	—	—
	—	—	—	(0.94)	—	—

*$p < .05$, **$p < .01$, on comparisons between members and disenrollees.

impaired this relationship was statistically significant in Equation 1. Those reporting any of six serious health conditions within the past year also had a significant negative coefficient. Having used either a hospital or chronic care services was also significantly (and negatively) associated with disenrollment. S/HMO plan membership, with these other attributes held constant, had no significant association with disenrollment.

The remaining five columns in Table 5.8 show how the basic results are affected by the incremental consideration of each of the satisfaction dimensions. Each scale is considered separately because they are correlated. The addition of satisfaction scales generally had little effect on the coefficients for the predisposing, enabling, health status, or health service use measures discussed in reference to Equation 1. Age became a significant (and negative) correlate of disenrollment when interpersonal and finances/benefits satisfaction was entered. The coefficient for persons living alone remained relatively constant regardless of the satisfaction dimension considered. The same is true for those with access to employer-paid insurance and those with other insurance. The influence of the presence of health problems, functional impairment, and the use of hospitals or chronic care services was also unaffected by satisfaction measure controls. S/HMO health plan never becomes significantly associated with disenrollment. Of the satisfaction dimensions, global satisfaction, interpersonal relations, and finances/benefits each produced significant associations with disenrollment. Higher satisfaction scores on these items were associated with lower rates of disenrollment.

Discussion and Conclusion

The social/health maintenance organization, in concept, couples the health and medical care features of an HMO with coverage for additional chronic care benefits. By providing improved benefits, S/HMOs are expected to have lower disenrollment rates than Medicare HMOs, and a greater propensity to retain members who have functional impairments and other health problems. A presumed factor contributing to such performance is that health plan satisfaction levels would be high among members. S/HMOs were found to have annual disenrollment rates that were generally lower than those of Medicare Competition Demonstration plans. S/HMOs were also found to have lower disenrollment rates in every health status group when compared to HMO "joiners" in their market areas. Disenrollment rates were lower at the S/HMOs that were sponsored by mature HMOs than at S/HMOs sponsored by newly formed HMO organizations.

While S/HMOs performed as well as or better than HMOs in retaining members, the results relative to fee-for-service plans were consistent with the experience of HMOs more generally. S/HMOs were better able to retain healthy members. Acutely ill and chronically impaired members—including those with ADL impairments—all showed a tendency for higher disenrollment. Among newly formed plans, the major reasons for disenrollment concerned dissatisfaction with physicians and inconvenience. Among the more mature plans, the major reasons involved cost and moving from the area.

These results are consistent with differences in price competition among the S/HMO market areas, and with differences between newly formed and mature organizations in medical group membership and practice.

Health plan satisfaction scores parallel the disenrollment results. S/HMOs were generally successful in meeting their continuing member needs and expectations for access, quality, interpersonal relationships, and finances/benefits. Satisfaction was highest among functionally *unimpaired* members. Satisfaction scores among this group were generally higher than the scores for Medicare beneficiaries in FFS systems. Functionally *impaired* S/HMO members, with the exception of finances/

benefits, had lower rates of satisfaction than either unimpaired S/HMO members or impaired persons receiving FFS care. These results are consistent with the assumption and experience of HMOs that they must be very satisfying to their "healthy" members to retain them. It also suggests that the chronic care benefit package, as limited as it is, may be serving to retain impaired members—even when satisfaction levels are relatively low.

The two newly formed S/HMOs generally performed as well as the two more mature organizations in achieving member satisfaction (among those continuing in the plans). The main area of difference was that both of the newly formed S/HMOs tended to have somewhat more problems in interpersonal relations. Controlling for case mix and other characteristics, plan membership by itself did not have a significant effect on the prediction of disenrollment. Low satisfaction scores on interpersonal relations and finances/benefits had strong effects on disenrollment.[14]

Retention in the plans was enhanced by experience in using services such as the chronic care benefits and hospital care. The effects of health status are more ambiguous. Within the logit regression, simple dummy variable representations of functional status and the presence of health problems reveal a modest but significant association with continued plan participation. More complex case-mix adjustments applied to the whole sample (Table 5.2) found similar rates of disenrollment among most of the health status classes. The very frail had a slightly higher disenrollment rate. The predisposing and enabling characteristics had limited effects on disenrollment. Most notable was that having other insurance, and having a former employer available to pay for other insurance had strong positive relationships with disenrollment.

Satisfaction analyses are biased by the "self-selection" of those who choose to become and then remain as members. The relatively high satisfaction scores among those continuing in the plan (and those in FFS) when compared with satisfaction levels among those who disenroll illustrate this. S/HMOs must be highly satisfying to members, particularly unimpaired members (90 percent or more in most dimensions) to retain them. If satisfaction drops below these levels, members are highly likely to leave. The competitiveness of the market area and the access members have to other insurance may affect the satisfaction thresholds that trigger disenrollment. The results suggest that members have to be more satisfied in highly competitive areas than in less competitive areas, or the likelihood of disenrollment increases.

This limited tolerance for dissatisfaction among the functionally unimpaired has important health policy implications. Plans have the potential of improving their operations to meet the expectations of these members, or of selectively reducing benefits to stimulate the departure of "high-cost" or high-risk" cases. But should the high-option benefits (e.g., prescription drugs, eyeglasses) fail to distinguish a S/HMO from its competition, or should premiums continue to rise relative to this competition, it is likely that a member's satisfaction may lessen over the levels seen here. This could precipitate an erosion of the plan's enrollment base.

With respect to the functionally impaired, the S/HMOs seemingly have a wide tolerance for dissatisfaction. Impaired members generally have rates of satisfaction (except in costs/benefits) that are between 5 and 15 percent lower than those among the unimpaired members. Functionally impaired disenrollees tend to have satisfaction levels another 5 to 15 percent below those who remain. This occurs in spite of the fiscal limitations on the S/HMOs' current chronic care benefits. Such results suggest the potential for an even wider tolerance if the chronic care benefit package is enhanced. Not fully explained in these analyses is why impaired continuing members of S/HMOs are less satisfied with their health plan than any other group. Perhaps this results from unfulfilled expectations about the plan. Perhaps, too, satisfaction would be greater if increased attention could be given to improving the interpersonal relationships between this group and their doctors, and to requiring less restrictive eligibility for the chronic care benefits.

Acknowledgments

Data collection and analysis supported by HCFA contract number 500-85-0042. The authors remain responsible for the content.

Notes

1. For further discussion of the Social/HMO concept and its differences from Medicare HMOs, see Newcomer, Harrington, and Friedlob (1990).
2. See, for example, Pascoe (1983); Ware, Snyder, and Wright (1976); Zastowny, Roghmann, and Hengst (1983); and Cleary and McNeil (1988) for extensive reviews.
3. The HMO members included in this table are from a probability sample (within each of the S/HMO market areas) of persons who had enrolled in an HMO during the S/HMOs initial enrollment build-up period (between January 1985 and March 1986). The fee-for-service sample consists of a probability sample of Medicare beneficiaries not enrolled in HMOs during this period. Both samples are described more fully later on.
4. These health status classes were extensively tested for predictive reliability relative to mortality. Comparisons were also made to sociodemographic attributes and prior service use.

5. The HSF was adapted from the screening interview used in the National Long Term Care Survey (NLTCS). The CAFs were developed by Brandeis University and the consortium of S/HMO demonstration health plans. Impaired persons were reassessed semiannually, usually by telephone.

6. Persons with functional impairments were oversampled in each community to compensate for their relatively fewer number and to permit a subgroup analysis of these cases. The impaired sample represents virtually all impaired members in the S/HMO and comparison group samples at that time. An exception occurs in Portland, where about 50 percent of the impaired group was drawn. Approximately equal sample sizes of unimpaired cases were selected from each plan to prevent the experience of one health plan or market area from dominating the results obtained.

7. Separate analyses, not shown, considered only those with ADL limitations, rather than combining the ADL- with IADL-impaired cases. This was done since the ADL-impaired were the more likely recipients of the "chronic care benefits" offered by the S/HMOs. Mean levels of satisfaction among the ADL-impaired are not affected by this, but there is a loss of statistical power because of the reduced sample size.

8. All cases were screened to update their health plan status at the time of the satisfaction interview. Unimpaired cases confirmed as having had a change to functionally impaired status ($n = 44$) were assigned to the impaired group for the present analysis. Panel members stratified as "impaired," but who were found to have improved in their health status (becoming "unimpaired") 12 months or more before the satisfaction interview date ($n = 92$) have been deleted from the analysis as ineligible respondents. This was done to retain the probability design for the unimpaired sample. Similar status changes did not change eligibility in the disenrollee group, but it did affect the subgroup placement. Health plan enrollment status was verified using Medicare group health plan membership files. S/HMO member sample cases found to have disenrolled have been deleted from the S/HMO sample as ineligible, and assigned to the disenrollee sample ($n = 74$). Any disenrollee found to have re-enrolled in the S/HMO has been excluded from the analysis. Appendix 5A shows the sample size and response rate by site and sample.

9. A sample size of 500 or more completed interviews among each of the unimpaired and impaired panels, was expected to be large enough to detect an effect size of .20 or more between the functional status groups in the S/HMO; and between the comparison group and S/HMO members in each functional status group. These calculations were based on a two-tailed alpha level of .05 and a power analysis beta of .80.

10. The PSQ in its more recent versions uses 30 items. These collapse into the dimensions of technical quality/competence, continuity/choice, communication/interpersonal care, outcomes or efficacy of care, and general satisfaction.

11. The PSQ domains omitted in these analyses are the efficacy of care (a section of the PSQ which has been greatly modified in revisions to the original instrument), and the availability of resources (which is not in recent PSQ versions). Continuity/choice (seeing the same physician at each appointment, freedom

to choose or change physicians) has been incorporated into interpersonal relations in our domains. Four items (general satisfaction, convenience of the MD office location, emergency care available, and hospital quality) did not load into either individual scales or global satisfaction.

12. This shortened version of the original PSQ was used to reduce respondent burden and facilitate the use of the instrument in a telephone interview. In most circumstances the deleted items were from parallel questions where one version of the question was a negative statement, the other positive. A balance of negative and positive statements was retained to avoid acquiescence bias. Wording changes were made, when necessary, to tailor the questions' appropriateness for the S/HMO model. Each item was recorded in an agree/disagree format, using a neutral middle option. The PSQ was originally developed with a five-option Likert format ranging from strongly agree to strongly disagree. Versions of the PSQ published after our field work began ask for ratings from poor to excellent (Davies and Ware 1988). The scoring of the satisfaction items followed the procedures used in other applications of the PSQ. Both positive and negative statements were rescored into a common direction: dissatisfaction was coded as 1, satisfaction was coded as 3, the neutral position or no opinion was coded as 2. Raw domain scale scores are computed by simple summation. All scales have been tested for reliability and internal consistency. They all have acceptable Cronbach coefficient alpha levels: access (.894), quality (.938), interpersonal relations (.595), benefit and cost (.493) and overall satisfaction (.916). These results are shown in Appendix 5B.

13. Disenrollment can either be voluntary (self-selected) or involuntary (required when one moves out of the S/HMO service area). Nineteen percent (92) of the disenrollees were considered to be involuntary because they moved out of the area. Although some of these individuals may have made a voluntary decision to move because of dissatisfaction with the S/HMO, others were true involuntary disenrollees who may have wanted to continue with the plan. Since it was not possible to distinguish between these two groups of movers, all those who moved were considered involuntary disenrollees.

14. Health status was not considered as an outcome in this analysis. As discussed previously, the impaired and unimpaired groups were initially stratified at baseline. Persons improving from an impaired status at least one year before the satisfaction interviews were deleted from the impaired sample. Anyone found to have become impaired was brought into the impaired sample. More than 97 percent of the impaired group as analyzed here had been impaired for at least one year prior to the survey. Identical procedures were applied to both comparison and treatment groups.

References

Boxerman, S. B., and V. D. Hennelly. "Determinants of Disenrollment: Implications for HMO Managers." *Journal of Ambulatory Care Management* (May 1983): 12–23.

Cleary, P. D., and B. J. McNeil. "Patient Satisfaction as an Indicator of Quality Care." *Inquiry* 25 (Spring 1988): 25–36.

Davies, A. R., and J. E. Ware. *GHAA's Consumer Satisfaction Survey and User's Manual.* Newton, MA: GHAA/Davies & Ware, 1988.

Friedlob, A. S., and J. A. Hadley. "Marketing Medicare in a Competitive Environment." Health Care Financing Special Report. Baltimore, MD: Health Care Financing Administration, 1985.

Harrington, C., R. J. Newcomer, and A. Friedlob. "S/HMO Organization and Management." In *Report to Congress: Evaluation of the Social/Health Maintenance Organization Demonstration.* Prepared for the Health Care Financing Administration, contract no. 500-85-0042. Baltimore, MD: Health Care Financing Administration, 1989.

Hennelly, V. D., and S. B. Boxerman. "Disenrollment From a Prepaid Startup Plan: A Multivariate Analysis." *Medical Care* 21 (December 1983): 1154–67.

Luft, H. *Health Maintenance Organizations: Dimensions of Performance.* New Brunswick, CT: Transition Books, 1987.

Manton, K., G. Lowremore, R. J. Newcomer, and C. Harrington. "Mortality and Attrition in Four Social/Health Maintenance Organizations." Durham, NC: Duke University, 1992b.

Manton, K., G. Lowremore, R. J. Newcomer, and C. Harrington. "Assessment of Selection Bias in Four Social/Health Maintenance Organizations." Durham, NC: Duke University, 1992b.

Mechanic, D., N. Weiss, and P. D. Cleary. "The Growth of HMOS: Issues of Enrollment and Disenrollment." *Medical Care* 21 (March 1983): 338–47.

Newcomer, R., C. Harrington, and A. Friedlob. "Social Health Maintenance Organizations: Assessing Their Initial Experience." *Health Services Research* 25, no. 3 (1990): 425–54.

Pascoe, G. C. "Patient Satisfaction in Primary Health Care: A Literature Review and Analysis." *Evaluation and Program Planning* 6, no. 2 (1983): 185–210.

Pope, C. R., D. K. Freeborn, and S. Marks. "Perceived Access to Care and Patient Satisfaction in a Prepaid Group Practice HMO." *The Group Health Journal* (Fall 1984): 22–28.

Rossiter, L., T. Wan, K. Langwell, J. Hadley, A. Tucker, M. Rivnyak, K. Sullivan, and J. Norcross. "National Medicare Competition Evaluation: An Analysis of Patient Satisfaction for Enrollees and Disenrollees in Medicare Risk-Based Plans. Final Analysis Report." Richmond, VA: Williamson Institute for Health Studies and Mathematica Policy Research, Inc., 1988.

Rossiter, L. F., K. Langwell, T. T. H. Wan, and M. Rivnyak. "Patient Satisfaction among Elderly Enrollees and Disenrollees in Medicare Health Maintenance Organizations: Results from the National Medicare Competition Evaluation." *Journal of the American Medical Association* 262, no. 1 (1989): 57–63.

Sorenson, A. A., and R. P. Wersinger. "Factors Influencing Disenrollment from an HMO." *Medical Care* 19 (July 1981): 766–73.

Tucker, A. M., and K. Langwell. "Disenrollment Patterns in Medicare HMOS: A Preliminary Analysis." Washington, D.C.: Mathematica Policy Research, Inc., 1989.

Ward, R. A. "HMO Satisfaction and Understanding among Recent Medicare Enrollees. *Journal of Health and Social Behavior* 28 (December 1987): 401–12.

Ware, J. E., M. K. Snyder, and W. R. Wright. *Development and Validation of Scales to Measure Patient Satisfaction with Health Services.* Volume I of a Final Report: Review of Literature, Overview of Methods, and Results Regarding Construction of Scales. NTIS No. PB.288–329. Springfield, VA: National Technical Information Service, 1976.

Ware, J. E., Jr., M. K. Snyder, W. R. Wright, and A. R. Davies. "Defining and Measuring Patient Satisfaction with Medical Care." *Evaluation and Program Planning* 6, no. 2 (1983): 247–63.

Zastowny, T. R., K. J. Roghmann, and A. Hengst. "Satisfaction with Medical Care: Replications and Theoretic Reevaluation." *Medical Care* 21 (March 1983):294–321.

Appendix 5A   Satisfaction Sample Response Rate

Site	Number Complete*	Percent Complete†	# Status Change‡
Brooklyn			
S/HMO	290	91.8%	5
Disenrollees	140	83.3	NA§
Comparison	298	88.4	13
Long Beach			
S/HMO	287	92.9	7
Disenrollees	118	83.5	NA
Comparison	320	91.4	6
Minneapolis			
S/HMO	353	93.6	6
Disenrollees	106	94.6	NA
Comparison	338	93.1	12
Portland			
S/HMO	318	93.0	4
Disenrollees	109	87.2	NA
Comparison	410	93.6	14
Total			
S/HMO	1248	92.9	22
Disenrollees	473	87.1	NA
Comparison	1366	91.4	45

*The sample was drawn in June 1988 from all the presumed surviving members of the S/HMO and comparison panels, and all known S/HMO disenrollees in the prior 12 months. Any disenrollees found in the S/HMO satisfaction sample were reassigned into the disenrollee sample. Completion rates include the number of interviews completed with the eligible sample members. The number eligible excludes all sample members who were found to have died, and from the S/HMO sample only, persons who disenrolled. Also excluded from S/HMO and comparison samples were those who changed from impaired to unimpaired status.

†Calculated as the number completed divided by the number eligible.

‡Number of unimpaired S/HMO and comparison sample persons found to have become impaired at the time of the satisfaction interview.

§Not applicable.

Appendix 5B   Satisfaction Scale Reliability Analysis*

Satisfaction Items	Mean (n = 2614)	s.d.	Scale Mean if Item Deleted	Alpha if Item Deleted
Access				
Appointment wait	2.79	.57	5.59	.84
Office waiting	2.81	.55	5.78	.85
Convenience of hospital	2.79	.58	5.59	.86
Standardized Item Alpha = .894				
Physician Quality				
MD continuity	2.80	.58	8.31	.91
MD thorough	2.79	.55	8.32	.93
MD attends previous problems	2.75	.58	8.36	.92
MD knowledgeable	2.77	.58	8.34	.91
Standardized Item Alpha = .938				
Interpersonal Relations/Courtesy				
MD spends enough time	2.78	.60	14.45	.54
All needs are met	2.90	.41	14.34	.52
Can get questions answered	2.80	.54	14.43	.51
Staff friendly and courteous	2.94	.33	14.30	.52
Freedom to change physician	2.89	.39	14.34	.56
Tests and treatment available	2.92	.32	14.31	.51
Standardized Item Alpha = .595				
Benefits and Cost				
Happy with benefits	2.73	.62	7.98	.49
Saving money	2.59	.64	8.12	.45
Cost of premiums	2.67	.58	8.03	.33
Copays and deductibles	2.71	.57	8.00	.37
Standardized Item Alpha = .493				
Overall Satisfaction				
General satisfaction	2.80	.57	30.61	.91
MD continuity	2.80	.58	30.62	.91
MD thorough	2.79	.55	30.63	.91
Appointment wait	2.79	.57	30.63	.91
MD attends previous problems	2.75	.58	30.67	.91
Convenience of hospital	2.79	.58	30.63	.91
Cost of premiums	2.67	.58	30.74	.92
MD knowledgeable	2.77	.58	30.64	.91
Can get questions answered	2.80	.54	30.62	.94
Copays and deductibles	2.71	.57	30.71	.92
Staff friendly and courteous	2.94	.33	30.48	.94
Office waiting	2.80	.55	30.61	.91
Standardized Item Alpha = .916				

*The maximum value for each scale is three times the number of items in that scale.

Chapter 6

Responses and Discussion

Haya R. Rubin

This discussion reviews three topics concerning patient satisfaction with HMOs and managed care: (1) factors promoting increased use of patient evaluations or judgments to compare the quality of care in different health plans; (2) what we know about the level of patient satisfaction with HMOs based on the papers by Newcomer and associates and Clement and associates, as well as the rest of the literature; and (3) why state-of-the-art measurement of patient judgments of quality of care will be important regardless of which health reforms are adopted.

Factors promoting the use of patient judgments to compare health plans

Three factors that have led to the increasing use of patient judgments to compare health plans are: (1) the rise of corporations as the major providers of medical care, and increasing competition among providers; (2) pioneering research by psychologists, sociologists, and health care researchers that has developed accurate ways of obtaining patient judgments, and has therefore made it practical enough to move them from research instruments to routine quality monitoring tools; and (3) the increasing power of private and public sector health care purchasers, often working together in coalitions, who are demanding information about the quality of the product they are buying.

Corporations and competition

The health care industry and its regulators have become increasingly interested in getting the patient's perspective on quality of care (Cleary and McNeil 1988; Moloney and Paul 1991). This mirrors a larger industrial interest in the customer perspective in the United States. In health care, the banner has been carried by Berwick (1989, 1990) and his colleagues, who have brought to the attention of the health care industry the writings of Deming (1986), Juran (1988), and other quality improvement gurus who invented and refined Japanese industrial quality management techniques (Ishikawa 1985; Imai 1986). The health care industry is now interested in this form of evaluation because of corporate and competitive forces. The highly competitive environment is only likely to increase under managed competition, which seems to be the health care reform proposal of political choice. Therefore, health care organizations need information for marketing purposes about their quality of care. The other factor is that health care organizations increasingly have corporate administrative structures controlled more by business and administrative leaders than by clinical staff, resulting in more emphasis on marketing in this competitive environment. Consumer satisfaction has been a desired outcome easier for administrators to work on than the quality of clinical services—a concept much harder to measure, especially within an organization, and less accessible to administrators without a clinical background. Technical quality standards are more changeable, depend on clinical staff to measure them, and have results that are harder to determine. More than other quality measures, consumer satisfaction results from things common to many service industries, like image, patient expectations, staff interpersonal skills, environmental comfort, and the quality of food, parking, and other services. Administrators can work on such issues without using physician time to do so.

Research transforming patient judgments into routine administrative measures

Clarification of important domains. Studies like those by Newcomer et al. and Clement et al. presented here have benefited from years of groundwork by psychometricians and health care researchers determining how to measure the quality of care. In the outpatient setting, the measurement of satisfaction began with the work of Barbara Hulka and her colleagues (1970). John Ware and his various coworkers over the years (Ware et al. 1976, 1981) refined this to develop the Patient Satisfaction Questionnaire, a version of which was used by Newcomer et al. in the paper evaluating Social/HMOs. This was derived from careful exploratory studies in the early 1970s clarifying the major dimensions of concern to patients, as the Newcomer and Clement investigating teams have reviewed. This extensive exploratory work can define which aspects are most important to patients. When we try to come up with brief, practical instruments for monitoring, we can turn to work that indicates which specific areas are most highly related to patients' overall satisfaction with their health plans. It used to be that patients' impressions of the quality of care by their physician were most important. We are now seeing that cost and finances have become much more prominent, especially for healthy enrollees. When designing brief measures, we must still try to include at least a single item in each of the important domains.

Similar work has been done measuring patient judgments of hospital care, and there are now studies that clarify domains of interest from the patient point of view, including the background work done to develop the 45-item Patient Judgments of Hospital Quality rating questionnaire (Meterko and Rubin 1990), and work performed by Cleary and colleagues as part of the Picker-Commonwealth Program for Patient-Centered Care (Cleary, Edgman-Levitan, Roberts, et al. 1991). The Newcomer and Clement papers did not incorporate patient evaluations of hospital care delivered by different types of health plans, and this is an important area for future monitoring.

Toward brief, yet sensitive and accurate measures. A second point that has moved measures of patient satisfaction from research into routine is that measurement advances have made brief measures much more feasible. A major advance in measurement in the 1980s was the discovery that patient evaluations or judgments that use ordinal rating scales are more sensitive to important differences in care than agreement or disagreement with evaluative statements (Ware and Hays 1986). An important insight is that it works better to vary the evaluative strength within the response scale than to rely on the strength written into the item stem. An example of this is an item that says "My care was excellent," and the respondent must indicate strength of agreement, versus an item that says "How would you rate your care: excellent, very good, good, fair, poor?" Thus excellent to poor and other evaluative rating scales have become popular. Using such scales makes single items more sensitive to differences and allows reduction of longer scales of items that used to be necessary with agree-disagree response scales, in order to incorporate a spectrum of items of different strength. Because of this advance, short measures using single items or two-item scales to represent a domain of interest have become possible, allowing us to evaluate how patients judge outpatient visits in 10 to 15 items instead of 65 to 100 items. To see this in practice, one need only compare the length of questionnaires in the Clement and Newcomer papers. We would all agree that although not quite as detailed, the measures used by Clement and associates would be easier to administer to large populations in comparing different health plans on an ongoing basis.

Recent years also have provided advances in statistical testing that facilitate data analysis by making these results more accurate and less prone to bias. The most important advance has been the availability in computerized statistical packages of ordinal logistic regression programs allowing tests of ordinal trend across several categories (*STATA Reference Manual* 1992). Clement and associates could confirm the results of the dichotomous analyses they have presented using such a technique, as ordinal models utilizing information from all categories will be more sensitive to differences than a logistic model based on a binary variable that combines the information in the good, fair, and poor categories. This will allow single-item measures to be as sensitive as possible. When multi-item measures are used, as is done in the Newcomer paper, linear models are reasonable approximations to the distribution of responses, and one can compare group means. However, ongoing monitoring of how patients judge care in different health plans will increasingly require single-item measures if it is to be practical to implement in regular beneficiary surveys by monitoring agencies, by industry consortia, or by independent watchdog groups.

Purchaser/Payer power: creating independent monitoring in the public interest

Currently popular models of health care reform will give purchasers of health care great importance. Buying cooperatives are likely to represent large groups of consumers and, as such, they will be able to afford expert staff who can understand more than an individual employer's benefits manager, much less an individual consumer, about how to distinguish between better- and worse-value health care (Starr 1992). Such groups are likely to exert influence to make sure that quality of care is monitored, and that accurate and independent information about patient judgments and other measures of quality of care is available.

How should patient judgments be incorporated in plans for monitoring quality of care if health care reforms are implemented? It matters a great deal who does the survey. Just as with political polling, different results are obtained depending on which questions are asked, which procedures are followed, and how data are presented. These in turn depend on the interest of those who commission the survey. Would a government effort be best? It is doubtful that such an effort could be truly independent of the huge federal and state government interests as health care payers. Other payers likewise have conflicts of interest.

When we perform this work for payers, we would like to demonstrate that organizations can spend less and still provide as high a quality of care. Individual providers are biased, because they would like to portray themselves in the best light for marketing. A happy medium is a regulatory mechanism that provides for an independent auditing agency to conduct surveys with strict controls to prevent conflicts of interest. While it is not out of the question that this auditor could be a government agency, safeguards are necessary to protect it from undue influence by payers to find the lowest cost option the best. Employer, payer, and health care provider information about the quality of health insurance and health providers—all are likely to have important biases.

The Newcomer paper signals the need to monitor the experience of large enough samples of sick people who use and need services in order to understand how well a plan meets this group's needs. This is particularly important for managed care plans, as providers as well as payers have incentives to underuse services with this type of payment arrangement.

Prepaid or managed care versus fee-for-service health plans

What do we know about prepaid or managed care compared with fee-for-service health care payment from the Clement and Newcomer papers as well as from other studies of patient judgments under different payment conditions (Davies et al. 1986; Rossiter et al. 1989; Rubin et al. 1993)?

Almost all of our knowledge comes from comparisons of fee-for-service patients with capitated HMO patients, rather than with patients in other forms of managed care. Compared with FFS patients, HMO patients have generally given better ratings of financial arrangements, including out-of-pocket costs, paperwork, and coverage for preventive services. They have given poorer ratings than FFS patients of their choice of providers, waits for an appointment, care by providers (time spent, interpersonal behavior, perceived competence), access to emergency and hospital services (especially out-of-plan services), and telephone consultation. Also, problems with HMOs appear to be worse for sick patients who need many services. None of these findings are unique to elderly patients in capitated managed care programs, but these problems appear to be worse for the sick elderly than for healthy patients.

Little is known about how managed care providers can find feasible ways to improve patient experience. The removal of conflict of interest at the physician and nurse level is an important issue, as stressed by *Consumer Reports* (1992), in an issue that rated HMOs around the country. Positive incentives for high quality of care, like bonus systems for improved patient satisfaction, are another. Identifying mechanisms that work will take much experimentation.

Incentives to improve quality of patients' experience in managed care

How can the managed care industry be encouraged to offer improved quality of care from the patients' point of view without destroying cost-containment incentives?

Setting standards and ideal goals for patient-judged quality will give the managed care industry some yardsticks against which it can judge its progress and with which comparisons among plans can be made. Dissemination of information about patient judgments and other quality of care measures using a uniform yardstick is critical both for individual consumers and consumer groups, and for health care purchasing cooperatives, to give competing plans incentives to improve quality of care. Purchasing agents on behalf of large groups of consumers must represent the consumer's interest in cost and quality rather than payers' or providers' interests. Finally, we need to make sure that both well and ill patients are surveyed about their care, and the prevalence of well and ill patients in a given health plan must be determined. If there is good information about quality, better providers will stay in the market—those that provide better care at the same cost.

Rather than paint a dismal picture of cost-containment efforts necessarily resulting in reduced patient satisfaction, being able to measure how patients judge care gives us a way to choose the best value for what we can spend. We need to be more realistic about what we can buy, and until we learn how to save money by reducing overuse of services, we can neither improve access to needed care nor improve its quality, including patient judgments. Although managed care in its current forms doesn't give the patient as much, moving to managed competition may be a politically acceptable way to get meaningful health care reform. If we monitor health care reforms as they are implemented, we will be able to see which plans are doing the best job in cost-cutting while maintaining patient satisfaction. Such monitoring will also move plans to experiment with low-cost ways to improve patient satisfaction, and I believe we have only begun to scratch the surface of what is possible here. The federal government can also do a great deal to make the public aware of real trade-offs in health care, demonstrating that there are real choices between low-cost coverage in one's healthy years and excellent care when one is ill. Only through increased interaction with the public can we achieve the greatest value for our health care dollars.

References

Berwick, D. M. "Continuous Improvement as an Ideal in Health Care." *New England Journal of Medicine* 320, no. 1 (1989): 52–66.

———. *Curing Health Care.* San Francisco: Jossey-Bass, 1990.

Cleary, P. D., and B. J. McNeil. "Patient Satisfaction as an Indicator of Quality Care." *Inquiry* 25, no. 1 (1988): 25–36.

Cleary, P. D., S. Edgman-Levitan, M. Roberts, T. W. Moloney, W. McMullen, J. D. Walker, and T. L. Delbanco. "Patients Evaluate Their Hospital Care: A National Survey." *Health Affairs* 10 (Winter 1991): 254–67.

Consumer Reports. "Health Care in Crisis: Are HMOs the Answer?" (August 1992): 519–53.

Davies, A. R., J. E. Ware, R. H. Brook, J. R. Peterson, and J. P. Newhouse. "Consumer Acceptance of Prepaid and Fee-For-Service Medical Care: Results from a Randomized Controlled Trial." *Health Services Research* 21, no. 4 (1986): 429–52.

Deming, W. E. *Out of the Crisis.* Cambridge, MA: MIT-CAES, 1986.

Hulka, B. S., S. H. Zyzanski, J. C. Cassel, and S. J. Thompson. "Scale for the Measurement of Attitudes Toward Physicians and Primary Medical Care." *Medical Care* 8, no. 5 (1970): 429–36.

Imai, M. K. *Kaizen: The Key to Japan's Competitive Success.* New York: Random House, 1986.

Ishikawa, K. *What is Total Quality Control?* Englewood Cliffs, NJ: Prentice-Hall, 1985.

Juran, J. M. *Juran's Quality Control Handbook,* 4th ed. New York: McGraw-Hill, 1988.

Moloney, T., and B. Paul. "The Consumer Movement Takes Hold in Medical Care." *Health Affairs* 10 (Winter 1991): 268–79.

Meterko, M., and H. R. Rubin. "Patient Judgments of Hospital Quality: A Taxonomy." In *Patient Judgments of Hospital Quality: Report of a Pilot Study,* edited by M. Meterko, E. C. Nelson, and H. R. Rubin. *Medical Care* 28, no. 8 (1990, Supplement): S10–S14.

Rossiter, L. F., K. Langwell, T. T. H. Wan, and M. Rivnyak. "Patient Satisfaction among Elderly Enrollees and Disenrollees in Medicare Health Maintenance Organizations: Results from the National Medicare Competition Evaluation." *Journal of the American Medical Association* 262, no. 1 (1989): 57–63.

Rubin, H. R., B. Gandek, M. Kosinski, C. McHorney, W. H. Rogers, and J. E. Ware. "Patient Ratings of Outpatient Visits in Different Practice Settings." *Journal of the American Medical Association* 270, no. 7 (1993): 835–40.

Starr, P. *The Logic of Health Care Reform.* Knoxville, TN: Grand Rounds Press, Whittle Direct Books, 1992.

STATA Reference Manual: Release 3, 5th ed. Santa Monica, CA: Computing Resource Center, 1992, pp. 77–85.

Ware, J. E., and R. D. Hays. "Methods for Measuring Patient Satisfaction with Specific Medical Encounters." *Medical Care* 26, no. 3 (1986): 393–402.

Ware, J. E., M. K. Snyder, and W. R. Wright. *Development and Validation of Scales to Measure Patient Satisfaction with Health Care Services: Volume I, Part B.*

Results Regarding Scales Constructed from the Patient Satisfaction Questionnaire and Measures of Other Health Perceptions. Springfield, VA: National Technical Information Service, 1976.

Ware, J. E., M. K. Snyder, W. R. Wright, and A. R. Davies. "Defining and Measuring Patient Satisfaction with Medical Care." *Evaluation and Program Planning* 6, no. 2 (1983): 247–63.

Sheila Leatherman, Deborah Chase, and Cynthia Polich

The satisfaction surveys conducted by Clement et al. and Newcomer et al. show the importance of analyzing the effectiveness of managed care delivery systems in serving the elderly. These studies serve to crystallize many issues related to evaluating managed care delivery systems which, in general, are held accountable for patient satisfaction while fee-for-service delivery systems are not.

If satisfaction surveys are to be useful, certain criteria must be observed. First, if these surveys are to be one measure of success, they must be designed rigorously enough to produce salient results. Second, detailed analyses on the overall perceived value of managed care systems must draw conclusions on which populations are served and which are not by discretely characterized managed care models. Third, satisfaction is not a sufficient measure of performance to determine overall effectiveness of managed care delivery systems—other measures must complement it. If satisfaction data are to be useful for policy and managerial decisions, they should be supplemented by other critical performance data on cost, access, appropriateness, and outcomes. Studies of managed care delivery systems should also take into account the evolution of and variation in managed care.

This discussion paper begins with specific comments on the two scientific papers and then provides a general perspective on patient satisfaction surveys and their usefulness in determining the success of managed care in serving the elderly as well as other populations. It concludes with a discussion of the importance of evaluating other components of health care delivery systems, in addition to patient satisfaction.

Medicare HMO study

The paper by Clement et al. provides useful information regarding patient satisfaction surveys, and it illustrates what may be the limited contribution that satisfaction surveys play in evaluating the effectiveness of health care delivery systems when using a singular measure.

A few comments on design and methods must precede discussion of the findings. The study design chosen by the authors makes the findings difficult to interpret. The study contrasts one HMO (of undefined model, size, age, and market) to 44 fee-for-service market areas, but differences in these market areas are not analyzed even though their characteristics could have significant effect on perceptions. A market-to-market comparison could have yielded more useful data. In the examination of the relationship between member satisfaction and disenrollment, it is unclear whether Clement controlled for disenrollment due to factors beyond a health plan's control. For example, an effective analysis of reasons for disenrollment must control for the following: death, relocation, transfer to another Medicare HMO, maturity of plan, system nonusers, and utilization. The results of Clement's analysis may be misleading if these factors were not controlled. Another difficulty presented by the study method is that the paper assumes all HMOs to be the same. As Newcomer points out in his paper on S/HMOs, the maturity, model, and market area of an HMO all affect enrollee satisfaction. Therefore, researchers should attempt to control for, or at least explain, these differences.

Clement's analysis focuses on comparing the rate of excellents, which may be misleading in terms of overall satisfaction and may not be the most appropriate focus. For instance, in Table 4.2 (the only table where excellent, good, fair, and poor are provided), overall quality of care is reported as excellent by 44.9 percent of enrollees and 51.7 percent of nonenrollees, which Clement points out shows a negative difference of 6.8. However, if excellent and good are grouped together, the difference is only 1.4. Grouping excellents and goods together may be a more helpful approach because it will then be easier to assess what percentage of members express overall satisfaction with the health care system. From a public policy and managerial perspective, it seems more significant to look at those who rated overall quality as fair or poor rather than focusing on those who did not rate quality as excellent. Concern would be more appropriately focused on the 8 percent of enrollees and 5 percent of nonenrollees who rate the quality of care as fair or poor. It is the concerns of those who are dissatisfied that could provide us with needed information about what is lacking in the Medicare HMO delivery model and how to make meaningful improvements.

The paper is useful in that it raised for us the issue of why the trade-offs of a Medicare managed care system are not examined. Although one general question was asked: "Would you recommend it to a friend?", the study does not address the overall value of what is received—whether the trade-offs are worth it. This seems to be a common occurrence in studies of patient satisfaction. In the Clement study, only 45 percent responded that overall quality of care was excellent, but fully 92 percent rated it as good or excellent. Also, 53 percent of enrollees responded that they were satisfied with out-of-pocket costs compared to 40 percent of nonenrollees. Furthermore, 94 percent said they would recommend the HMO to a friend. It is this final decision—whether members would choose managed care—that should be emphasized when evaluating Medicare managed care delivery systems. Rather than placing such heavy emphasis on government oversight through such mechanisms as enrollee surveys, it seems more appropriate to let individual consumers exercise their right to choose health care. It would then be a constructive policy action to make an assessment of the success of different models based on predominating choices. The final analysis of a plan's success should be in its perceived overall value.

The study also calls attention to the emphasis placed on patient satisfaction surveys and recommends that "surveys should be done on a more regular basis." Medicare HMOs already conduct surveys regularly, and sufficient resources are already used for conducting surveys. A more important contribution could be made by analyzing already conducted HMO surveys in a more rigorous fashion to detect patterns of strengths or deficiencies in serving the elderly. In addition, the Medicare HMO program could be analyzed more comprehensively if resources were dedicated to analyzing additional dimensions of performance to supplement satisfaction data. Analysis could be conducted in terms of realized cost savings and utilization to shape policy recommendations. Purchasers increasingly are demanding data that will allow them to evaluate health care systems on more than just price. Patient satisfaction is one dimension that purchasers are demanding, but they, like policymakers, also need salient information that measures other dimensions of health care delivery, such as clinical outcomes and appropriateness.

S/HMO study

The paper by Newcomer et al. offers new information on the S/HMO demonstrations and provides substantive data; however, it could make further contributions if more emphasis were placed on interpreting these data and drawing conclusions. Further analysis of the results of the Newcomer study provides significant insight into pinpointing an appropriate service delivery model for the elderly, especially the frail elderly.

The paper presents significant findings. In particular, it explains that enrollees in the newly formed plans, Elderplan and SHP, had higher dissatisfaction levels than enrollees in the preexisting HMOs, SeniorPlus and Medicare Plus II. The study points to the new plans' difficulties in establishing and maintaining their acute and physician service networks and to the fact that Elderplan was the only HMO in its market area. This is a highly significant finding in terms of policy decisions as it points to the importance of maturity and stability of an HMO as a success indicator for enrollee satisfaction. It also demonstrates the importance of understanding the different attributes of individual managed care systems and the characteristics of individual market areas before launching new HMO initiatives. In addition, the findings seem relevant for other populations besides the elderly. As managed care delivery systems expand, it is important for health plans to understand their market area and for consumers to be informed about the characteristics of individual health plans so that they can make educated choices.

Another significant finding in the Newcomer paper was that those who had health problems, who had functional impairments, and who used chronic care services were slightly more likely to remain in the plan. Also those unimpaired who disenrolled were more satisfied overall than any other group. The authors conclude: "By providing improved benefits, it is expected that S/HMOs will have lower disenrollment rates than Medicare HMOs and a greater propensity to retain members having functional impairments and other health problems." However, there seems to be even more to their findings. The data presented in the paper suggest that enhancing benefits will not address the real problems with S/HMOs. Those members who are impaired, and thus making the most use of benefits, are not the ones most likely to disenroll. It is possible that the impaired do not disenroll because they have no other option for chronic care services outside of a nursing home. Furthermore, the unimpaired were the most likely to disenroll, presumably because they were most dissatisfied with costs and benefits, which suggests that they like the S/HMOs but do not perceive them as a good value.

These findings suggest a possible flaw in the S/HMO demonstration design, which requires that each site have a certain percentage of healthy and unhealthy members. The S/HMOs receive 100 percent of the AAPCC, and this, coupled with member premiums, is supposed to enable them to increase benefits to include chronic care services. With the overall premiums kept so low, it is impossible to expand benefits without enrolling a substantial proportion of healthy members. However, as the Newcomer paper infers, the healthy members are satisfied but do not perceive S/HMOs as a value due to high premium costs. This suggests the prudence of considering policies to change the design of the S/HMOs so that they serve *only* the chronically ill and frail elderly. In order to accomplish this, the reimbursement system for S/HMOs must be changed. The AAPCC is not an appropriate reimbursement calculation for this population.

Moving beyond satisfaction surveys

The Clement and Newcomer papers demonstrate the importance of analyzing how effective health care delivery systems are in serving the elderly. Patient-reported measures are a critical aspect of the analysis, and satisfaction is one of these measures. However, satisfaction should not be the only measure of an HMO's success, particularly in an era of reform. To assess the effectiveness of any health care delivery system, satisfaction may have to be weighed in relation to affordable price and improved access to high-quality, appropriate services.

The Clement paper states that "measures of satisfaction serve as indicators of the perceived quality of care delivered by HMOs, and can be used to assess various aspects of the structure, process, and outcome of care." It is true that satisfaction should be measured as *one* indicator of success. Satisfaction is an appropriate proxy for concerns about adequate access and utilization—particularly given suspicions that underutilization is a feature of HMOs. However, satisfaction surveys should not be weighed in isolation from broader medical outcomes information. Patient dissatisfaction with a health care delivery system does not imply automatically that the delivery system is performing poorly. For instance, a study should not perpetuate the notion that more medical care is necessarily better and, further, that if members of a health plan feel they are being denied services, this automatically means that insufficient care is being provided. In fact, it has been demonstrated that this is not the case with the frail elderly, who receive too much acute care when less intensive primary or support care is often what is needed. For S/HMOs in particular, providing appropriate and continuous chronic care (versus service-intensive episodic care) as a way of avoiding unnecessary acute care services is an extremely important approach and deserves heavy weight when contextualizing satisfaction levels.

In general, lower satisfaction levels must be put into the context of broader medical information. Evaluations of the health care system beyond satisfaction surveys are needed, including increased emphasis on performance evaluation regarding quality of care, cost and efficiency of care delivery, and appropriateness of services rendered. Although such evaluations have taken place to some degree, these efforts have been scattered, and rarely is one HMO described and evaluated in all of these dimensions. Among existing studies one HMO may be evaluated in terms of price, another in terms of quality, and then still another in terms of customer satisfaction. Then conclusions are drawn about the effectiveness of managed care delivery systems in general. This approach does not allow us to assess the effectiveness of any delivery system, especially given the fact that all managed care systems, as with delivery systems in general, are not the same.

As the elderly population continues to grow in record proportions and as the number of people 85 and older (who typically suffer from more chronic conditions) grows even faster, it becomes all the more important to address the needs of this population. Since the appropriateness of much of the care currently provided to the elderly is unclear, rigorous evaluation is necessary to assess which aspects of this care are adequate and to identify areas for improvement.

Scrutiny of delivery systems

Managed care delivery systems are held accountable for patient satisfaction, while fee-for-service delivery systems are not. Other Medicare programs that involve financial incentives that can affect quality are not subject to this evaluation. For example, Medicare hospital patients are not asked how satisfied they are with their length of stay although this may be relevant to the evaluation of impact for the DRG system of payment, and the impact of RBRVS (Medicare's Resource-Based Relative Value Scale of payment to physicians) is not evaluated in terms of patient satisfaction.

Is it appropriate to continue heavy scrutiny of managed care without commensurate attention to nonmanaged care? In the 1970s and early 1980s, when HMOs were experimental or alternative forms of care, such a biased focus was probably necessary. However, with 20 years of experience and more than half of all employees enrolled in some form of managed care, these delivery systems have become mainstream and are accepted as appropriate forms of care. It is no longer necessary to question whether they offer acceptable services compared to fee-for-service. It is not a question of whether evaluation of managed care systems should occur but whether they should be the sole delivery systems evaluated. In fact, nonmanaged care systems are plagued with problems of inadequate access and inappropriate utilization. Continuous evaluation that focuses on measuring and then improving the health care system is indeed needed; this means a more inclusive approach to evaluating health care services for the elderly.

Recognizing the diversity of managed care

There is a pervasive lack of knowledge about the evolution and status of managed care. For instance, one paper refers to HMOs as "a closed system of providers on a prepaid basis." This is a common misconception. Managed care includes many more models than staff-model, closed-panel HMOs. One important distinction is that not all managed care delivery systems directly employ physicians. For instance, in the Minneapolis–St. Paul metropolitan area, Group Health, a staff-model HMO; Medica Primary, a gatekeeper, network-based HMO; and Medica Choice, a fee-for-service, open panel HMO, all have had a Medicare risk contract. Each has a different arrangement with its physicians in terms of direct ties between service delivery and payment. This demonstrates that the utility of HMO patient satisfaction surveys for generalized purposes of evaluation and improvement are potentially quite limited. It also calls attention to the fact that to evaluate managed care accurately, studies must account for the diversity of managed care.

When designing studies to evaluate managed care systems, it is important to avoid misguidedly lumping all HMOs and other forms of managed care together. A rigorous research design must incorporate methods to distinguish among the many different types of HMOs now in existence. Efforts should be made to control for discrepancies in satisfaction due to model types, and to explain strengths or weaknesses (or both) of certain models. This misunderstanding of the nature of managed care permeates the health policy community and even the nation as a whole. There is a critical need for education about the evolution of and variation in managed care in order to recognize the different models and then analyze their performance in providing care to various population groups.

Conclusion

The Clement and Newcomer studies of patient satisfaction surveys highlight many issues surrounding surveys and the evaluation of managed care in general. The heavy focus on surveying managed care enrollees in an oversight fashion is no longer the appropriate focus. It is time to leave behind the notion that HMOs are anomalies or interesting experiments that require special vigilance, and concentrate on improving, not just passively monitoring, the performance of these managed care systems. This will necessitate evaluating other aspects of health care delivery, including quality and appropriateness of care and cost/value. Once delivery systems are measured (both managed and nonmanaged care), the next step will be focusing on improving areas that are identified as needing change. Such an approach holds considerable potential for helping to ameliorate some of the problems we face in this country regarding health care delivery.

General Discussion

A participant opened the discussion with a question for the authors: "Is the goal of this effort to attract the 85 percent of the population that is not in HMOs, or is it to ask how we integrate the total health care needs of all populations?" A response was that one goal of the government is to increase the HMO enrollment of Medicare beneficiaries. If HMOs are able to do a better job at lower cost, then they ought to be encouraged.

Susan Palsbo commented on the difficulty of measuring satisfaction in various populations. Someone who is employed, has a spouse and dependents, and does not tend to use a lot of health services may be more concerned about out-of-pocket costs than about having access to a particular provider. As people become older and develop chronic diseases such as hypertension and diabetes, then the choice of physician becomes more important, and the criteria used in selecting health delivery systems begins to shift. We are just now at a stage in our research that we recognize this, but we do not know much about what triggers the shift.

It was pointed out by Edward Wagner that some of the discussion at this conference is based on the premise that there is a satisfaction "price" to pay in HMOs. He suggested that the data do not tell us that. What we are looking at is people who have fairly recently experienced a disruption in their health care relationship. Other literature tells us that people who have gone through this tend to have lower levels of satisfaction. They are coming into a new system and struggling to accommodate themselves. Evidence from the RAND study tells us that satisfaction does improve with time, a factor that should not be underestimated. After all, what we are talking about is the process of establishing a doctor/patient relationship. So it is not fair to compare patients who are newly relocated with those who have a long-standing, stable relationship.

Haya Rubin responded that that is an important point, and that some studies have looked back to when people had a relationship with a provider. There are studies in progress that have controlled for the time frame of the patient-provider relationship. As we move toward a system where we are comparing plans in a more detailed way, we will have better data about the timing, and it will be easier to see if there are real differences.

Louis Rossiter said that he sometimes calls it the "grumpiness factor." When people have just changed plans, they usually complain a little more. But it is difficult to compare across a whole decade. Very early on there was a study of satisfaction across three plans, and the investigators found that HMO enrollees were more satisfied than those in FFS. After these findings were reported, Rossiter did a study that indicated that HMO enrollees and those in FFS had overall the same levels of satisfaction. Now Clement, Retchin, and Brown are reporting that perhaps satisfaction among HMO enrollees is a little lower. That is contrasted with Brown's findings that started with 20 percent favorable selection, and it is now down to about 10 percent, and maybe in some areas it's even adverse selection. The programs are maturing and enrollment is growing; people have switched plans, so some dynamics are occurring, and what we observe is that the programs are changing before our eyes.

The authors were asked if they have looked at the difference between expectations and experience. One can manipulate expectations, and this will change the satisfaction scores. In the same way, one can manipulate experience and change the satisfaction scores. Thus, the satisfaction score does not really tell us what is going on.

A conference participant pointed out that some studies demonstrate that dissatisfaction with HMOs is frequently shown by people who have had no contact with the plan. In addition, there are degrees of satisfaction and degrees of expectation. If someone is looking for the perfect doctor who is available 24 hours a day and does not charge a fee—that is the ultimate expectation. What level of expectation is implicit when they are responding to a satisfaction survey? What experience have they had with the plan? Fifty percent of people who dropped out of one HMO had never been seen in the plan. It may be that they lost their job or moved away. It was noted that in this study questions about satisfaction were asked of those who had used services.

Susan Palsbo commented that there is a tendency for policymakers to think that satisfaction is equivalent to quality. That is definitely not the case. The patient's standards may not be directly related to the quality of care provided.

A comment was raised about Table 4.4 in the paper by Clement, Retchin, and Brown. It indicates that only 49 percent of enrollees are satisfied with the availability of emergency care. For those with a bona fide emergency, the care was available. Possibly the people who were dissatisfied were expecting to use emergency care inappropriately. Or they might have been answering a question on something they had no experience with. In regard to the same table, it would be interesting to know how much of the dissatisfaction about ability to see the physician of choice actually led to a disenrollment. If a physician should drop out of an HMO or otherwise become unavailable, that person's patients might be dissatisfied about the loss, but that does not necessarily mean that they will disenroll.

Haya Rubin commented that it is very important to look at contact with the plan. Thus, if you want to have a comprehensive understanding of people's judgment of the plan, you want to sample people who are enrolled; you want to sample people who have made visits; and you want to sample people who have been hospitalized. Neither of these papers dealt with satisfaction of the subset of people who had been hospitalized. This is an important factor to measure. Another important patient variable that should be included in any model is people's mental health, because this affects the rating. People who are depressed have much lower ratings of care and are strongly influenced by this in their satisfaction with care. In fact, this is the most powerful predictor of patient satisfaction.

Louis Rossiter asked whether it would be fair to say that the 10 percent of enrollees who indicated that they are dissatisfied were saying, "I'm paying a little less and I'm getting a little less for it"? But for 90 percent, that is not true. They are very satisfied. This raises another question. What do you make of the 10 percent difference? What is the policy or management relevance of a 10 percent difference? This raises a lot of methodological issues.

Dr. Rubin responded that that is a very important point concerning the calibration of these scales, which is within the very high positive end of the spectrum. For example, in the Clement paper, if we see something that the patient thinks is very important at a level of 90 percent satisfaction, that may translate to a relatively high level of disenrollment. It is at a high point on the curve. People tend to give their medical care the benefit of a doubt, and when a problem arises, it causes a small decrement. Therefore, one needs to expand the spectrum of the scales. A difference between 90 percent and 95 percent satisfied may correspond to a much larger difference in the percentage who would go back to that doctor if given a choice, who would take medications as directed, or who would drop the plan. All of these important distinctions occur at the top of the scale between the excellent, the very good, and the good, as well as all the way down to the fair and the poor. One needs to look across the whole spectrum and not limit oneself by saying that policy relevance occurs only at the bottom of the scale.

Jan Malcolm brought up the idea that two different dynamics are going on. We have talked about the importance of measuring expectations as well as whether those expectations are fulfilled. Yet, it may be the case that expectations are higher in the HMO setting than in FFS, perhaps because that is what HMOs are selling. They are selling convenience and access. They are saying, "Come here and your needs will be met." HMOs are creating high expectations. The second and confounding factor is the difference of having a system that you can hold accountable for satisfaction versus a nonsystem. If you are in an HMO you know you are involved with a big corporate entity. FFS is not accountable; who does one complain to? We cannot measure the accountability of the FFS system.

Harold Luft remarked that relatively few people really like the process of medical care—the medical encounter itself. One is at the mercy of the system, and we are socialized into not verbalizing complaints about that kind of experience. Most people complain about the cost, but they love their doctor. It seems to be the case in both these studies and in other studies that when you're in an HMO you do not have cost to complain about anymore. The process may not have changed very much, and you still do not enjoy your doctor visits, but not being able to attribute dissatisfaction with the visit to cost factors brings out the grumpiness factor.

Sheldon Retchin commented that there are two reassuring points in the results of these two papers. One is that we see differentiation. The differentiation in the Clement paper was fairly consistent across the board. This is a static measure for this paper, but it does represent a continuum of satisfaction for a decade. In that sense, it is telling a story. The story is not at an end, and thus the paper represents a dynamic process of looking at satisfaction. It is reassuring that there is a differentiation, that there is a consumerism, and that that consumerism can be measured with these instruments. As Haya Rubin pointed out, the more sensitive the measures the better, but there has to be a trade-off somewhere. On the opposite side, there has to be a certain level of dissatisfaction as we go through this process of switching from indemnity plans to lower-cost services.

Bryan Dowd referred to some work he and others at the University of Minnesota have done with the under-age-65 employed population, looking at what may be another methodological problem. That is, how important people consider each aspect of these health plans to be; not whether they are satisfied, but how important it is to them that they be satisfied with each aspect. On a simple variable like paperwork, there are large differences in how important paperwork is to people, and it is exactly what you would expect. The people who hate paperwork are in HMOs, and people who get some perverse enjoyment out of tracking every dollar they spend are in FFS. Both groups are satisfied with the level of paperwork in their plan. Dr. Dowd did not know what to do with the wide variance of personal preferences or utility weights, but wanted to add a strong caution to all of these results: when you learn something about the satisfaction of one group in a particular type of health plan, you cannot conclude anything about the likely level of satisfaction of another group not selecting that plan if they were to be moved into such a plan.

One participant commented that in surveying the results presented thus far in the conference, whether they concern costs or satisfaction, there does not appear to be a big difference among HMOs. On the other hand, there also are not a lot of results here to indicate that HMOs save a lot of money.

Haya Rubin remarked that this cautions us to preserve choice in the system. We no longer have the kinds of choices we once did in the United States. We now have 52 percent of American workers covered by managed care plans. In the last two years, the percentage of large firms with over 1,000 employees offering nonmanaged care to their workers has gone from 90 percent to 62 percent. That is a huge drop in those kinds of choices. She suggested that maybe we should be thinking about a lot of different kinds of models. If there are different expectations out there and different utility weights, we need to have a pluralistic group of models that offer the option, for example, to pay more and receive certain services. These data argue for that.

Jan Malcolm commented that investigators have focused great energy on evaluating the effects of HMOs over the last few years, and rightfully so, while the non-HMO system goes largely unexamined. There are many presumptions that choice equals quality, and yet the ability to choose to see a provider is something of an empty choice when you know virtually nothing about the quality of care provided. She suggested that if we are going to preserve that kind of a choice, it is essential that the same kind of evaluative measures be placed on the nonsystems as the systems. This is not easy to do because there is no one to hold accountable. This is especially true for evaluations of PPOs, because that is where most people who are not in managed care are going.

Dolores Gurnick Clement thanked the participants for their helpful comments. She mentioned that in her study investigators ran the data for good and excellent as well as fair and poor, and that basically the results come out the same. The differences are smaller but still statistically significant. The choice for the paper was a matter of looking at the one category where there was a larger difference.

Robert Newcomer pointed out that when one talks about the homogeneity of managed care, the one characteristic that is common is that for the most part it is not managing problem cases, it is managing well cases or relatively well, nonfrail cases. In the S/HMO demonstration, which has a very limited conceptualization of management, other than the HMO model itself, these data show that those plans essentially failed relative to the FFS system in providing an adequate interpersonal relationship resource for those members. It may be inferred that that is primarily because the HMOs have continued to serve these high-risk people in the same manner that they serve their average enrollment.

Using "standard procedures," including a cookie-cutter notion of hourly appointments, has not met the needs of this special group.

Dr. Newcomer continued that in attempting to assess managed care more generally, one is considering the ability of HMOs to differentiate their services to the subsegments in their membership that have particular kinds of management needs. That is the challenge that we have to look forward to, and the S/HMOs in their second generation have the opportunity to address this issue.

In response to these remarks, Sheila Leatherman of United Health Care suggested that if Dr. Newcomer were to look at the S/HMOs now as opposed to S/HMOs at the time of his study, he would see that that evolution has taken place.

In reference to the study by Newcomer et al., Dr. Luft said that it pointed out the enormous differences between the mature plans and the newer plans with respect to whether they had prior experience in long-term care. He suggested that this could also be flipped around the other way. The two mature plans may not have had nearly enough experience with long-term care populations and services. That was new for them, and everybody has problems starting up with something new. This points up the need to look at plans once they mature and learn to deal with the kind of clientele they have.

In response, Dr. Newcomer said that the fact that there is low satisfaction is the criticism that he wanted to emphasize. Managed care must be tailored to different groups.

According to Sheila Leatherman, it appeared that the Newcomer paper did not show that those plans failed in terms of FFS; it showed that they succeeded relative to other HMOs. So they did do something very positive for that population.

Dr. Newcomer qualified this, saying that this was true in terms of disenrollment but not in terms of satisfaction. The fact that there is a lower satisfaction rate for members is in some ways a positive finding, because it shows that members are remaining in the plan, but it is also true that the satisfaction levels were much lower than those for their FFS counterparts. The major finding that came out of the study is that managed care must be tailored to subgroups.

Ms. Leatherman countered that the dichotomy between HMOs and FFS does not really exist. Patients have access to FFS care although they are in an HMO structure. It would not serve anyone if we line up on different sides of the table here and take sides without solid information. One thing that might move this debate ahead is to look at individual managed care interventions, whether they be in an HMO, an indemnity plan, a PPO, or anything else. For example, the ability to identify and manage high-risk populations: this is an intervention that can be examined to determine how it contributes to the health status of a particular subset of enrollees.

Dr. Wagner suggested that instead of looking at this as a dichotomy, it is helpful to think of this as a continuum beginning with unadulterated FFS care at one end and the traditional, totally capitated staff model HMO at the other end. One can array a set of characteristics related to physician payment and a variety of other things. He said that unless we think of this as a continuum and start to consider the context of individual plans and interventions on that continuum, the comparisons don't make any sense.

Dr. Luft seconded the notion of a continuum, but with different labels. For example, capitation is not economically neutral; salary is neutral. Other possible dimensions are group versus individual practice settings.

Part **III**

Quality of Care for Selected Conditions

Chapter 7

Care of Patients Hospitalized with Strokes under the Medicare Risk Program

Sheldon M. Retchin,
Dolores Gurnick Clement,
and Randall S. Brown

Under the Tax Equity and Fiscal Responsibility Act (TEFRA) of 1982, HMOs are allowed to enroll Medicare beneficiaries and receive fixed, predetermined monthly payments from HCFA. With TEFRA contracts, HMOs are responsible for providing comprehensive health care services that parallel those provided to beneficiaries in fee-for-service (FFS) settings. The TEFRA program was designed to contain the rising costs of caring for the Medicare population, while expanding the choice of health care services offered to the beneficiaries.

This work includes data from an evaluation of the Medicare risk program, with a specific focus on the care of patients hospitalized with strokes. We include discussion on background, choice of study areas, research design, sample selection, data collection, and results. Finally, we discuss the results in the context of health policy, and furnish our views on future areas for research and monitoring for the program.

Background

The increasing longevity of Americans, together with medical advances, have greatly contributed to rapid growth in the rate of health care consumption among the elderly (Rice et al. 1983). Principally because of mounting costs of care for the elderly, recent federal policies have turned toward managed care initiatives aimed at containing expenditures in the Medicare program.

Systems of care that place the physician at risk for financial payments related to patient care are likely to affect medical decisions, particularly those that are resource-intensive. While HMOs have incentives to reduce all health services among elderly enrollees, the majority of the reductions are in expensive health services such as hospitalizations (Nelson et al. 1986; Manning et al. 1984). These incentives have raised concerns about the quality of care enrollees may receive in HMOs (Gillick 1987).

Most studies on the quality of care in HMOs indicate that access to selected services is equal to or better than that provided by FFS or indemnity plans (Davies et al. 1986; Gaus, Cooper, and Hirschman 1976; Retchin et al. 1992). However, in efforts to contain the expense of hospitalizations, providers with HMO patients may discharge enrollees prematurely. Poor outcomes of care may result from premature discharge and may necessitate readmissions. To compensate for earlier discharges, HMOs may be expected to provide more frequent posthospital services, such as physical therapy, or furnish less expensive environments, like nursing homes, for recuperation.

Although the incentive structure may lead to concerns about quality of care for enrollees, there are several reasons why HMOs might be likely to provide superior quality of care. First, HMOs frequently use primary care gatekeepers to manage the care of enrollees and monitor their utilization of medical services. The gatekeeper is usually required to authorize nonprimary care services, such as hospital admissions and referrals to specialists (Nelson et al. 1990). This case management approach is often advocated for the complex health care needs of older persons as a means to assure better coordinated care. Further, HMOs often provide coverage for medical expenses frequently required by the elderly that are not covered routinely by Medicare. These special benefits, which HMOs frequently offer to attract beneficiaries, could improve the quality of care and outcomes for enrollees. The benefits fall into five categories (Nelson et al. 1990): preventive care, such as routine physical examinations and flu shots; prescription drug coverage; refractions or visual exams, including free eyeglasses by some; hearing exams; and dental care. In addition, HMOs are more likely than FFS settings to introduce careful discharge planning activities designed to prevent costly and untoward events, such as readmission (Rubenstein and Kane 1985). These administrative efforts in HMOs may improve treatment for elderly enrollees who need more effective management of multiple medical and social problems. HMOs may also improve access to care by eliminating or reducing copayments and deductibles.

Because of concerns regarding quality of care in the Medicare risk program, a comprehensive evaluation was undertaken. This study included the evaluation of two tracer conditions, colon cancer and cerebrovascular accident (strokes). We report on the latter in this chapter.

Methods

For this evaluation of the Medicare risk program, cerebrovascular accident (CVA) was selected as a tracer condition for several reasons. First, as a serious illness with disabling and life-threatening consequences to the patient, it virtually always requires hospitalization immediately after the onset of symptoms. The urgency of hospitalization arises from the need for diagnostic specificity: the consequences of neurologic signs and symptoms commonly seen with CVA patients include rapid deterioration, urgent therapeutic decisions, and diagnostic/therapeutic steps to exclude other comorbid, potentially life-threatening illnesses that can be associated with a CVA. Second, CVAs are primarily a disease of the elderly, usually having onset after age 65. Third, CVAs are not uncommon, and their prolonged sequelae lead to a high prevalence of residual impairments. Finally, because CVA patients often suffer a relatively poor prognosis, and frequently require expensive resources for rehabilitation, systems of care designed to contain costs might be prone to limit access to care inappropriately, or to withhold therapy.

To assess the differences between the quality of care delivered in HMOs and FFS, we targeted comparable samples of patients that were sufficiently large and unclustered to yield a high probability of detecting important differences. To achieve these objectives, we used a three-stage sampling approach. This section describes this approach.

HMO sample

The HMO sample was selected in the fall of 1989, based on the enrollment of Medicare risk plans as of September 1989. The set of eligible plans was limited to the 82 plans having 1,000 or more members. Plans were selected by *interval sampling*, a pseudo-random procedure that yields a higher probability of selection for large HMOs but ensures that each individual patient has an equal probability of selection. The 82 HMOs in the Medicare risk program were listed in descending order by size, and the cumulative enrollment total was calculated. The total enrollment in the 82 plans (N = 1,095,623) was divided by the number of plans to be selected to determine the sampling interval. Four plans had total enrollment larger than this interval, and these plans were automatically included in the sample. The other 16 plans were selected by calculating the total enrollment in the remaining 78 plans and recomputing the sampling interval by dividing this new total by 16.

The 20 HMOs selected were geographically dispersed and included 62 percent of the total Medicare risk enrollment as of September 1989. One of the 20 selected plans declined to participate in the study, so the sample was reallocated over the 19 participating plans. The 19 participating plans had a distribution by model type similar to that of the full set of 82 plans. Thus, nine plans were Independent Practice Associations (IPAs), six were group model HMOs, and four were staff model HMOs. The 19 HMOs that agreed to participate provided lists of enrollees who had been hospitalized during 1989 for CVAs, along with the name of the hospital where each had been admitted. Seventy-one hospitals were selected for the HMO sample. Two of the plans had too few CVA cases (< 16), and all of the eligible cases in these small HMOs were included in the sample. The shortfall in cases from these plans and from the nonparticipation of one plan was spread across the other plans.

FFS sample

The FFS sample was drawn from the same market areas as the HMO plans, and allocated across market areas to match the distribution of the enrollee sample. Thus, the total number of cases to be selected from a given market area was equal to the number of HMO cases allocated to that area. Cases were also allocated across counties within the market area to match the geographic distribution of HMO enrollees in the sample. The counties included in the FFS sample were limited to those containing at least 10 percent of the corresponding HMO plan's total enrollment as of September 1989. The number of cases to be drawn from each county was determined, and MEDPARS files were used to rank order hospitals by the number of CVA patients in 1989 who resided in each county. A total of 60 hospitals was selected for the FFS sample.

Both samples were heavily concentrated in California and Florida, each of which accounts for 20 to 25 percent of the cases and 25 percent of the sample HMOs. All hospitals contacted agreed to participate. The 100 percent participation rate of hospitals was attributed to an advance letter from HCFA requesting the hospital's participation and to the study design, which minimized both the number of cases drawn from a hospital and the burden on hospital staff and facilities.

Eligibility

To select appropriate samples for evaluation of care in HMO and FFS settings, eligibility requirements were selected to reflect a clinically homogeneous population. Patients admitted to target hospitals with the diagnosis of CVA, stroke, or cerebral thrombosis during the selected time interval were chosen for study. Patients not having significant neurologic deficits affecting vision, speech, movement, alertness, or mental status, were ineligible for the study.

Patients were also excluded if they were not considered to have a completed CVA or if their neurologic deficits were secondary to another condition. Thus, patients whose symptoms disappeared within 24 hours or whose symptoms had first appeared more than 14 days prior to the admission were considered ineligible. Patients were also considered ineligible with the following diagnoses: subdural bleed, multiple sclerosis, skull fracture, meningitis, encephalitis, brain abscess, and primary or metastatic cancer involving the brain, as well as those who were on chronic dialysis or who had a history of kidney transplant. Patients with evidence of definite, probable, or possible new myocardial infarction on day one of the admission were also ineligible for study.

Instrument development

For this study we modified an instrument developed by the RAND Corporation for assessing the quality of care for patients with CVAs (Rubenstein et al. 1985). The instrument was intended to measure the complexity of the case, the process of care, and the outcomes experienced by patients with CVAs. Because our purpose differed somewhat from that of the RAND study, we performed modest alterations in the instrument. Thus, a number of items were deleted, others were added, and changes were made to lessen the burden on hospitals and time required for abstractors to complete their work. The most substantial modification involved designating specific items not documented in the medical record as "documentation problems," rather than assuming they were not performed.

Data collection

All abstractors were registered nurses, and many had additional experience in quality assurance, utilization review, medical records abstracting, or other research projects. All but one of the 22 nurses who participated had a baccalaureate degree in nursing, and most had ten years experience. All abstractors attended a five-day training session that included a thorough review of the instruments and procedures, along with practice abstracting exercises. These sessions were led by the project staff experienced in medical records abstraction, and included presentations by the principal investigator. The abstractors were encouraged to share their hospital-based experiences to resolve potential regional differences in terminology. To reinforce the training, teams of abstractors visited hospitals in the training area on the last day of the session to abstract cases for that market area. These abstracts were reviewed with the nurse abstractors prior to the close of the session. Group discussions were held to resolve any general problems.

Data collection took place over the period September 1990 through February 1991. A weekly telephone conference was scheduled with each of the abstractors to resolve field problems and review comments. All problems were resolved by a survey specialist, and any questions that required medical expertise were referred to the principal investigator. The proportion of ineligible cases ranged from 10 to 17 percent, with rates of ineligibility being higher for HMO than for FFS (means = HMO 14.6%; FFS 9.9%). This discrepancy was due primarily to the poorer quality of the data supplied by HMOs on patients' ICD-9 codes. Ineligibility was typically due to the onset of symptoms more than 14 days prior to admission, or cases where symptoms resolved within 24 hours after admission, and our rates compared favorably with those reported by others using the identical instrument (Kahn 1992). Thus, most of these cases represented a transient ischemic attack (TIA), or a reversible ischemic neurologic deficit (RIND). We did not choose to study the care for these cases because the amount of inpatient care would have been too sparse to evaluate. In addition to the ineligible cases, about 6 percent of the cases were not abstracted, either because records were not found or were not available. Abstracting took about 1.75 hours per case.

Interrater reliability

To assess the reliability of the instruments, we photocopied 5 percent of the medical records, and a second nurse completed the abstraction form from the photocopied record. Each of the 22 abstractors photocopied medical records, excluding laboratory reports, for two eligible CVA cases in their sample of cases. No more than two records were copied at any one hospital, and records of stays shorter than 2 days or longer than 30 days were excluded. The total of 44 photocopied cases was then randomly assigned to other abstractors. In general, interrater agreement was high. For example, abstractors generally agreed on the presence or absence of neurologic deficits (kappa = .47–1.0), nursing care (kappa = .80–1.0), use of physical restraints (kappa = .917), and functional status at discharge (kappa = .80–.95 for individual activities).

Analysis

For bivariate comparisons between groups, Student's *t*-test and the chi-square statistic were used for continuous variables and categorical variables, respectively. For comparisons between HMO plans and FFS settings regarding utilization of echocardiography, the Cochran-Mantel-Haenszel statistic (Landis, Heyman, and Koch 1978) was used to control for differences in cardiac indications (presence of atrial fibrillation or other cardiac arrhythmias). For evaluation of the use of intensive care units by HMOs and FFS, logistic regression analysis was used to control for multiple variables that could influence medical decision-making, such as age, stroke severity, and presence of comorbid illnesses, and 95 percent confidence intervals were constructed around each odds ratio.

Results

The demographic characteristics and principal diagnoses are shown in Table 7.1 for enrollees and nonenrollees who were admitted with the primary diagnosis of CVA during the sample period. As shown, there were significant differences in the ages of the two groups, with nonenrollees being slightly older than enrollees. There were no significant differences between the two groups regarding gender; however, enrollees were significantly more likely to be married than nonenrollees. Neither race nor residence prior to hospitalization was different between enrollees and nonenrollees. In both groups the vast majority of patients were admitted through the hospital emergency room; however, more enrollees were admitted through another hospital's emergency room. In Table 7.2, data on selected comorbid illnesses are shown. A history of hypertension was present in the majority of patients in both groups, and approximately one-fifth had a history of atrial fibrillation or flutter. A previous history of CVA, stroke, or TIA was present in approximately one-third of patents. Enrollees were less likely to have experienced a myocardial infarction more than three months prior to admission, were half as likely to have valvular heart disease, and were less likely to have a history of arrhythmias. However, there were no other statistically significant differences seen among more than 25 comorbid illnesses examined.

Neurologic symptoms

Neurologic symptoms and deficits present on admission for both groups are shown in Table 7.3. Only the presence of visual deficits and confusion was significantly different between groups, and both were more likely to be present in nonenrollees. Low proportions of both groups presented with coma or unresponsiveness (enrollees 8.2 percent, nonenrollees 9.8 percent), and fewer than one-fifth of admitted patients with CVAs were unable to follow commands. Approximately 60 percent of patients had an onset of symptoms and/or deficits on the day of admission. Fewer

Table 7.1   Personal Characteristics of Enrollees and Nonenrollees

Characteristic	Enrollees	Nonenrollees
Age Categories		
65–69	45 (11.2)†	59 (14.5)
70–74	108 (26.9)	84 (20.6)*
75–79	127 (31.6)	99 (24.3)
> 80	132 (32.8)	159 (39.0)
Sex		
Male	199 (49.5)	181 (44.4)
Female	203 (50.5)	227 (55.6)
Marital Status		
Single	161 (40.8)	217 (54.3)**
Married	234 (59.2)	183 (45.8)
Race		
White	329 (86.8)	329 (87.7)
Black	25 (6.6)	31 (8.3)
Hispanic	23 (6.1)	11 (2.9)
Residence Prior to Hospitalization		
Home alone	78 (19.8)	95 (23.6)
Home, with others	273 (69.1)	253 (62.8)
Home, unspecified	15 (3.8)	10 (2.5)
Nursing home	16 (4.1)	30 (7.4)
Retirement home	12 (3.0)	13 (3.2)
Transfer from another acute care hospital	15 (3.7)	6 (1.5)*
Admitted through hospital emergency room	346 (86.1)	349 (85.5)
Admitted through another hospital's emergency room	33 (8.2)	10 (2.5)**

*Significant at the .05 level; **Significant at the .01 level. The test statistic used is the Chi-square test of the equivalence of the distributions for enrollees and nonenrollees.
†Percent of sample given in parentheses.

than 7 percent of either group had an onset greater than three days prior to admission. More importantly, there were no differences in the two groups that might have indicated a delay in access to timely care. CT scan findings at admission revealed similar proportions of enrollees and nonenrollees with hemorrhagic CVAs or infarcts. Where listed in the medical record, hemispheric involvement indicated fairly equal distribution between left and right hemispheres. Slightly fewer than 20 percent of patients with CVAs in both groups had lacunar infarcts as

Table 7.2 Proportion of Enrollees and Nonenrollees with CVAs Who Had Comorbid Illnesses at Admission or during Hospitalization

Illness	Enrollees	Nonenrollees
Number with valvular heart disease prior to admission	17 (4.2)	35 (8.6)**
Number with angina prior to admission	37 (9.2)	51 (12.5)
Number with chest pain of unknown origin prior to admission	12 (3.0)	12 (2.9)
Number with myocardial infarction within three months of admission	1 (0.3)	2 (0.5)
Number with myocardial infarction ≥ four months prior to admission	49 (12.2)	71 (17.4)*
Number with congestive heart failure prior to admission	59 (14.7)	72 (17.7)
Number with history of coronary artery bypass surgery	10 (2.5)	19 (4.7)
Number with history of hypertension on admission	239 (59.5)	237 (58.1)
Number with history of atrial fibrillation or flutter on admission	81 (20.3)	83 (20.5)
Number with history of other arrhythmias besides atrial fibrillation or flutter	28 (7.0)	52 (12.8)**

*$p < .05$; **$p < .01$.

the principal type. While nonenrollees were slightly more likely to have increased intracranial pressures according to CT scan findings, the differences were not significant. Mental status and more detailed descriptions of speech deficits are also shown, and no important differences were found.

Medications

Common medications often used for anticoagulation, or "blood thinning" in the treatment of nonhemorrhagic CVA, were evaluated. These medications can be expensive to use, particularly since they may require prolonged hospitalization while the patient is being anticoagulated. As shown in Figure 7.1, approximately half of the patients received some antiplatelet medication (i.e., aspirin or persantine). While heparin or coumadin use was much rarer, in both cases there were no meaningful differences between the two systems of care. Further, both also used other regimens such as mini-dose heparin schedules, equally often.

Table 7.3   Symptoms, Signs, X-Ray Results, and Laboratories of
Enrollees and Nonenrollees with CVAs at Admission

Variable (% with Symptoms)	Enrollees	Nonenrollees
Onset of symptoms		
Day of admission	243 (60.5)	261 (64.0)
Day prior to admission	74 (18.4)	70 (17.2)
2–3 Days prior to admission	55 (13.7)	42 (10.3)
4–14 Days prior to admission	25 (6.2)	28 (6.9)
Visual deficits	114 (28.4)	162 (39.7)**
Sensory or facial motor deficits	234 (58.4)	232 (57.0)
Speech deficits	272 (67.7)	268 (66.0)
Motor deficits in extremities	348 (86.6)	362 (88.7)
Peripheral sensory deficits	129 (32.2)	109 (26.7)
Coma or unresponsiveness	33 (8.2)	40 (9.8)
Obtundation or stupor	82 (20.4)	99 (24.3)
Decerebrate or decorticate posturing	9 (2.2)	14 (3.4)
Unresponsive to touch or tactile stimuli	21 (5.2)	27 (6.6)
Unable to follow commands	70 (17.4)	81 (19.9)
Confusion	94 (23.4)	124 (30.4)*
Seizure on admission	9 (2.2)	11 (2.7)

Variable	Enrollees	Nonenrollees
Hemisphere involved†		
Right	147 (36.8)	175 (43.1)
Left	170 (42.5)	160 (39.4)
Type of CVA		
Hemorrhagic	43 (10.7)	40 (9.8)
Lacunar	79 (19.7)	70 (17.2)
Mean systolic blood pressure on admission	160.5 (32.0)	158.9 (31.8)
Mean diastolic blood pressure on admission	86.8 (16.0)	85.6 (17.6)
CT scan findings:		
Increased intracranial pressure	17 (4.6)	27 (7.1)
Infarct	129 (34.6)	147 (38.5)
Hemorrhage‡	36 (9.7)	35 (9.2)
Proportion with CPK cardiac enzyme		
> 150 on admission	28 (7.0)	42 (10.3)
Cognitive impairment prior to admission	49 (35.5)	80 (39.2)

Condition	Enrollees	Nonenrollees
Mental status at admission§		
Oriented to "person"	247 (61.4)	242 (59.3)
Oriented to "place"	223 (55.5)	204 (50.0)

Continued

Table 7.3 Continued

Condition	Enrollees	Nonenrollees
Oriented to "time"	193 (48.0)	180 (44.1)
Recall or recent memory	47 (11.7)	63 (15.5)
Language intact	60 (14.9)	79 (19.4)
Attention and calculation	40 (10.0)	58 (14.2)
Speech Deficits¶		
Aphasia	78 (34.7)	54 (26.0)
Unable to speak	21 (9.3)	21 (10.1)
Dysarthria	121 (53.8)	128 (61.5)
Normal speech	1 (0.44)	1 (0.5)

*Significant at the .05 level; **Significant at the .01 level.
†Chi-square may not be a valid test. Some cells contain less than five observations.
‡Chi-square may not be a valid test. Some cells contain less than five observations.
§Numbers and proportions refer to patients where mental status component was "intact," indicating "no deficit."
¶According to physician's assessment.

Figure 7.1 Medications Used for Enrollees and Nonenrollees during Hospitalizaton for CVAs

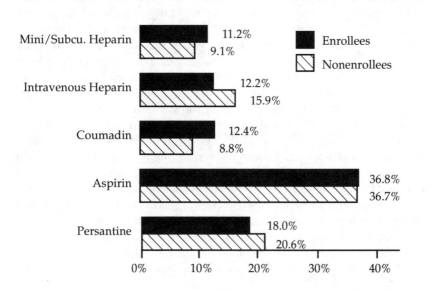

Test and procedure ordering

To examine test and procedure ordering, we attempted to analyze the findings either by established criteria for the test or by stratifying by stroke severity. By these methods we attempted to determine if differences in ordering rates between HMOs and FFS settings were attributable to more efficiency, differences in care, or severity of illness.

As shown in Table 7.4, diagnostic criteria were used for ordering echocardiography. Echocardiograms are often used for stroke patients to assess ventricular function and whether or not an intracardiac thrombosis may be the source of an embolic stroke. In particular, echocardiograms have been suggested for patients with recent strokes and cardiac arrhythmias (Sherman 1990; Dunbabin and Sandercock 1991; Hofmann et al. 1990). Once these clinical criteria were controlled for, the differences in utilization rates of this test virtually disappeared. For instance, since cardiac arrhythmias can lead to embolic events, most physicians would recommend an echocardiogram for patients with a recent CVA and atrial fibrillation, or those with specific arrhythmias. Table 7.4 supports this view: for both enrollees and nonenrollees, those with atrial fibrillation or the other expanded indications were more likely to receive an echocardiogram. Therefore, once the sample had been stratified for the presence of atrial fibrillation, the enrollee-nonenrollee differences in test-ordering were mostly confined to those without the arrhythmia. This pattern persisted when the sample was controlled for multiple clinical indications.

Other areas of utilization of hospital services were also examined for differences between FFS and HMOs: length of stay, intensive care unit stays, physical therapy, and speech therapy; we also evaluated the use of another diagnostic test, carotid doppler ultrasound (to assess the presence of plaques in the carotid artery) and echocardiograms. Because utilization of selected cardiac and neurovascular tests by HMO physicians may not always be indicated, we were also interested in whether the severity of the patient's stroke at admission was related to utilization of specific services. We used available guidelines in the literature to establish two groups related to severity based on neurologic deficits and symptoms at admission, including: presence of coma, decerebrate or decorticate posturing, unresponsiveness (Levy et al. 1981; Caronna and Levy 1983). Any of the preceding symptoms or signs were assumed to indicate a high severity. Conversely, the lack of any of these symptoms or signs indicated a low severity. Since we used fairly demanding criteria for determining severity, the grouping variable was skewed in favor of most patients having a low severity.

The results, as shown in Table 7.5, indicate several patterns. First, length of stay remained significantly different between enrollees and

Table 7.4 Utilization of Echocardiography According to Selected Indications

Diagnostic Test	Enrollees	Nonenrollees
Echocardiogram performed		
Patient had atrial fibrillation		
Yes	33 (40.7)†	34 (41.0)
No	83 (26.0)	111 (34.5)*
Multiple clinical indications§		
Yes	53 (39.6)	56 (38.1)
No	64 (23.9)	89 (34.1)**

*$p < .05$; **$p < .06$.

†Numbers in parentheses correspond to proportions of enrollees and nonenrollees, respectively, with *cardiac indications*, who received echocardiography.

‡Mantel-Haenzel test was used for testing significance of differences in proportions between enrollees and nonenrollees, controlling for the presence of cardiac indications.

§Includes the diagnosis of atrial fibrillation or flutter, as well as other cardiac arrhythmias (e.g., supraventricular tachycardia, multifocal atrial tachycardia, paroxysmal atrial tachycardia), or congestive heart failure.

nonenrollees with low-severity strokes, but the gap narrowed slightly with high-severity strokes (relative difference −18.4 percent versus −14.3 percent), and the absolute difference was no longer significantly different from zero (although this difference in significance was due solely to the smaller sample size for high-severity cases). The difference was more striking for the number of days in an intensive care unit—42.7 percent reduction for enrollees with low stroke severity versus 11.1 percent reduction for enrollees with high-stroke severity—and the proportion with any ICU stay, a 30 percent relative reduction for low-severity strokes, compared to a small and statistically insignificant reduction for high-severity cases. However, for rehabilitative care such as physical therapy and speech therapy, the results indicate little evidence of differential reductions for high- and low-severity cases. Although relative differences were sometimes greater and sometimes smaller for the low-severity cases, only the difference in the number of physical therapy days was statistically significant. And while the relative difference on this measure was larger for the high-severity cases, the absolute difference was identical for the two subgroups (1.8 days). For echocardiography and doppler ultrasound, two expensive, high-tech procedures, the results showed very strong differences between high- and low-severity cases. While enrollees and nonenrollees with high-severity were equally likely (about 25 percent) to receive these tests, enrollees with low-severity strokes were much less likely than comparable nonenrollees to receive them.

Table 7.5 Comparison of Utilization of Services for Enrollees and
Nonenrollees

Variable	Enrollees† (n = 287)	Nonenrollees† (n = 263)	Relative Difference Estimated‡
Low Stroke Severity§			
Length of stay (days)	8.0 (0.5)	9.8 (0.6)	−18.4%**
Number of days in intensive care unit (ICU)	0.9 (0.1)	1.5 (0.2)	−42.7%**
Proportion of hospital stay in ICU	10.3 (1.3)	14.8 (2.4)	−30.4%*
Number of days of physical therapy	3.8 (0.2)	4.6 (0.3)	−17.4%*
Proportion of hospital days receiving physical therapy	50.1 (2.9)	49.1 (4.5)	+2.0%
Number of days of speech therapy	1.4 (0.2)	1.2 (0.2)	+16.7%
Proportion of hospital days receiving speech therapy	17.1 (1.5)	12.3 (1.3)	+43.9%**
Proportion receiving echocardiograms	30.7 (2.7)	40.2 (2.9)	−23.6%**
Proportion receiving Doppler ultrasound	37.9 (2.8)	50.7 (3.0)	−25.2%***

Variable	Enrollees (n = 90)	Nonenrollees (n = 109)	Relative‡ Difference
High Stroke Severity§§			
Length of stay (days)	10.2 (0.9)	11.9 (1.0)	−14.3%
Number of days in intensive care unit (ICU)	2.4 (0.4)	2.7 (0.4)	−11.1%
Proportion of hospital stay in ICU	29.3 (4.5)	32.2 (4.3)	−9.3%
Number of days of physical therapy	4.0 (0.6)	5.8 (0.8)	−31.0%*
Proportion of hospital days receiving physical therapy	35.7 (3.7)	39.8 (3.4)	−10.3%
Number of days of speech therapy	1.5 (0.3)	1.6 (0.3)	−6.3%
Proportion of hospital days receiving speech therapy	14.9 (3.0)	10.9 (1.7)	+36.7%
Proportion receiving echocardiograms	24.2 (4.3)	24.2 (3.9)	0
Proportion receiving Doppler ultrasound	19.2 (4.0)	18.3 (3.5)	+4.9%

$*p < .10; **p < .05; ***p < .01.$
†Values represent means, with standard errors in parentheses.
‡(Enrollees − Nonenrollees) ÷ (Nonenrollees).
§Low Stroke Severity was based on neurologic signs at admission. If one of the signs was present, the patient was excluded from the analysis. The following mental status deficits at admission were used for exclusion: presence of coma, decerebrate or decorticate posturing, unresponsiveness.
§§High Stroke Severity was based on neurologic signs at admission. If one of the signs was present, the patient was included in the analysis. The following mental status deficits at admission were used for exclusion: presence of coma, decerebrate or decorticate posturing, unresponsiveness.

Since it represents one of the more expensive resources for hospitalized patients, we also examined the utilization of intensive care units (ICUs) for patients with CVAs in both groups. There were 120 enrollees (29.9 percent) and 142 nonenrollees (34.8 percent) with CVAs who were admitted to ICUs at some time during their hospitalization. We used logistic regression analysis to control for age, stroke severity, cormobidity, race, history of prior CVA, history of dementia, abnormal mental status, and vital sign instability. As shown in Table 7.6, after controlling for other factors, enrollment status was not associated with ICU admissions. Stroke severity was, by far, the strongest predictor of an ICU stay. A history of cancer and mental status impairment on admission were significantly "protective" factors, and patients with these characteristics were less likely to have an ICU stay during their hospitalization.

Aside from conventional medical interventions, rehabilitative services are conventionally offered to improve the functional status of stroke patients. As shown in Figure 7.2, patients with speech deficits on admission were tracked from admission to discharge to determine the relative frequency of speech therapy sessions, and the functional status at discharge. As shown, the number and proportion of patients with speech deficits on admission were approximately the same in the two settings. Further, the mean number of hospital days when each group received speech therapy was similar for enrollees and nonenrollees with speech deficits. Nonetheless, there was much higher prevalence of residual speech deficits among enrollees at discharge. This may indicate that,

Table 7.6 Logistic Regression Model for ICU Utilization According to Enrollment

Characteristic	Odds Ratio	95% Confidence Interval
Enrollment status = HMO	0.81	0.59, 1.11
Age > 75	0.79	0.56, 1.11
High stroke severity	2.72	1.81, 4.07***
Comorbidity	1.35	0.98, 1.86
Race white	0.70	0.44, 1.12
Prior CVA	0.74	0.52, 1.05*
Prior hospitalization	0.81	0.52, 1.25
History of cancer	0.42	0.23, 0.74***
History of dementia	0.64	0.40, 1.01*
Impaired mental status	0.71	0.51, 0.99**
Vital sign instability	1.40	0.97, 2.03*

*$p < .10$; **$p < .05$; ***$p < .01$.

despite an equivalent amount of speech therapy, the length of stay for enrollees may not have allowed for the same degree of recovery for speech as for the nonenrollees. It is noteworthy that, despite having a substantially higher prevalence of speech deficits at discharge (53.7 percent HMO versus 34.7 percent FFS), enrollees did not have a higher rate of planned speech therapy post-hospitalization compared to nonenrollees. As shown in Figure 7.3, the prevalence of motor deficits at admission was similar among enrollees and nonenrollees. However, the mean number of days of physical therapy was higher for nonenrollees compared to enrollees, and there was a higher rate of persistent motor deficits among enrollees (58.6 percent) compared to nonenrollees (49.5 percent) at discharge. Despite the higher prevalence of motor deficits at discharge, the proportion of enrollees with these deficits who had physical therapy planned as an outpatient (64.2 percent) was not significantly higher than among nonenrollees (62.5 percent).

Figure 7.2   Speech Therapy for Enrollees and Nonenrollees with Speech Deficits (Numbers refer only to enrollees and nonenrollees who were discharged alive)

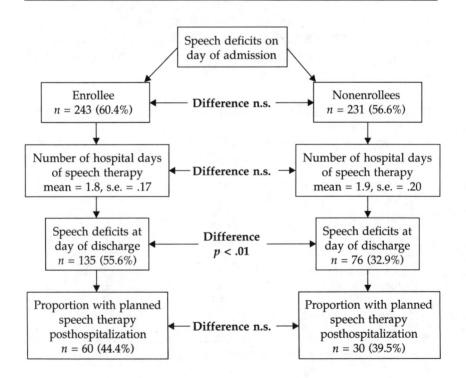

Figure 7.3　Physical Therapy for Enrollees and Nonenrollees with Motor Deficits (Numbers refer only to enrollees and nonenrollees who were discharged alive)

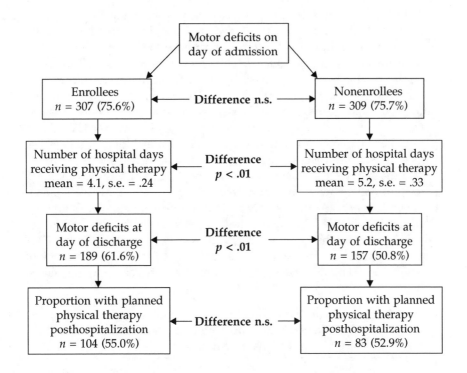

Outcomes

Several outcomes were observed for the hospitalization. First, comparisons between neurologic symptoms on admission with signs and symptoms on discharge were performed. As shown in Table 7.7, for several of the deficits that occurred with moderate frequency, there were significant differences in residual deficits. For example, although there were no differences between groups regarding speech deficits at admission, with two-thirds of both groups exhibiting difficulties, at discharge a much higher proportion of enrollees had continued deficits (enrollees 53.7 percent, nonenrollees 34.7 percent, $p < .01$). Similarly, motor deficits were more likely to persist among enrollees than nonenrollees at discharge (enrollees 58.6 percent, nonenrollees 49.5 percent). A higher prevalence of residual deficits among enrollees compared to nonenrollees also existed for other neurologic symptoms such as facial motor deficits and sensory deficits at the time of discharge, although statistical significance was marginal.

Lengths of stay and readmissions post-hospital discharge for patients in both groups are displayed in Table 7.8. Enrollees had significantly shorter LOS for the target hospitalization (approximately 18 percent lower than nonenrollees). This trend was true as well for post-target hospitalizations. There were no significant differences in the mean number of post-target hospitalizations. There were also no significant differences in the number of readmissions less than 31 days, less than 61 days, or less than 91 days after the target hospitalization for CVA.

Other outcomes for patients with CVAs are included in Figure 7.4. No significant differences were found in the continence status at admission or discharge for enrollees and nonenrollees. Overall, approximately 8 percent of patients who were admitted with continent status were incontinent at discharge. A surprisingly high proportion of patients, about two-thirds, were classified as "bedbound" at admission, but only 25 percent remained so at discharge. However, approximately one-third of the CVA patients required a cane or walker at discharge for ambulation. One of the more important adverse outcomes, pressure sores or decubitus ulcers,

Table 7.7 Neurologic Symptoms and Signs of Enrollees and Nonenrollees at Discharge among Those with Similar Symptoms and Signs on Admission

Variable (% with symptoms)‡	Enrollees	Nonenrollees
Visual deficits	27 (23.7)†	37 (22.8)
Sensory or facial motor deficits	61 (26.1)	45 (19.4)*
Speech deficits	146 (53.7)	93 (34.7)***
Motor deficits in extremities	204 (58.6)	179 (49.5)**
Peripheral sensory deficits	39 (30.2)	22 (20.2)*
Coma or unresponsiveness	17 (51.5)	16 (40.0)
Obtundation or stupor	21 (25.6)	24 (24.2)
Decerebrate or decorticate posturing	7 (77.8)	2 (14.3)***
Unresponsive to touch or tactile stimuli	8 (38.1)	6 (22.2)
Unable to follow commands	25 (35.7)	22 (27.2)
Confusion	26 (27.7)	23 (18.6)

*$p < .10$; **$p < .05$; ***$p < .01$.

†The numbers in parentheses in each column represent the proportion of patients with the deficit at admission, who had the same deficit persist at discharge.

‡The test statistic used is the Chi-square test of the equivalence of the distributions for enrollees and nonenrollees.

Table 7.8 Length of Stay, Readmissions, and Deaths among Enrollees and Nonenrollees Admitted with the Diagnosis of CVA

Length of Stay	Enrollees	Nonenrollees
Target LOS	8.6 (8.1)†	10.5 (10.5)**
Mean number of readmissions	0.5 (0.9)	0.4 (0.7)
Readmissions		
< 31 days of hospital discharge	33 (09.3)	43 (12.4)
< 61 days of hospital discharge	51 (14.4)	52 (14.9)
< 91 days of hospital discharge	61 (17.3)	60 (17.2)
In-hospital deaths	49 (12.2)	60 (14.7)

*$p < .10$; **$p < .05$; ***$p < .01$.

†Numbers in parentheses represent standard deviations of means for continuous variables (i.e., LOS, mean number of readmissions) and percentages for categorical variables (i.e., proportion with < 31, < 61, and < 91 days postdischarge) and number of in-hospital deaths; t-tests and Chi-square tests used, respectively.

were present at discharge in fewer than 5 percent of the patients, with no differences between groups. Not unexpectedly, there were substantial functional impairments at discharge, with more than half of the patients requiring assistance with at least one activity of daily living. However, no clinically meaningful differences were found between enrollees and nonenrollees. Finally, 109 patients died during the hospitalization, 12.2 percent of the HMO patients and 14.7 percent of the FFS patients, a difference that was not statistically significant.

Discussion

Enrollment in HMOs for Medicare beneficiaries has been enthusiastically supported by the federal government since the early 1970s (Iglehart 1982). With passage of TEFRA, HMOs were encouraged to enroll Medicare recipients and provide medical care on a capitated basis. In the initial demonstrations, studies evaluating the care of beneficiaries who enrolled in HMOs suggested that outcomes of care, including functional status and survivorship, were similar (Retchin et al. 1992). Recommended elements of routine and preventive care were more likely to be performed for enrollees in HMOs than for nonenrollees in FFS settings (Retchin and Brown 1990). Other studies have indicated that HMO enrollees receive care similar to that received by nonenrollees for a variety of conditions (Retchin and Brown 1990; Preston and Retchin 1991; Retchin and Brown 1991; Retchin and Preston 1991).

Figure 7.4   Outcomes for Enrollees and Nonenrollees with CVAs at Discharge

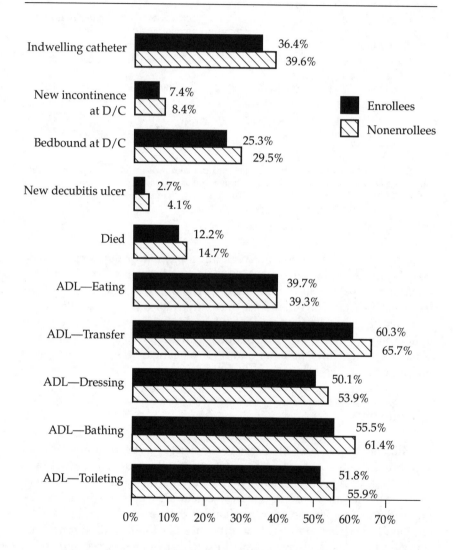

This study of the Medicare risk program included evaluation of HMO enrollees and FFS nonenrollees hospitalized with strokes. Although patients with CVAs selected for study in the two settings were drawn from different target populations, the samples were comparable in many important personal characteristics, such as age, race, and place of residence, that might have importance regarding access to care or patient delay in presentation. There was also no compelling evidence that patients in the two groups were markedly different with respect to either the severity of the CVA or the presence of comorbidity. While isolated differences were present regarding the presence of selected neurologic deficits at admission, the two groups were virtually identical on indicators of a life-threatening event (presence of coma, obtundation, stupor, or unresponsiveness). These similarities in both neurologic deficits and comorbidity are important to emphasize for the study since HMO enrollment was not randomized. Further, numerous studies have demonstrated that the severity of early neurologic deficits from CVAs is highly correlated with functional, as well as medical outcomes (Abu-Zeid et al. 1978; Allen 1984; Britton et al. 1980; Dove, Schneider, and Wallace 1984).

One of the principal areas of concern for the care of elderly Medicare beneficiaries in HMOs is the potential for delay in urgent hospitalization. HMOs often require at least administrative approval prior to hospital admissions, and these delays could have serious consequences for patients with a dynamic condition like CVA. However, in this study, CVA patients in both settings had the onset of neurologic signs and symptoms in similar proximity to the time of hospital admission. More than 90 percent of both groups were admitted to the hospital within three days of the onset of symptoms relevant to the occurrence of the CVA. Had delays in diagnosis been present, it seems likely that these delays would have been evident at the time of admission.

Although the proportion of patients first seen in other hospitals was small, HMO patients were much more likely to have either been transferred from another hospital, or to have been admitted through another hospital's emergency room. While this is not surprising, and most likely represents HMO policies regarding reimbursement for care in other hospitals, the transfer of patients with a critical condition raises important policy questions. For instance, a survey of HMO policies regarding access to emergency departments found that more than 90 percent of HMOs require enrollees to gain permission from gatekeepers prior to emergency room visits for "non-life-threatening" problems (Kerr 1989). However, the relatively high rate of transfers from other hospitals' emergency rooms in this study should be reassuring in that HMO policies regarding emergency access do not appear to deter enrollees from seeking care at the nearest emergency room for a life-threatening problem. If true delays in transfers had occurred, this should have produced differences in the "evolution" of CVA symptoms and neurologic deficits. Yet the detailed effort to assess these deficits failed to detect a pattern of differences in severity or number of deficits.

After controlling for stroke severity among patients admitted for CVAs, the differences in length of stay between HMO and FFS settings for those with high stroke severity were slightly less. One would expect that reductions in hospital LOS would be difficult to achieve with elderly Medicare enrollees in HMOs. Thus, the briefer LOS between HMO and FFS settings for CVA patients is even more remarkable, particularly in view of concurrent efforts in the FFS sector for reducing LOS through prospective payment. The differences must be largely due to the fact that physicians in FFS have more control over discharges than do hospitals, and they have less incentive to shorten a patient's stay. In HMOs, physicians and hospitals have similar financial incentives for reducing utilization and, therefore, length of stay. HMOs also perform more extensive discharge planning and case management of post-hospital care, which can shorten LOS (Hurley and Bannick 1992; Kramer, Fox, and Morgenstern 1992). The data from other studies on LOS are mixed. Several investigators have found little or no difference between HMO and FFS settings (Luft 1978; Wilner et al. 1981; Arnold, Debrock, and Pollard 1984). However, most studies that have found no difference in lengths of stay between prepaid and FFS settings, have either been limited to single market areas, have failed to control for patient characteristics, or have predated changes in FFS payment systems. More recent studies have found hospital stays to be substantially shorter in HMOs for certain diagnostic groups (Stern et al. 1989; Bradbury, Golec, and Stearns 1991; Dowd, Johnson, and Madson 1986).

The most powerful predictor of stroke recovery is function at admission (Ahlsio et al. 1984). However, these two FFS and HMO groups had equivalent prevalence rates of neurologic deficits at admission. Since the trend was consistent in that HMO enrollees had a higher prevalence of persistent neurologic deficits on discharge, it may be that the recuperative period had simply not been completed. Thus, the differences in length of stay seen between HMOs and FFS in this study may have been chiefly responsible for the poor neurologic status at discharge observed in HMOs. Conversely, the decrease in utilization of selected services, such as rehabilitation, could have adversely affected these outcomes. Whether discharging CVA patients "sicker and quicker" is poor care or more efficient care is not clear from this study.

After controlling for neurologic status on admission, some of the deficits persisted more frequently in enrollees at discharge. In particular, there were three neurologic deficits that are especially related to functional recovery and are amenable to therapy: speech, motor, and sensory deficits. For two of these, there were important differences in specific therapeutic services, and inpatient differences in therapy may have contributed to the observed differences in neurologic outcomes. Despite the higher prevalence of speech and motor problems at discharge among enrollees, there was no evidence of a higher rate of planned speech therapy or physical therapy post-hospitalization in HMOs for those with these problems. HMOs and HMO providers may be reducing the utilization of stroke rehabilitative services because of the lack of convincing data on its effectiveness. Among the clinical trials that have been performed, few have consistently demonstrated better outcomes or faster recovery rates with rehabilitation services (Harris 1990; Ernst 1990). Furthermore, the outcomes at discharge are probably insufficient to make valid conclusions regarding stroke recovery for these two groups. Follow-up at six months and longer is required before judgments can be made regarding the appropriateness of stroke rehabilitation (Smith 1990).

As with length of stay, we also examined the influence of stroke severity on utilization of other resources. After using available guidelines to establish stroke severity, the gap between HMO and FFS settings narrowed both for the number of days in an intensive care unit and the number of days of physical therapy. Further, for most differences seen in utilization of procedures, such as echocardiography, severity heavily influenced their use. Therefore, for patients who had low-severity strokes, echocardiography and doppler ultrasounds were used more frequently among nonenrollees. However, for high-severity strokes, the procedures were used with similar frequency. Furthermore, we used logistic regression to control for such other factors as stroke severity and comorbidity, which might influence ICU decisions, and found that enrollment status was not associated with ICU utilization. These patterns of care suggest that HMOs conserve on resources when the severity of the stroke is relatively low. However, when the severity of the stroke is high, they appear to have equivalent utilization of some expensive diagnostic services, as well as of high-intensity settings such as intensive care units.

There are several limitations to this study worth noting. First, it was not possible to randomly assign Medicare recipients to HMOs and FFS care. This can lead to biases in inferences about effects of the HMO style of care on quality of care if patients in the HMOs are not similar to those in the FFS sector. Nonetheless, we limited the evaluation to patients with CVAs in HMOs and FFS settings, both of whom satisfied similar eligibility requirements. Further, HMO enrollees and FFS nonenrollees were similar on presenting conditions and severity of illness. Second, the comparison groups of FFS nonenrollees were drawn from the same geographic location as the HMO groups of enrollees, for hospital admission occurring over the same time period (1989). Third, where appropriate, we controlled for differences in the two groups by estimating enrollee-nonenrollee differences separately by subgroups of patients defined by important characteristics at admission, on which enrollees and nonenrollees differed. Last, because of sample size limitations, this study could have missed important differences between groups. However, with samples of this size, we had 80 percent power to detect effects of 10 percentage points on binary outcome variables with a mean of .50, using a two-tailed test at the .05 significance level. For binary variables with a very high mean value, such as .90, the detectable difference at 80 percent power is about 5 percentage points. Thus, this sample size provides a high level of confidence that our analysis could detect modest differences between HMOs and FFS care.

Another limitation of the study is that the samples drawn may not have been representative of HMOs, or of patients who enroll in HMOs, especially since small HMOs were underrepresented. However, the HMO sample was randomly selected with a probability proportional to the plan size. Also, the large HMOs represent the largest share of the program; those included in this study accounted for approximately 60 percent of the total HMO enrollment at the time the samples were drawn. Further, since this study was based on evaluation of care for a single condition, there may also be concern that the results are not reflective of the overall quality of care for HMOs or FFS. While this is true, the care of patients with strokes was specifically chosen because it represents acute care of a chronic illness, such as CVA. As such, findings from the study of strokes should reflect a broad range of care through the spectrum of medical and rehabilitative elements studied. Further, this study used a medical record review to determine performance rates for items of routine care of the CVA patient. It thus can be categorized as a study of the process of care and record-keeping. However, studies of the reliability and validity of medical records have established that technical aspects of medical care, such as procedure-ordering and medications, are likely to reflect actual performance. For elderly patients, the medical record itself is an especially important component of care, since their complex medical needs often call for multiple providers (Hofmann et al. 1990).

Since many outcomes of care for CVA patients require long-term follow-up, it is difficult to conclude with certainty that the financial incentives of prepaid care had any effect, positive or negative, on outcomes. However, selected outcomes that could be determined during hospitalization, or could be examined through other methods, such as readmissions, were evaluated. First, there were no significant differences between groups for in-hospital mortality or readmissions following hospital discharge for the CVA patients studied. Further, there were no significant differences in functional status at discharge. On the other hand, several neurologic deficits, including speech and motor deficits, appeared to persist more among HMO enrollees with CVAs at discharge, compared to FFS nonenrollees with CVAs. The early discharge rate in HMOs was likely responsible for these differences in resolution of neurologic deficits, but longer follow-up periods will be necessary to confirm this. Finally, there were no differences in the proportion of CVA patients with new ambulation difficulties or new urinary incontinence at discharge.

These data provide evidence that HMOs provide quality of care equal to that furnished in FFS settings. While HMOs appear to economize on inpatient care by limiting access to resource-intensive services, such as intensive care, diagnostic tests, and rehabilitative therapy, the results suggest that outcomes are not affected by these reductions in services. HMO providers appear to use clinical judgment to determine which patients are severely ill and thus most critically in need of scarce resources. Furthermore, while HMO enrollees with strokes are discharged earlier with a higher prevalence of neurologic deficits, this is most likely due to the shorter length of stay, on average, in HMOs. Thus, although longer follow-up of functional status for these patients is needed to provide confirmation that HMO efforts to contain costs do not lead to more morbidity, these data provide reassuring evidence that short-term outcomes are comparable to those found in FFS settings.

Acknowledgments

Supported, in part, by a contract with the Health Care Financing Administration.

The authors gratefully acknowledge the programming assistance of Ms. Barbara Abujaber. Ms. Anne Brooks provided help and guidance in the preparation of this manuscript. Ms. Rhoda Cohen was instrumental in the training and supervision of data collection efforts. Finally, consultation with Dr. Lisa Rubenstein regarding the instrument development and its use was appreciated.

References

Abu-Zeid, H. A. H., N. W. Choi, P. Hsu, and K. K. Maini. "Prognostic Factors in the Survival of 1484 Stroke Cases Observed for 30 to 48 months: Part 2, Clinical Variables and Laboratory Measurements." *Archives of Neurology* 35 (1978): 213–18.

Ahlsio, B., M. Britton, V. Murray, and T. Theorell. "Disablement and Quality of Life after Stroke." *Stroke* 15 (1984): 886–90.

Allen, C. M. C. "Predicting the Outcome of Acute Stroke: Prognostic Score." *Journal of Neurology, Neurosurgery, and Psychology* 47 (1984): 475–80.

Arnould, R. J., L. W. Debrock, and J. W. Pollard. "Do HMOs Produce Specific Services More Efficiently?" *Inquiry* 21, no. 3 (1984): 243–45.

Bradbury, R. C., J. H. Golec, and F. E. Stearns. "Comparing Hospital Length of Stay in Independent Practice Association HMOs and Traditional Insurance Programs." *Inquiry* 28, no. 1 (1991): 87–93.

Britton, M., U. de Faire, C. Helmers, and K. Miah. "Prognostication in Acute Cerebrovascular Disease." *Acta Medica Scandinavica* 207 (1980): 37–42.

Caronna, J. J., and D. E. Levy. "Clinical Predictors of Outcome in Ischemic Stroke." *Neurological Clinician* 1, no. 1 (1983): 103–17.

Davies, A. R., J. E. Ware, R. H. Brook, J. R. Peterson, and J. P. Newhouse. "Consumers Acceptance of Prepaid and Fee-For-Service Medical Care: Results from a Randomized Controlled Trial." *Health Services Research* 21, no. 2 (1986): 429–52.

Dove, H. G., K. C. Schneider, and J. D. Wallace. "Evaluating and Predicting Outcome of Acute Cerebral Vascular Accident." *Stroke* 15 (1984): 858–64.

Dowd, B. E., A. N. Johnson, R. A. Madson. "Inpatient Length of Stay in Twin Cities Health Plans." *Medical Care* 24, no. 4 (1986): 294–310.

Dunbabin, D. W., and P. A. Sandercock. "Investigation of Acute Stroke: What is the Most Effective Strategy?" *Postgraduate Medical Journal* 67 (1991): 259–70.

Ernst, E. "A Review of Stroke Rehabilitation and Physiotherapy." *Stroke* 21 (1990): 1081–85.

Gaus, C. R., B. S. Cooper, and C. G. Hirschman. "Contrasts in HMO and Fee-For-Service Performance." *Social Security Bulletin* 39, no. 5 (1976): 3–14.

Gillick, M. R. "The Impact of Health Maintenance Organizations on Geriatric Care." *Annals of Internal Medicine* 106, no. 1 (1987): 139–43.

Haldane, J. B. S. "The Estimation and Significance of the Logarithm of a Ratio of Frequencies." *Annals of Human Genetics* 20, no. 4 (1956): 309–14.

Harris, J. M. "Stroke Rehabilitation: Has it Proven Worthwhile?" *Journal of Florida Medical Association* 77 (1990): 683–86.

Hofmann, T., W. Kasper, T. Meinertz, A. Geibel, and H. Just. "Echocardiographic Evaluation of Patients with Clinically Suspected Arterial Emboli." *The Lancet* 336 (1990): 1421–24.

Hurley, R. E., and R. R. Bannick. "Utilization Management Practice in HMOs with Medicare Risk Contracts." Draft report submitted to Health Care Financing Administration, 1992.

Iglehart, J. "The Future of HMOs." *The New England Journal of Medicine* 308 (1982): 451–56.

Kahn, K. L., D. Draper, E. B. Keeler, et al. *The Effects of the DRG-Based Prospective Payment System on Quality of Care for Hospitalized Medicare Patients.* Publication no. R-3931-HCFA. Washington, DC: Government Printing Office, 1992, pp. 15–17.

Kerr, H. D. "Access to Emergency Departments: A Survey of HMO Policies." *Annals of Emergency Medicine* 18 (1989): 274–77.

Kramer, A. M., P. D. Fox, and N. Morgenstern. "Geriatric Care Approaches in Health Maintenance Organizations." *Journal of American Geriatric Society* 40, no. 10 (1992): 1055–67.

Landis, R. J., E. R. Heyman, and G. G. Koch. "Average Partial Association in Three-Way Contingency Tables: A Review and Discussion of Alternative Tests." *Internal Statistical Review* 46 (1978): 237–54.

Levy, D. E., D. Bates, J. J. Caronna, et al. "Prognosis in Nontraumatic Coma." *Annals of Internal Medicine* 94 (1981): 293–301.

Luft, H. S. "How Do Health Maintenance Organizations Achieve Their "Savings?" *The New England Journal of Medicine* 298, no. 24 (1978): 1336–43.

Manning, W. G., A. Leibowitz, G. A. Goldberg, W. H. Rogers, and J. P. Newhouse. "A Controlled Trial of the Effect of a Prepaid Group Practice on Use of Services." *The New England Journal of Medicine* 310, no. 23 (1984): 1505–11.

Nelson, S., K. Langwell, R. Brown, et al. *Organizational and Operational Characteristics of TEFRA HMOs/CMPs.* Princeton, NJ: Mathematical Policy Research, Inc., 1990.

Nelson, L., L. W. Rossiter, K. W. Adamache, and K. Berman. "The National Medicare Competition Demonstrations Evaluation: A Preliminary Analysis of the Use and Cost of Services–Aggregate HMO Data." Report prepared under contract no. 500-83-0047 for DHHS, HCFA, 1986.

Preston, J. A., and S. M. Retchin. "The Management of Geriatric Hypertension in Health Maintenance Organizations." *Journal of the American Geriatric Society* 39, no. 7 (1991): 683–90.

Retchin, S. M. and B. Brown. "Management of Colorectal Cancer in Medicare Health Maintenance Organizations." *Journal of General Internal Medicine* 5, no. 1 (1990): 110–14.

Retchin, S. M. and B. Brown. "Quality of Ambulatory Care in Medicare Health Maintenance Organizations." *American Journal of Public Health* 80, no. 4 (1990): 411–15.

Retchin, S. M., and B. Brown. "Elderly Patients with Congestive Heart Failure under Prepaid Care." *American Journal of Medicine* 90, no. 2 (1991): 236–42.

Retchin, S. M., D. A. Gurnick, L. F. Rossiter, B. Brown, R. Brown and L. Nelson. "How the Elderly Fare in Health Maintenance Organizations: Outcomes from the Medicare Competition Demonstrations." *Health Services Research* 27, no. 5 (1992): 651–69.

Retchin, S. M., and J. A. Preston. "The Effects of Cost Containment on the Care of Elderly Diabetics." *Archives of Internal Medicine* 151 (1991): 2244–48.

Rice, D. P., H. M. Rosenberg, L. R. Curtin, et al. "Changing Mortality Patterns, Health Services Utilization, and Health Care Expenditures, U.S. 1978–2003." In *Vital and Health Statistics*, Series 3–No. 23. DHHS Publication no. (PHS)83-1407. Public Health Service. Washington DC: Government Printing Office. 1983.

Rubenstein, L. Z., and R. L. Kane. "Geriatric Assessment Programs: Their Time Has Come." *Journal of the American Geriatric Society* 33, no. 9 (September 1985): 646–47.

Rubenstein, L. V., J. Kosecoff, L. Kahn, et al. "Medical Record Abstraction Form and Guidelines for Assessing Quality of Care for Hospitalized Patients with Cerebrovascular Accident." RAND publication no. N-2802-HCFA, Santa Monica, CA, December 1988.

Sherman, D. G. "Cardiac Embolism: The Neurologist's Perspective." *American Journal of Cardiology* 65 (1990): 32C–37C.

Smith, D. S. "Outcome Studies in Stroke Rehabilitation: The South Australian Stroke Study." *Stroke* 21, no. 2 (1990): 1156–58.

Stern, R. S., P. I. Juhn, P. J. Gertler, and A. M. Epstein. "A Comparison of Length of Stay and Costs for Health Maintenance Organization and Fee-For-Service Patients." *Archives of Internal Medicine* 149 (1989): 1185–88.

Wilner, S., S. C. Schoenbaum, R. R. Monson, R. N. Winickoff. "A Comparison of the Quality of Maternity Care Between a Health Maintenance Organization and Fee-For-Service Practices." *The New England Journal of Medicine* 304 (1981): 784.

Chapter 8

Do HMOs Provide Better Care for Older Patients with Acute Myocardial Infarction?

David M. Carlisle, Albert L. Siu,
Emmett B. Keeler, Katherine L. Kahn,
Lisa V. Rubenstein, Robert H. Brook, and
the HMO Quality of Care Consortium*

Health maintenance organizations (HMOs) have become a large, and still growing, component of our health care delivery system with over 31 million enrollees throughout the nation. Because of their observed operating efficiencies, they have attracted much interest from policymakers concerned with controlling medical costs and improving access to medical care. The Health Care Financing Administration of the United States Department of Health and Human Services has succeeded in increasing the number of elderly beneficiaries enrolled in HMOs from

*The HMO Quality of Care Consortium consists of 12 managed care plans seeking to establish a quality of care research agenda leading to the development of valid outcome- and process-related measures that can be utilized by differing health delivery systems. Consortium members are AV-MED, CIGNA Health Plans, Community Health Care Plan, Group Health Cooperative of Puget Sound, Harvard Community Health Plan, The Health Care Plan of Buffalo, The Health Plan of America, Kaiser-Permanente Colorado Region, Kaiser-Permanente Northwest Region, Kaiser-Permanente Southern California Region, MedCenters Health Plan, and United Healthcare Corp.

Reprinted, with permission, from Carlisle, David M., Albert L. Siu, Emmett B. Keeler, Elizabeth A. McGlynn, Katherine L. Kahn, Lisa V. Rubenstein, Robert H. Brook, and the HMO Quality of Care Consortium. "HMO vs Fee-for-Service Care of Older Persons with Acute Myocardial Infarction." *American Journal of Public Health* 82, no. 12 (December 1992): 1626–30. © 1992, American Public Health Association.

521,894 in 1979 to 1.7 million in 1987 (Marion Laboratories 1988). Yet, little is actually known about the quality of medical care received by enrollees of health maintenance organizations.

Enhanced competition within the health care delivery system has been encouraged as a strategy to control health care costs. Competition that has developed among health plans has historically been on the basis of differences in premiums and benefit packages and on public perceptions about differences in quality. While there is much desire on the part of health plans for competition based on actual quality differences, the lack of objective measures of quality of health care has hindered the development of such competition. Previous research has shown that the quality of the care delivered by HMOs has generally been found to be better than or comparable to fee-for-service care (Cunningham and Williamson 1980; Luft 1981). However, little evidence exists on the quality of care received by elderly individuals enrolled in HMOs or on differences in quality among individual health plans (Langwell and Hadley 1989; Shapiro et al. 1967).

This study compares the quality of medical care received by HMO and fee-for-service elderly persons hospitalized with a myocardial infarction. We selected acute myocardial infarction (MI) because it is relatively frequent in occurrence, it is associated with significant mortality and morbidity, and its outcome can be influenced by the quality of medical care a patient receives. Myocardial infarction is one of the most significant medical problems faced by Americans today. Over 1.3 million myocardial infarctions occur yearly in the United States. Of those stricken with acute MI, 50 percent die within one year. Although half of these deaths occur outside the hospital, the outcome in the remaining 50 percent of individuals is frequently affected by the quality of their medical care.

The relationship between the quality of the process of in-hospital medical care received by patients with acute MI and their eventual outcome has been aptly demonstrated by previous work performed by researchers at the RAND Corporation and UCLA using a large, multistate, fee-for-service Medicare population (the Evaluation of Quality of Care Under the Prospective Payment System (PPS) Project) (Kahn et al. 1990a). This study is designed specifically to answer some questions about the quality of in-hospital medical care received by HMO enrollees who are 65 years old and older relative to non-HMO patients of the same age group: How does the quality of care received by HMO patients compare to that received by a nationally representative sample of fee-for-service patients? How does the quality of care differ among HMOs? Do outcome and process measures of quality of care lead to similar conclusions?

Methods

To evaluate the quality of care received by Medicare patients, we selected and reviewed medical records of HMO and fee-for-service patients 65 years of age or older admitted between July 1, 1985 and June 30, 1986 with a principal diagnosis of acute myocardial infarction (International Classification of Diseases, Ninth Revision, codes 410.0 through 410.9). We selected three HMOs from a national consortium of 12 HMOs that had been organized to evaluate the feasibility, reliability, and validity of producing clinically meaningful measures that could be used to compare quality among health plans. The three plans were different in size, geographic region served, and selected organizational characteristics.

A total of 1,469 HMO patients were identified who met the criteria for initial inclusion in the study. After over-sampling records from the two smaller HMOs, 459 medical records were selected for review. Of these, 90 records were excluded for the following reasons: 39 patients received their initial care at and were transferred from a fee-for-service hospital; 12 patients had admission dates falling outside the sampling time frame; 2 patients died in emergency departments; 2 patients had incomplete records; and the records of 38 patients did not demonstrate signs or symptoms that were consistent with acute MI at the time of hospital admission (Table 8.1, further on). Three patients had more than one reason for being excluded. Actual rates of transfer varied among the HMOs. This resulted in a final sample of 369 hospital admissions.

The fee-for-service sample was obtained from a previously reported study (Draper et al. 1990). In that study a sample of Medicare fee-for-service admissions was drawn from 297 hospitals in five states that were selected to closely match the nation in terms of urban:rural mix, size, teaching status, ownership, patient demographics, and Medicare/Medicaid distribution. Fee-for-service patients from rural hospitals were excluded from the present analysis because none of our HMOs were in primarily rural areas. After excluding these patients 1,119 patients remained. Additional information about the fee-for-service sample is available in an earlier publication (Kahn et al. 1990b).

Data from hospital medical records were collected using an abstraction tool developed to collect process and outcome data for patients with acute myocardial infarction (Kosecoff et al. 1988). For the FFS group, contracted peer review organizations in each of the five states received photocopies of each of the admission records. Nurses and medical record abstractors specifically trained in the use of this abstraction tool then abstracted each of the admission records. For the HMO sample, medical records were photocopied by each HMO and sent to a nurse who had previously abstracted fee-for-service records. A non-physician reviewer checked all forms for completeness, legibility, and internal consistency. A physician reviewer then evaluated them to confirm the diagnosis of acute myocardial infarction.

Patient records provided information on the following patient characteristics: patient sex, age, length of stay, and the presence of a "do not resuscitate order" at any point during the hospital stay. Abstracted information was used to generate sickness at admission, instability at discharge, and quality of care scales designed to predict mortality at 30 and 180 days post-admission, respectively. The sickness at admission scales, previously developed and validated (Keeler et al. 1990), incorporate items from the Killip and Kimball (1967) and Norris et al. (1969) measures of the severity of acute myocardial infarction, the APACHE II severity of illness scale (Knaus et al. 1985), and measures of comorbidity. These scales are based on information obtained at the time of hospital admission including patient vital signs, laboratory values, and components of initial history and physical examinations. Markers such as patient age and the presence of chronic conditions were important predictors of long-term mortality and received greater weight when incorporated into the index predicting mortality at 180 days. Instability at discharge was assessed by a method previously developed which indicated the mean number of unstable conditions among patients with more than one instability (Kosecoff et al. 1990).

For the HMO group, post-discharge death data (30 and 180 days post-admission) were obtained from the National Death Index maintained by the National Center for Health Statistics. For the fee-for-service sample, similar data were obtained from HCFA's Health Insurance Master File. Mortality was adjusted for sickness at admission.

The quality of the process of in-hospital care was assessed by a recently developed and validated process of care algorithm (Kahn et al. 1990c) incorporating 93 specific process of care criteria. To generate these criteria, process measures were identified by literature review and by expert consultation. These criteria were then reviewed by an expert panel and by internists and cardiologists from each of the participating HMOs to see if they were clinically acceptable and to determine if they were reliably recorded in the medical record. Criteria were then grouped by clinical opinion and tested by psychometric analysis. This resulted in an overall process of care scale and five process subscales: (1) the MD Cognition subscale, which measures the physician's performance in the areas of the initial history and physical examination, and the repeated clinical assessment of the patient during the hospital course; (2) the RN Cognition subscale, which measures the performance of the nurse in the clinical assessment of the patient; (3) the Technical Diagnostic subscale, which evaluates the use of diagnostic tests and procedures; (4) the

Technical Therapeutic subscale, which evaluates the use of medications and therapeutic procedures; and (5) the ICU/Telemetry subscale, which measures the appropriate use of the ICU or telemetry monitoring.

Two additional scales are shown in Table 8.5 (further on), which were not incorporated into the overall process scale. These are the normal last lab scale and the abnormal labs rechecked scale. The normal last lab scale is an assessment of the presence of normal labs at the time of patient discharge and is a measure of the overall clinical status of patients prior to discharge. The abnormal labs rechecked scale reflects the extent to which abnormal lab results are confirmed and investigated and, therefore, is a measure of the overall care rendered to a patient.

Because patients differ in terms of the level of care they need, each scale contains criteria that are not applicable to all patients with a myocardial infarction. For example, using a Swan-Ganz catheter in myocardial infarction patients with severe congestive heart failure and hypotension was considered indicated, but invasive monitoring was not considered necessary in a patient without these complications. As a result, the number of applicable criteria varied from patient to patient. Performance on process scales was scored by calculating compliance with applicable criteria.[1] Process scores obtained in this manner have been shown to correlate with the probability of death (Kahn et al. 1990c).

Compliance with process scales and severity-adjusted death rates for the aggregated HMO population of 369 admissions were compared to the 1,119 fee-for-service admissions. Comparisons within the HMO group were also performed. All scales were normalized to have a mean of 0 and a standard deviation of 1 using the entire fee-for-service sample that included rural patients as the reference population. Therefore, if a process scale is reported as having a value of 0.71 in the HMO group and 0.42 in the fee-for-service group, the process score for the HMO is 0.71 standard deviations greater than the reference population (fee-for-service rural and urban patients) and 0.29 standard deviations greater than the fee-for-service comparison. Differences in process of care were tested for significance using two-tailed t-tests.

Results

There was a small difference in the proportion of HMO and fee-for-service patients excluded from the study: 21 and 16 percent, respectively (Table 8.1). However 26 percent of admissions sampled from HMO1 were excluded compared to 14 percent from HMO2 ($p < .05$) and 20 percent from HMO3. Most of the difference between HMOs 1 and 2 was produced by the exclusion of admissions that were transferred from a fee-for-service hospital to the HMO facility (a difference of 8.8 percent). HMO enrollees were twice as likely to be transferred during the hospital admission than were their fee-for-service counterparts. Additionally, 18 percent of admissions from HMO3 were excluded because they were erroneously coded with a discharge diagnosis of acute myocardial infarction.

HMO patients were slightly younger, were more likely to be male ($p < .001$), were discharged from the hospital earlier ($p < .01$), and were less severely ill ($p < .05$) than their fee-for-service counterparts (Table 8.2). Within the HMO group, no significant differences were found for these patient characteristics. No differences in either instability at discharge or the percentage of patients designated to not be resuscitated were found between the HMO and FFS groups. However, patients from HMO2 were more unstable at discharge (with an average of 1.46 instabilities) and more likely to be designated "do not resuscitate" (an average of 20.4 percent of MI admissions) than patients from HMO1 and HMO3.

Unadjusted mortality for in-hospital, 30-day, or 180-day follow-up periods tended to be lower among the HMO group although these differences never achieved statistical significance (Table 8.3). After adjusting for sickness at admission by using the FFS population as the referent group, mortality differences between the overall HMO and fee-for-service sample or among the HMOs diminished in magnitude and remained insignificant.

Compliance with overall process of care criteria (Table 8.4) was higher in the HMOs than in the fee-for-service sample (0.54 vs. 0.23; $p < .01$). The pooled HMO patients had higher process of care scores than

Table 8.1 Reasons for Record Exclusion (Percentage of records sampled by category)

	FFS (%)	HMO (%)	HMO1 (%)	HMO2 (%)	HMO3 (%)
Not hospitalized during study year	0.4	2.7*	4.4	2.0	0.0**
Not eligible	1.5	—	—	—	—
ICD-9 code = MI					
Age < 65	0.3	0.0	0.0	0.0	0.0
Transferred from another hospital	4.1	8.7*	14.6	5.8**	0.0**
No signs/symptoms of MI at admission	6.5	8.5	6.8	5.2	18.0**
Other competing conditions	2.2	—	—	—	—
Patient died in emergency room	—	0.4	0.0	0.7	1.1
Insufficient data	—	0.4	0.0	0.7	1.1
Total exclusions	16.1	20.7*	25.8	14.4**	20.2

*Significantly different from the FFS sample, $p < .05$.
**Significantly different from HMO1, $p < .05$.

Table 8.2 Selected Characteristics of the FFS and HMO Samples

Characteristics	FFS	HMO	HMO-FFS Difference and 95% C.I.	HMO1	HMO2	HMO3
Number	1119	369				
Sex (% female)	50.5	38.5	12.0*** (6.15,17.9)	34.1	43.2	39.4
Age (years)	76.2	75.5	0.7 (−0.10,1.50)	74.9	76.3	75.4
Length of stay (days)	11.1	9.7	1.4** (0.57,2.27)	10.0	8.8	10.5
Sickness (30)‡	25.2	23.6	1.6* (0.012,3.19)	23.0	24.7	22.7
Sickness (180)‡	39.9	37.6	2.3* (0.19,4.41)	37.4	38.7	36.2
Instability at discharge	1.07	1.13	0.06 (−0.16,0.30)	0.96	1.46†	0.93
% no code	11.6	13.5	1.9 (−2.0,5.9)	9.1	20.1†	11.3

*Significantly different from FFS mean, $p < .05$.
**Significantly different from FFS mean, $p < .01$.
***Significantly different from FFS mean, $p < .001$.
†Significantly different from HMO1. (Other Intra-HMO group differences are not statistically significant.)
‡Sickness at Admission scales predict mortality at 30 and 180 days postadmission. A higher number indicates a higher level of sickness at admission.

Table 8.3 Percent Mortality

	Percent Dead*				
	FFS Mean	HMO Mean	HMO1	HMO2	HMO3
In-hospital	22.7	20.8	17.3	25.3	20.0
30-day	24.2	23.8	22.3	27.1	20.9
180-day	35.4	35.3	34.4	35.1	37.5

*HMO:FFS and HMO:HMO differences in adjusted mortality are not significant ($p > .05$).

the fee-for-service patients on three of the five sub-scales (MD Cognitive, RN Cognitive, and ICU/Telemetry monitoring, $p < .01$). No significant differences were found between the HMO and FFS groups on the normal last lab results scale or the abnormal labs rechecked scale. However, fee-for-service patients had higher scores on the Technical Diagnostic sub-scale than did HMO patients ($p < .05$).

Compliance with process criteria varied among the HMOs (Table 8.5). Compliance with overall process of care criteria was greater in each of the three HMOs than in the fee-for-service population. However, HMO1 and HMO3 had greater compliance than HMO2 with the overall process of in-hospital care scale ($p < .05$). HMO2 had significantly lower compliance than either HMO1 or HMO3 on the normal last lab results scale. The greatest difference between the HMOs was seen on the Technical Diagnostic sub-scale, where HMO2 demonstrated markedly lower compliance.

Note that while actual means for the various scales may often appear to differ greatly, these differences may not achieve statistical significance while small differences do. For instance, a .17 standard deviation difference between HMO1 and HMO2 on the physician cognitive scale was significant while a .25 standard deviation difference between HMO2 and HMO3 on the technical therapeutic scale was not significant. These effects are due to loss of statistical power produced by either sample size differences or extreme variation in the distribution of scale values for a particular HMO.

Appendix 8A presents a summary of individual criteria from the initial evaluation phase (the first 48 hours of admission) for each of the HMOs individually as well as the HMO and FFS groups. Marked

Table 8.4 HMO and Fee-For-Service Comparison of Process Scales

Process Scales†	FFS Mean	HMO Mean	HMO-FFS Difference and 95% C.I.
ICU/Telemetry	.08	.28	.20(.10,.29)*
MD cognitive	.21	.49	.28(.18,.39)*
RN cognitive	.12	.67	.55(.45,.65)*
Technical diagnostic	.18	.04	−.14(.03,.24)*
Technical therapeutic	.06	.22	.16(−.01,.32)
Overall Process	.23	.54	.32(.23,.42)*
Normal last lab results	−.03	.02	.05(−.08,.17)
Abnormal labs rechecked	.10	.01	.09(−.30,.10)

*$p < .05$.

†Process scales have a mean of zero and a standard deviation of one. The scales were standardized using the entire FFS population (including rural patients). A higher number indicates greater compliance with items constituting the process scale.

Table 8.5 Intra-HMO Comparisons of Process Scales

Process Scales†	HMO1	HMO2	HMO3	HMO1–HMO2 Difference and 95% C.I.	HMO1–HMO3 Difference and 95% C.I.	HMO2–HMO3 Difference and 95% C.I.
ICU/Telemetry	.26	.27	.33	−.01(−.16,.15)	−.07(−.25,.11)	−.06(−.24,.12)
MD cognitive	.56	.39	.56	.17(.01,.19)*	.00(−.19,.19)	−.17(−.38,.04)
RN cognitive	.69	.61	.73	.08(−.05,.21)	−.04(−.19,.11)	−.12(−.29,.05)
Technical diagnostic	.44	−.34	−.11	.78(.58,.98)*	.55(.35,.74)*	−.23(−.50,.04)
Technical therapeutic	.18	.16	.41	.02(−.32,.38)	−.23(−.63,.17)	−.25(−.67,.17)
Overall Process	.70	.35	.59	.35(.19,.51)*	.11(−.06,.28)*	−.24(−.46,−.02)*
Normal last lab results	.10	−.16	.17	.26(.03,.49)*	−.07(.28,.14)	−.33(−.65,−.01)*
Abnormal labs rechecked	−.05	−.08	.31	.03(−.41,.47)	−.36(−.88,.16)	−.39(−.94,.16)

*$p < .05$.
†Process scales have a mean of zero and a standard deviation of one. The scales were standardized using the entire FFS population (including rural patients). A higher number indicates greater compliance with items constituting the process scale.

variation in compliance with individual criteria is apparent both within the HMO group and between the HMO and FFS groups.

Recent work applying these process criteria and process of care scales to a nearly identical population (combined rural and urban FFS) has demonstrated a highly significant relationship between process and 30-day postadmission mortality ($p < .001$) (Kahn et al. 1990c). We found the same relationship in this analysis. In our combined HMO and urban fee-for-service study population, patients in the lowest quartile of overall process were 1.8 times more likely to die within 30 days of admission as those in the highest quartile. More precisely, a 20 percent increase in compliance with overall process of care from a process score of .50 to .60 was associated with a 3.7 percent reduction in 30-day post-admission mortality. These findings illustrate the relationship between improved process and better outcome.

Discussion

We have demonstrated in this paper similar mortality, after adjustment for differences in level of sickness at admission, but greater compliance with process of care criteria for Medicare patients treated for acute myocardial infarction in three health maintenance organizations compared to a representative group of fee-for-service Medicare patients treated in urban hospitals. HMO physicians and nurses adhered significantly more closely with process of care criteria than did their fee-for-service counterparts. HMO physicians and nurses performed more appropriate physical examinations and took more appropriate histories. HMO patients more frequently received appropriate cardiac monitoring. Only in the area of diagnostic testing, such as receiving electrocardiograms and chest radiographs when appropriate, did fee-for-service compliance exceed that received by HMO patients.[2] Additionally, significant variation was noted among the HMOs themselves. HMO2 had significantly less compliance with process scales than did the other two HMOs. Finally, compliance with overall process of care criteria for patients with MI was associated with lower mortality when all results were pooled.

While certain limitations apply to our study, they are not likely to have a substantial effect on our overall conclusions. These limitations include out-of-plan use not reported to the HMO, the exclusion of HMO patients transferred from fee-for-service hospitals, selection bias, and changes in the management of patients with acute MI since the development of our criteria. Out-of-plan use, while important, has been shown to occur mainly for non-covered services, psychiatric care, or care received after accidents and injuries (Manning et al. 1984). Hence the effect of out-of-plan use for patients with myocardial infarction is likely to be small.

While we excluded HMO patients admitted to and then transferred from fee-for-service hospitals, this was a relatively small portion of our sample population. Additionally, patients transferred to HMO facilities were not initially managed by HMO physicians and, thus, may not be reflective of HMO quality. However, if HMO procedures led to treatment delays or inappropriate transfers, quality of care and outcome might be affected. While selection bias is a potential problem in any non-experimental study, its potential effect is minimized by our use of process criteria that take into account differences in level of sickness and by the use of a clinically detailed severity scale to adjust for differences in mortality. Finally, although the criteria were designed to be most relevant to the management of acute myocardial infarction during our study period of 1985–1986, most of the criteria apply equally well to current practice. The most significant change in the management of acute myocardial infarction patients in the last five years is the use of thrombolytic therapy. Three of the five process sub-scales (with the exception of the therapeutic and physician evaluation sub-scales) would be largely unaffected by the advent of thrombolysis.

This study does show greater compliance with process measures of quality in three different HMOs compared to a sample of urban fee-for-service care. Although the consistency of our findings across the three plans is noteworthy, we cannot generalize our results to all HMOs. Furthermore, given the proliferation of HMOs in number and type in the last decade, generalizing to the many newer, smaller, and hybrid HMO forms that are not included in the consortium of health plans participating in this study may not be particularly meaningful. In addition, inclusion of rural hospitals in the fee-for-service sample would only have increased the magnitude of the observed differences between the HMO and fee-for-service samples.

Our results strongly suggest that the process of care sub-scales, and the specific items that constitute them, can be of clinical importance to health plans and other providers in evaluating quality of care within their organizations. For example, by establishing a framework for the evaluation of myocardial infarction quality of care, continuous improvement programs (Laffel and Blumenthal 1989) can be undertaken by such organizations to monitor and improve selected areas of health care process. A health plan finding poor comparative performance on a given dimension of care (e.g. the use of diagnostic tests) could focus monitoring, feedback, and other continuous improvement activities on this aspect of care.

Other measures of quality have been developed and could be used by plans in a continuous improvement process. Patient judgments are a very good measure of how consumers assess the performance of their health care providers (Meterko, Nelson, and Rubin 1990), but they provide less information about the technical aspects of medical care. Thus patient judgments complement rather than substitute for the technical process measures discussed in this paper. Outcomes measurement (Ellwood 1988) has recently garnered much interest from the policy and medical community as a means of measuring quality. However, measuring outcomes alone, while attractive because it may be a more efficient means of assessing quality, cannot provide relevant clinical information on what variations in process might have led to the observed variations in outcome. Information linking process and outcome is essential in identifying strategies for improving the quality of medical care.

The findings presented in this paper have important policy implications. First, statistics about quality that are based on mortality obtained from administrative or claims data alone may not be sufficiently reliable or sufficiently sensitive to compare different health plans. Either the data need to be improved or other information needs to be collected. Perhaps both could be done by reviewing medical records to collect process data and to produce clinically adjusted mortality rates for patients confirmed to have a myocardial infarction. Second, the finding of greater process of care scores for each of our HMOs versus the fee-for-service system for a complex disease requiring expenditure of many resources provides substantial evidence suggesting that enrollment of Medicare recipients into HMOs will not necessarily harm their health. If care in these systems is also less expensive, such policies might be pursued. Third, we have demonstrated that quality of care varied among the HMOs. This finding provides an additional dimension for competition among health plans, raising the possibility of direct comparison of quality in addition to historic comparisons of costs, benefits, and premiums. If all HMOs in a given area would release such data to the public during open enrollment periods along with data on price, this might increase the efficiency and effectiveness of the health care system. Finally, collecting simultaneous process and outcome data from multiple plans might make it possible for continuous quality improvement activities to proceed at each plan in a more effective manner.

Acknowledgments

This work was supported by the John Hartford Foundation, the National Institute on Aging, and the members of the HMO Quality of Care Consortium. The opinions, conclusions and proposals in the text are those of the authors alone and do not necessarily represent the views of the Hartford Foundation, RAND Corporation, the University of California, Los Angeles, or the Robert Wood Johnson Foundation.

Notes

1. Process scores reflect the relationship between those actions that are necessary given a specific clinical scenario and those that are actually performed. Excessive, inappropriate, or unnecessary actions are not included in these scores.
2. Although this may be a reflection of a tendency for increased overall clinical activity, including unnecessary care.

References

Cunningham, F. C., and J. W. Williamson. "How Does the Quality of Health Care in HMOs Compare to That in Other Settings? An Analytic Literature Review: 1958 to 1979." *The Group Health Journal* 1, no. 1 (1980): 4–25.

Draper, D., K. L. Kahn, E. J. Reinisch, et al. "Studying the Effects of the DRG-Based Prospective Payment System on Quality of Care: Design, Sampling, and Fieldwork." *Journal of the American Medical Association* 264, no. 15 (1990): 1956–61.

Ellwood, P. M. "Shattuck Lecture—Outcomes Management." *The New England Journal of Medicine* 318 (1988): 1549–56.

Kahn, K. L., D. Draper, E. B. Keeler, L. Rubenstein, M. Sherwood, E. Reinisch, J. Kosecoff, and R. Brook. "The Effects of the DRG-Based Prospective Payment System on Quality of Care for Hospitalized Medicare Patients: Supplemental Design, Methods, and Results." RAND Publication no. N-3132-HCFA. Santa Monica, CA, 1990.

Kahn, K. L., L. V. Rubenstein, D. Draper, J. Kosecoff, W. Rogers, E. Keeler, and R. Brook. "The Effects of the DRG-based Prospective Payment System on Quality of Care for Hospitalized Medicare Patients: Introduction to the Series." *Journal of the American Medical Association* 264, no. 15 (1990): 1953–55.

Kahn, K. L., W. H. Rogers, L. V. Rubenstein, M. Sherwood, E. Reinisch, E. Keeler, D. Draper, J. Kosecoff, and R. Brook. "Measuring Quality of Care with Explicit Process Criteria Pre- and Post-Implementation of the DRG-based Prospective Payment System." *Journal of the American Medical Association* 264, no. 15 (1990): 1969–73.

Keeler, E. B., K. L. Kahn, D. Draper, M. Sherwood, L. Rubenstein, E. Reinisch, J. Kosecoff, and R. Brook. "Changes in Sickness at Admission Following the Introduction of Prospective Payment." *Journal of the American Medical Association* 264, no. 15 (1990): 1962–68.

Killip, T., and J. T. Kimball. "Treatment of Myocardial Infarction in a Coronary Care Unit." *American Journal of Cardiology* 20 (1967): 457–61.

Knaus, W. A., E. A. Draper, D. P. Wagner, et al. "APACHE II: A Severity of Disease Classification System." *Critical Care Medicine* 13 (1985): 818–29.

Kosecoff, J., K. L. Kahn, W. H. Rogers, L. Rubenstein, D. Draper, E. Keeler, E. Reinisch, M. Sherwood, and R. Brook. "Prospective Payment System and Impairment at Discharge: The 'Quicker-and-Sicker' Story Revisited." *Journal of the American Medical Association* 264, no. 15 (1990): 1980–83.

Kosecoff, J., L. V. Rubenstein, K. L. Kahn, D. Draper, E. Keeler, M. Sherwood, E. Reinisch, and R. Brook. "Medical Record Abstraction Form and Guidelines for Assessing Quality of Care for Hospitalized Patients with Acute Myocardial Infarction." RAND Publication no. N-2798-HCFA. Santa Monica, CA, 1988.

Laffel, G., and D. Blumenthal. "The Case for Using Industrial Quality Management Science in Health Care Organizations." *Journal of the American Medical Association* 262 (1989): 2869–73.

Langwell, K. M., and J. P. Hadley. "Evaluation of the Medicare Competition Demonstrations." *Health Care Financing Review* 11, no. 2 (1989): 65–80.

Luft, H. S. *Health Maintenance Organizations: Dimensions of Performance.* New York: Wiley, 1981.

Manning, W. G., A. Leibowitz, G. A. Goldberg, et al. "A Controlled Trial of the Effect of a Prepaid Group Practice on the Use of Services." *The New England Journal of Medicine* 320 (1984): 1505–10.

Marion Laboratories, Inc. *The 1988 Marion Managed Care Digest.* Kansas City, MO, 1988.

Meterko, M., E. C. Nelson, and H. R. Rubin, eds. "Patient Judgments of Hospital Quality: Report of a Pilot Study." *Medical Care* 28, no. 9 (1990, Supplement).

Norris, R. M., P. W. T. Brandt, D. E. Caughey, et al. "A New Coronary Prognostic Index." *The Lancet* 1 (1969): 274–78.

Shapiro, S., J. J. Williams, S. Yerby, P. M. Densen, and H. Rosner. "Patterns of Medical Care by the Indigent Aged, Under Two Systems of Medical Care." *American Journal of Public Health* 57 (1967): 784–90.

Appendix 8A Initial Assessment Criteria (Examples)

Initial Nurse Assessment

All Patients. Within the initial two days of hospitalization, the nurse should document each of the following in the medical record:

Criterion	HMO2	HMO1	HMO3	All HMO	All PPS
Chest Pain (presence or absence of patient complaint) Day 1	96.3 (100)	96.3 (100)	97.2 (100)	96.5 (100)	92.7 (100)
Chest Pain (presence or absence of patient complaint) Day 2	97.6 (94)	98.1 (98)	98.6 (97)	98.0 (96)	92.9 (95)
PVCs Assessed (presence or absence on monitor) Day 1	80.6 (100)	84.8 (100)	85.9 (100)	83.5 (100)	68.3 (100)
PVCs Assessed (presence or absence on monitor) Day 2	92.9 (94)	91.9 (98)	94.2 (97)	92.7 (96)	76.1 (95)
Admission Weight recorded, Day 1 or Day 2	42.5 (100)	65.2 (100)	56.3 (100)	55.3 (100)	43.8 (100)
Preadmission Residence Noted	97.8 (100)	98.8 (100)	100 (100)	98.6 (100)	94.0 (100)
Cardiac Monitor Rhythm Strips Documented (at least 3 placed in medical record on Day 1)	97.0 (100)	97.6 (100)	97.2 (100)	97.3 (100)	87.4 (100)

Initial Physician Assessment

All Patients. Within the initial two days of hospitalization, the physician should document each of the following in the medical record:

Criterion	HMO2	HMO1	HMO3	All HMO	All PPS
Previous Cardiac History	96.3 (100)	95.7 (100)	95.8 (100)	95.9 (100)	90.7 (100)
Time of Onset of AMI Symptoms	97.0 (100)	95.1 (100)	100 (100)	96.8 (100)	97.0 (100)
Social or Family History Noted	72.4 (100)	75.0 (100)	77.5 (100)	74.5 (100)	67.6 (100)
Current Medications Noted	92.5 (100)	92.7 (100)	95.8 (100)	93.2 (100)	89.0 (100)
Allergy History Noted	67.9 (100)	86.0 (100)	71.8 (100)	76.7 (100)	64.9 (100)

Continued

Appendix 8A   Continued

Criterion	HMO2	HMO1	HMO3	All HMO	All PPS
Alcohol and Smoking Habits Noted	59.7 (100)	83.5 (100)	71.8 (100)	72.6 (100)	67.7 (100)
Jugular Veins Examined	87.3 (100)	70.7 (100)	53.5 (100)	73.4 (100)	73.8 (100)
Heart Sounds Examined	88.8 (100)	79.9 (100)	83.1 (100)	83.7 (100)	84.5 (100)
Heart Murmurs Examined	89.6 (100)	90.2 (100)	80.3 (100)	88.1 (100)	85.0 (100)
Abdomen Examined	97.8 (100)	97.6 (100)	98.6 (100)	97.8 (100)	97.4 (100)
Lower Extremity Examined for Edema	88.1 (100)	88.4 (100)	87.3 (100)	88.1 (100)	84.6 (100)
Chest Pain (Presence or absence of patient complaint) Assessed Day 1	97.0 (100)	97.6 (100)	100 (100)	97.8 (100)	94.8 (100)
Chest Pain (Presence or absence of patient complaint) Assessed Day 2	81.0 (94)	82.3 (98)	91.3 (97)	83.7 (96)	72.4 (95)
Lungs Examined, Day 1	98.5 (100)	99.4 (100)	100 (100)	99.2 (100)	97.8 (100)
Lungs Examined, Day 2	77.8 (94)	88.2 (98)	87.0 (97)	84.3 (96)	73.1 (95)

Initial Chest X-Ray and Electrocardiographic Assessment

All Patients. Within the initial two days of hospitalization, order each of the following:

Criterion	HMO2	HMO1	HMO3	All HMO	All PPS
Chest X-ray on Day 1 or Day 2	92.5 (100)	93.3 (100)	93.0 (100)	93.0 (100)	93.9 (100)
EKG on Day 1	97.0 (100)	99.4 (100)	98.6 (100)	98.4 (100)	97.1 (100)
EKG on Day 2	92.1 (94)	96.3 (98)	98.6 (97)	95.2 (96)	90.9 (95)

Continued

Appendix 8A   Continued

Initial Laboratory Assessment

All Patients. Within the initial two days of hospitalization, order each of the following laboratory studies:

Criterion	HMO2	HMO1	HMO3	All HMO	All PPS
BUN	85.8	92.7	83.1	88.4	93.6
	(100)	(100)	(100)	(100)	(100)
Creatinine	70.2	92.7	84.5	82.9	82.7
	(100)	(100)	(100)	(100)	(100)
Bicarbonate (V)	90.3	98.2	25.4	81.3	91.6
	(100)	(100)	(100)	(100)	(100)
Sodium	88.1	98.2	91.6	93.2	96.2
	(100)	(100)	(100)	(100)	(100)
Potassium	88.1	98.2	94.4	93.8	96.5
	(100)	(100)	(100)	(100)	(100)
White Blood Cell Count	85.1	97.6	94.4	92.4	96.3
	(100)	(100)	(100)	(100)	(100)
Hematocrit or Hemoglobin	85.1	97.6	94.4	92.4	96.5
	(100)	(100)	(100)	(100)	(100)
Cardiac *Enzymes* or *Iso-enzymes*,	88.8	93.1	93.0	91.1	94.6
Day 1	19.4	81.7	38.0	50.7	54.4
	(100)	(100)	(100)	(100)	(100)
Cardiac *Enzymes* or *Iso-enzymes*,	88.9	91.3	95.7	91.3	90.3
Day 2	45.3	85.7	47.8	64.0	61.0
	(94)	(98)	(97)	(96)	(95)

Note: The upper number within the cell is the percentage of patients within each group meeting the process criteria. The number in parentheses is the percentage of patients to whom the criteria are applicable.

Appendix 8A Continued

Initial Technical Therapeutic Criteria

If	Then	HMO2	HMO1	HMO3	All HMO	All PPS
Patients Moderately or Very Sick (ASSC ≥ 5), Day 1 or 2	Obtain arterial blood gas, Day 1 or Day 2	62.3 (40)	75.0 (32)	40.0 (42)	62.2 (35)	79.7 (36)
Patients with Cardiogenic Shock with End Organ Damage, Arrhythmias, AND very sick (ASSC ≥ 7) Day 1 or 2	Place a Swan-Ganz catheter on Day 1 or Day 2	31.6 (14)	41.7 (7)	0.0 (13)	27.5 (11)	45.7 (8)
Patients with Cardiogenic Shock with End Organ Damage, Arrhythmias, AND very sick (ASSC ≥ 7) Day 1	Use pressors or IV unloading agents, Day 1	71.4 (10)	57.1 (4)	100 (11)	75.9 (8)	76.5 (6)
Patients with Cardiogenic Shock with End Organ Damage, Arrhythmias, AND very sick (ASSC ≥ 7) Day 2	Use pressors or IV unloading agents, Day 2	83.3 (4)	80.0 (3)	100 (1)	83.3 (3)	85.7 (4)
Patients with Ventricular Tachycardia, Day 1	Use Antiarrhythmics, Day 1	0 (0)	0 (0)	0 (0)	0 (0)	87.5 (1)
Patients with PVCs, Day 1	Use Antiarrhythmics, Day 1	73.9 (34)	76.5 (31)	86.4 (31)	77.3 (32)	68.0 (23)
Patients with Ventricular Tachycardia, Day 2	Use Antiarrhythmics, Day 2	0 (0)	0 (0)	0 (0)	0 (0)	80.0 (1)

Patients with PVCs, Day 2	Use Antiarrhythmics, Day 2	84.0 (19)	61.3 (19)	100 (21)	77.5 (27)	63.4 (17)
Patients with 3rd Degree Heart Block, Day 1 or 2 and Anterior MI	Use pacemaker, Day 1 or 2	100 (2)	0 (1)	0 (0)	75 (1)	63.6 (1)
Patients with 3rd Degree Heart Block, Day 1 or 2 and NO Anterior MI	Use pacemaker, Day 1 or 2	40 (4)	0 (1)	0 (3)	22.2 (2)	80.6 (3)
Patients given Streptokinase	Document bleeding history (presence or absence)	25 (3)	40 (3)	33.3 (13)	33.3 (5)	13.0 (4)
Patients given Streptokinase	Start streptokinase within 6 hours of the time symptoms were first noted	75 (3)	80 (3)	55.6 (13)	66.7 (5)	73.2 (4)
Patients with Congestive Heart Failure but No Hypotension, Day 1	Give loop diuretics, Day 1	50 (15)	57.1 (13)	57.1 (10)	54.2 (13)	52.9 (19)
Patients with Congestive Heart Failure but No Hypotension, Day 1	Give loop diuretics, Day 2	100 (4)	75 (5)	71.4 (10)	81.0 (6)	69.6 (11)

Note: The upper number within the cell is the percentage of patients within each group meeting the process criteria. The number in parentheses is the percentage of patients to whom the criteria are applicable.

Chapter 9

Responses and Discussion

Patrick S. Romano

With increasing interest in managed care as a method to reduce the cost of health care for elderly Medicare beneficiaries, quality of care in risk HMOs is an important concern. As of November 1, 1992, there were 95 such risk HMOs participating in the Medicare program, with over 1.5 million enrollees (Office of Operations 1992). Applications were pending from an additional 15 plans, as well as 20 proposed service area expansions for existing plans. As risk HMO enrollment increases, we must demonstrate to the satisfaction of both policymakers and Medicare beneficiaries that switching from fee-for-service to managed care does not compromise quality. The papers by Carlisle et al. and Retchin et al. represent important contributions to this discussion.

To summarize the results of these elegant studies, Medicare beneficiaries enrolled in HMOs appear to experience outcomes of hospital care for acute medical conditions similar to the outcomes of beneficiaries in the fee-for-service system. Although Retchin et al. found a higher prevalence of residual speech and motor deficits at discharge among HMO enrollees, this difference is more likely attributable to shorter hospital stays or larger infarcts than to poorer quality of care. Given the limited short-term benefit associated with speech therapy and physical therapy (Ernst 1990), it seems unlikely that the modest reported differences in utilization could account for the impressive disparity in neurologic status at discharge. Using a sophisticated and well-validated risk adjustment tool, Carlisle et al. were unable to demonstrate a difference in either in-hospital or postdischarge mortality. Both of these studies had reasonably large HMO samples ($n = 369$ in Carlisle et al., $n = 402$ in Retchin et al.), but Type II error may still be a concern given the large amount of residual variance attributable to unmeasured determinants of mortality. Both studies also had consistent findings related to the process of care, although that consistency is somewhat obscured by the authors' discordant approaches to presenting and interpreting their data.

Carlisle et al.'s paper places greatest emphasis on the "MD cognitive" and "RN cognitive" subscales, which are precisely the measurements most sensitive to documentation bias. In other words, higher scores among HMO enrollees may reflect better documentation in the history and physical or in the nursing assessment rather than true differences in the process of care. These two subscales appear to explain most of the difference in the overall process measure between HMO enrollees and nonenrollees. Yet quality improvement programs that involve auditing records are probably more prevalent in managed care systems than in the fee-for-service setting. HMO physicians and nurses may therefore face greater pressure to document everything that they do during their patient encounters. In addition, physicians practicing in HMOs tend to be younger and more recently trained than physicians in fee-for-service practice. Young physicians may have superior knowledge of current standards of care, but may also have been warned about the liability implications of inadequate documentation. Physicians in fee-for-service practice may have easier access to outpatient records than physicians in staff model HMOs, so fee-for-service physicians may feel less compelled to record all relevant data in hospital charts. For these reasons, the inpatient records of HMO enrollees may more likely reflect the cognitive services that were actually provided than the records of nonenrollees.

By contrast, Retchin et al. modified the RAND assessment tool by designating informational items not found in the medical record as documentation errors rather than as deficiencies in physician or nurse assessment. They did not report the relative prevalence of these documentation errors among HMO enrollees and nonenrollees. Instead, they focused on the utilization of diagnostic and rehabilitative services. Their finding that HMO enrollees with low-severity strokes were less likely than similar nonenrollees to undergo echocardiography or carotid ultrasound is consistent with Carlisle et al.'s finding that compliance with process criteria for "technical-diagnostic" care was better in the fee-for-service setting. Retchin et al.'s finding that stroke patients with motor deficits received fewer physical therapy sessions if they were in an HMO, while those with speech deficits received comparable numbers of speech therapy sessions, is also consistent with Carlisle et al.'s finding that overall compliance with process criteria for "technical-therapeutic" care was similar in the two settings. Indeed, HMO patients with myocardial infarction were more likely than fee-for-service patients to receive some potentially appropriate therapeutic services (e.g., arterial blood gas) but less likely to receive several others (e.g., antiarrhythmics).

Several potential biases affect both of these studies, despite the best efforts of the authors. These biases do not undermine the results of either study, but simply suggest the need for careful interpretation. First, the organizations selected for participation may not adequately represent the population of Medicare risk HMOs. This concern is particularly relevant in the RAND study, which included only three Medicare HMOs, all of which were large members of a national consortium. Because these HMOs were largely self-selected, they may differ in important respects from the entire population of Medicare HMOs. The participating HMOs may have had better quality improvement programs and more skilled physicians than the HMOs that did not participate. Retchin et al.'s study included a far broader group of HMOs, although small plans were unavoidably underrepresented.

Another concern follows from the observed differences in clinical characteristics between HMO enrollees and nonenrollees in both studies. HMO patients were more likely to be male (although not significantly so in Retchin et al.'s analysis) and were less severely ill, as measured by a sickness-at-admission scale or by comorbidity burden, than their fee-for-service counterparts. Although HMO enrollees and nonenrollees presented with similar neurologic signs and symptoms in Retchin et al.'s study, this finding is not convincing because of striking differences in neurologic status at discharge. For example, it is inconceivable that the higher proportion of HMO enrollees with persistent decerebrate or decorticate posturing is due to a difference in medical care. The disparity in the prevalence of persistent speech deficits (54 percent versus 35 percent) also suggests an underlying difference in stroke characteristics that was not apparent on admission. These clinical characteristics could confound the apparent associations between HMO enrollment and quality of care, if documentation errors occur more frequently among severely ill patients than among moderately ill patients (and technical-diagnostic errors occur more frequently among moderately ill patients). This hypothesis is supported by the observation that the HMO with the sickest patient profile in Carlisle et al.'s study resembled the fee-for-service group more closely than did the other two HMOs, according to several process measures.

Another possibility is that the quality of care for myocardial infarction and stroke may not be representative of the overall quality of care provided to Medicare beneficiaries enrolled in risk HMOs. Myocardial infarctions and strokes occur frequently among elderly Americans and are associated with significant morbidity and mortality (e.g., 26 percent mortality within 30 days of admission for MI) (Udvarhelyi et al. 1992). However, the treatment of myocardial infarction is concentrated in special inpatient units and is typically supervised by cardiologists. Neurologists are often involved in the care of stroke patients. Findings regarding quality of care for these conditions may not generalize to other settings, where practice standards may be less clear and physicians may have less specialized training. Fortunately, several previous studies of other conditions by Retchin's group have generated similar results, in that Medicare beneficiaries enrolled in HMOs receive equal or better-quality care than similar nonenrollees. These conditions include hypertension (Preston and Retchin 1991), colorectal cancer (Retchin and Brown 1990a), and congestive heart failure (Retchin and Brown 1991). Screening tests for breast cancer, colorectal cancer, and gynecologic cancer appear to be performed more often in Medicare HMOs than in the fee-for-service system; this advantage was greater for staff model HMOs than for IPAs (Retchin and Brown 1990b). The general health status outcomes of Medicare HMO enrollees (e.g., changes in instrumental activities of daily living, bed days, restricted activity days) also appear similar to those of nonenrollees (Langwell and Hadley 1989).

One important issue that neither of the studies in this volume addresses is the possible interaction between sociodemographic characteristics and the effectiveness of HMO care. The RAND Health Insurance Experiment reported that low-income, initially sick persons who were randomly assigned to a staff model HMO in Seattle had significantly more bed days per year due to poor health and more serious symptoms than those assigned to free fee-for-service care (Ware et al. 1986). This difference was not observed among high-income persons or among persons who were not chronically ill at enrollment. Although this finding has been criticized as a chance association (Wagner and Bledsoe 1990) and was not corroborated in a more detailed analysis of health status measures in the RAND Health Insurance Experiment (Sloss et al. 1987), one observational study also suggests that low-income Medicare HMO enrollees are at risk for deficient care (Heller, Larson, and LoGerfo 1984). Because equity in the health care system is an important goal, we cannot ignore the possibility that low-income enrollees experience particular difficulty getting their health needs met in the HMO environment.

How can we reconcile the observed differences in process measures of quality with the lack of differences in outcome measures? Sisk and colleagues (1990) argue that "process measures gain validity as quality indicators only to the extent that they have been associated with changes in patient outcomes, and outcome measures gain validity only to the extent that they have been linked to the prior medical care process" (p. 265). Outcome measures represent the "bottom line" for assessing the performance of any health care system, but there are several limitations to the outcome measures used in these studies.

First, there is too much unexplained variability (e.g., "random noise") in patient outcomes because many important psychosocial and medical characteristics are not measured. Adverse outcome rates are low for most conditions, thereby compromising statistical power. Assessment of many adverse outcomes requires long-term follow-up, which is difficult to achieve with budgetary and time constraints. To assess the appropriateness of rehabilitative services, for example, Retchin et al. would have needed to collect functional outcomes data 6 to 12 months after discharge. The outcome measures used were too crude and too short-term to reflect the full impact of observed process differences. Some outcomes are difficult to measure with optimal reliability and validity (e.g., chronic pain). For these reasons, it is more difficult to discern meaningful differences across systems of care using outcome criteria than using process criteria.

Yet outcome criteria remain the gold standard for quality assessment, because the specific aspects of process that affect outcomes are often unclear. For instance, does limiting the use of echocardiography among HMO enrollees with strokes endanger the lives of patients with intracardiac thrombi, or does it demonstrate cost-effective practice? Retchin et al. do not report how many of these echocardiograms were normal. Does constrained utilization of rehabilitative services permit neurologic deficits to linger, or does it reflect sober appraisal of the limited effectiveness of such services? Does the greater frequency of documentation deficiencies among fee-for-service patients reflect careless history-taking or abbreviated note-writing? If the same information is elicited from fee-for-service patients but not recorded, does that documentation failure adversely affect patients when no other physicians are involved in management? Perhaps HMO physicians spend too much time documenting all of their findings and interpretations; patient outcomes could conceivably improve if this administrative burden were lifted. The principal value of process criteria is that they elucidate the link between medical care and outcomes, so that providers can identify the weak components of their systems and design corrective interventions. Process criteria are therefore well suited to continuous quality improvement because they foster a dialogue among clinicians and administrators over how to enhance outcomes. In the absence of outcome differences, process differences become difficult to interpret.

This recent work of Carlisle et al. and Retchin et al. confirms that the overall quality of hospital care for Medicare enrollees with acute medical conditions is essentially unrelated to HMO enrollment. Although HMO physicians and nurses may be more likely to document their historical and physical findings, these differences are modest and have questionable clinical significance. Utilization of diagnostic and therapeutic services is less in the HMO setting, but this difference essentially disappears among the most severely ill patients. There is little evidence that constrained utilization among HMO patients has a deleterious effect on postdischarge outcomes, although it may increase the risk of transfer to a nursing home. Longer follow-up studies with outcome measures other than mortality may expose previously unrecognized differences between HMO enrollees and nonenrollees. Nonetheless, the evidence accumulated to date suggests that risk HMOs are able to provide cost-effective care of adequate quality to Medicare beneficiaries. Further studies are necessary to establish the appropriate indications for services that are utilized less often in the HMO setting than in fee-for-service practice. Continuous quality improvement programs are needed to ensure that process aspects of care, and ultimate outcomes, are optimized for all Medicare beneficiaries, regardless of where they receive their health care.

References

Ernst, E. "A Review of Stroke Rehabilitation and Physiotherapy." *Stroke* 21 (1990): 1081–85.

Heller, T. A., E. B. Larson, and J. P. LoGerfo. "Quality of Ambulatory Care of the Elderly: An Analysis of Five Conditions." *Journal of the American Geriatric Society* 32, no. 11 (1984): 782–88.

Langwell, K. M., and J. P. Hadley. "Evaluation of the Medicare Competition Demonstrations." *Health Care Financing Review* 11, no. 2 (1989): 65–80.

Office of Operations, Office of Prepaid Health Care Operations and Oversight, Health Care Financing Administration. "Medicare Coordinated Care Contract Report." Washington, DC (Data as of 1 November 1992).

Preston, J. A., and S. M. Retchin. "The Management of Geriatric Hypertension in Health Maintenance Organizations." *Journal of the American Geriatric Society* 39, no. 7 (1991): 683–90.

Retchin, S. M., and B. Brown. "Elderly Patients with Congestive Heart Failure under Prepaid Care." *American Journal of Medicine* 90, no. 2 (1991): 236–42.

Retchin, S. M., and B. Brown. "Management of Colorectal Cancer in Medicare Health Maintenance Organizations." *Journal of General Internal Medicine* 5, no. 1 (1990a): 110–14.

Retchin, S. M., and B. Brown. "The Quality of Ambulatory Care in Medicare Health Maintenance Organizations." *American Journal of Public Health* 80, no. 4 (1990b): 411–15.

Sisk, J. E., D. M. Dougherty, P. M. Ehrenhaft, G. Ruby, and B. A. Mitchner. "Assessing Information for Consumers on the Quality of Medical Care." *Inquiry* 27, no. 3 (1990): 263–72.

Sloss, E. M., E. B. Keeler, R. H. Brook, B. H. Operskalski, G. A. Goldberg, and J. P. Newhouse. "Effect of a Health Maintenance Organization on Physiologic Health." *Annals of Internal Medicine* 106, no. 1 (1987): 130–38.

Udvarhelyi, I. S., C. Gatsonis, A. M. Epstein, C. L. Pashos, J. P. Newhouse, and B. J. McNeil. "Acute Myocardial Infarction in the Medicare Population: Process of Care and Clinical Outcomes." *Journal of the American Medical Association* 268, no. 18 (1992): 2530–36.

Wagner, E. H., and T. Bledsoe. "The Rand Health Insurance Experiment and HMOs." *Medical Care* 28, no. 3 (1990): 191–200.

Ware, J. E., R. H. Brook, W. H. Rogers, E. B. Keeler, A. R. Davies, C. D. Sherbourne, G. A. Goldberg, P. Camp, and J. P. Newhouse. "Comparison of Health Outcomes at a Health Maintenance Organization with Those of Fee-For-Service Care." *The Lancet* 1 (1986): 1017–22.

Edward Wagner

The central question about health care reform is no longer whether it will happen, but the form it will take. Will reform simply try to put an expenditure lid on the pot we call the delivery system, ignoring the mess bubbling underneath, or will it try to stir the pot? Moving more and more of the population into managed care systems through managed competition or other approaches remains a favored pot-stirring approach. Since federal Medicare policy for the past decade has encouraged enrollment of older adults into managed care organizations, this review of that experience and its impact on patient health could not be better timed. Cross-system comparisons of quality and cost furnish the essential grist for the policymakers' mill. Certainly, early studies of HMO quality (Cunningham and Williamson 1980; Luft 1981) and the RAND Health Insurance Experiment (Ware et al. 1986; Sloss et al. 1987; Wagner and Bledsoe 1990) offered succor in the mid-1980s to those advocating managed care for Medicare and Medicaid.

The Carlisle et al. and Retchin et al. papers contribute important new information about the relative quality of hospital care rendered to older patients with major vascular events treated in HMOs versus fee-for-service. The studies have several advantages over earlier examinations of comparative quality, most notably in the larger number of HMOs examined. Both groups of investigators used well-grounded criteria established by the RAND group, rigorous sampling, and meticulous data collection, which make it especially interesting that their findings do not entirely agree.

Both of these post-PPS studies show that HMO patients with myocardial infarction (MI) and stroke remained in the hospital one to two days less than similar patients cared for under FFS, and that these shorter hospital stays included less time in the ICU, at least for stroke patients. These shorter hospital stays almost certainly would translate into lower costs. The reductions in hospital stay with HMO care were not associated with differences in hospital or posthospital mortality or readmission rates. And for MI patients, services required by the quality of care criteria were performed more frequently among HMO patients so that an overall measure of the quality of the process of care was significantly better—higher quality at lower cost. Of note, one of the three HMOs under study (HMO2) exhibited significantly worse process measures, and discharged patients in less stable condition a day or two earlier than the other two HMOs.

The situation for stroke patients was more complicated. On the one hand, HMO stroke patients of low severity received fewer diagnostic services like echocardiograms and Doppler ultrasounds, while those with high severity or specific indications received these tests as often as in FFS. This appeared to the authors to be a rational conservation of expensive resources.

On the other hand, HMO stroke patients also received fewer rehabilitative services, were more often discharged with neurological deficits, and more often went from the hospital to a nursing home. This practice style concerns the authors even though there were no differences in functional status at discharge, hospital mortality, or readmission rates. Their data suggest that discharge to a nursing home may have resulted in less intensive rehabilitation. If full recovery depends on intensive rehabilitation, then this pattern of early discharge of stroke patients to nursing homes by HMOs could be dangerous and result in a higher rate of long-term disability and institutionalization. There is some precedent for this unfortunate sequence of events. Fitzgerald et al. (1987) studied hip fracture patients treated in an Indianapolis hospital before and after institution of the prospective payment system. After PPS, patients stayed six fewer days in the hospital, but over twice as many were discharged to nursing homes (48 percent versus 21 percent before PPS), and three times as many were still in the nursing home six months later (39 percent versus 13 percent).

Forgoing intensive rehabilitation in the acute care hospital or a rehabilitation hospital would indeed constitute a serious deficiency in care if there were clear evidence in the literature that rehabilitation services enhanced functional recovery and return to home. But the authors acknowledge "the lack of convincing evidence" supporting the effectiveness of rehabilitation services for stroke patients. Without data assuring us that long-term functional outcomes did not suffer, HMO care appears deficient because it varies from the standard in many communities—a standard for which, in this case, there is a "lack of convincing evidence." Is this underservice or efficient care?

To what standards will we hold health systems? Many criteria sets reflect prevailing community standards, which most often emanate from the predominant FFS sector with its excess hospital and specialist capacity, domination by subspecialists, and incentives to overserve because of payment for piece work. Information on medical effectiveness may play a subordinate role. Thus, community standards often include unproved or even ineffective services. As a result, organizations that attempt to limit services to those with a demonstrated positive effect on patients will be viewed by some as substandard. This fact of American medical life keeps HMOs and other conservative, data-driven practice organizations on the defensive against the charge that they are harming patients by denying them needed service. Why is similar attention not given to the health and economic consequences of overservice?

This dilemma is evident in comparisons of care quality between HMOs and fee-for-service care even when performed by proponents of HMO care. The policy question of interest generally seems to be whether HMOs are a health hazard. For example, Carlisle and associates concluded that their findings showing that HMOs gave better care in fewer hospital days "provide substantial evidence that enrollment of Medicare recipients into HMOs will not harm their health"—not exactly a ringing endorsement.

At the heart of this discussion and at the heart of most comparisons of care quality between HMOs and FFS, is the orientation of American medicine and most criteria sets toward detecting errors of omission, rather than errors of commission. For example, the lists of criteria for MI care included in the Appendix to the Carlisle paper include only tests and treatments to be performed, not ones to be avoided. This bias in quality of care standards precludes the detection of overservice, which in the case of patients with myocardial infarction might be life-threatening if catheterization, angioplasty, or bypass grafting were done needlessly.

This bias may be contributing to the difficulty that HMOs are having in controlling their rates of cost inflation. Certainly HMOs or other health care providers that deviate from so-called community standards should carefully monitor outcomes and change protocols if there is evidence that patients suffer. But HMOs must also be prepared to challenge standards for which effectiveness data are lacking if they are going to control their own costs and contribute to a more generally cost-effective practice style in the community.

A current example of the community run amuck is screening for prostate cancer using prostate-specific antigen (PSA). Pressures to screen from the urology community, the industry marketing the test, and other well-intentioned agencies have become intense. At Group Health Cooperative, we have carefully reviewed the literature on the efficacy of PSA screening, consulted with experts, and concluded that the regular use of PSA screening in asymptomatic men is unjustified. We are aggressively educating consumers and physicians, studying the impacts of PSA use in our system, and debating local and national proponents of screening (Stuart et al. 1992). It is distressing to consider the energy and resources required to justify *not* doing just one unproved procedure.

Although Carlisle and his associates did not report the organizational characteristics of the HMOs they studied, one can assume that more traditional staff/group model HMOs predominate. If so, his positive findings would appear to confirm older evidence that traditional HMOs provide care of comparable or better quality (Cunningham and Williamson 1980; Luft 1981; Ware et al. 1986; Sloss et al. 1987; Wagner and Bledsoe 1990). Retchin and colleagues studied a larger number of plans, nearly one-half of which were IPAs. In reviewing the literature on HMOs and quality in 1988, Luft warned that the medical environment is changing in ways that make the available data increasingly irrelevant to the policy questions facing HCFA and other payers. These questions concern the performance of newer managed care models, like IPAs, in which FFS physicians provide care to a portion of their patients under some form of capitated arrangement. Did Retchin and associates find greater evidence of early discharge of disabled patients and lower rates of rehabilitation in the traditional group/staff model HMOs in their sample, or were these effects concentrated among newer organizational models?

This is the critical research question. Does the alphabet soup of newer managed care arrangements provide care of equal or better quality than that of either traditional staff/group model HMOs or FFS care? More recent comparisons suggest the hypothesis that the more a managed care organization resembles a staff/group model HMO, the better its performance. I do not know whether Retchin and colleagues have a sufficient sample to examine this hypothesis in their data, but it would be a valuable contribution if they do.

Studies of clinical and financial performance must begin to disaggregate the very heterogeneous group of organizations loosely called HMOs. The disaggregation should be based on characteristics that have been shown or postulated to affect physician performance. If one believes that traditional HMOs have consistently performed well, then the organizational characteristics of particular importance would include: methods of physician selection, methods of physician payment, proportion of each physician's patients enrolled in the HMO, strength of the clinical culture, and care management strategies employed. Older designations like staff, group, or IPA may no longer capture the important differences in organizations.

Traditional HMOs have carefully considered the cultural congruity of physician prospects. This intense selection has been eroded recently somewhat by market forces that have reduced availability and increased the price in some specialties. Recent comparative studies may be corroborating the prejudice of the traditional HMO community that patients are best served when economics is removed from the bedside (Hillman, Pauly, and Kerstein 1989). Financial incentives to reduce tests or referrals might result in potentially deleterious undertreatment. Organizations that place the well-compensated provider on a neutral economic playing field would seem optimal.

The noneconomic influence of HMOs on individual providers will obviously increase as the number of enrollees per provider increases (Hillman, Pauly, and Kerstein 1989). How this influence, whether as "clinical culture" or specific care management strategies, affects care delivery is an area acutely in need of further research. Case-by-case micromanagement strategies such as precertification review and mandatory second opinions appear to exert small effects on utilization, but we know precious little about their impact on care quality or provider quality of life. It would be interesting to know whether HMO2 in the Carlisle paper achieved its potentially dangerous reductions in length of stay through such micromanagement.

Thus, we are left with two well-executed studies using similar methods and criteria developed by the same group yielding somewhat contradictory assessments of the relative quality of HMO and FFS inpatient care. They provide additional evidence that HMOs reduce utilization without short-term adverse consequences. The Carlisle paper also showed that HMOs vary widely in quality and utilization. This observation punctuates the urgent need for studies comparing the different organizational characteristics of HMOs in order to identify characteristics predictive of higher or lower quality of care. However, we cannot expect that those who continue to believe that HMOs are harmful to health will have their minds changed.

References

Cunningham, F. C., and J. W. Williamson. "How Does the Quality of Care in HMOs Compare to That in Other Settings? An Analytic Literature Review: 1958 to 1979." *The Group Health Journal* 1, no. 1 (1980): 4–25.

Fitzgerald, J. F., L. F. Fagan, W. M. Tierney, and R. S. Dittus. "Changing Patterns of Hip Fracture Care before and after Implementation of the Prospective Payment System." *Journal of the American Medical Association* 258, (1987): 218–21.

Hillman, A. L., M. V. Pauly, and J. J. Kerstein. "How Do Financial Incentives Affect Physicians' Clinical Decisions and the Financial Performance of Health Maintenance Organizations?" *New England Journal of Medicine* 321, no. 1 (1989): 86–92.

Luft, H. S. *Health Maintenance Organizations: Dimensions of Performance.* New York: John Wiley and Sons, 1981.

Luft, H. S. "HMOs and the Quality of Care." *Inquiry* 25, no. 1 (1988): 147–56.

Sloss, E. M., E. B. Keeler, R. H. Brook, B. H. Operskolski, G. A. Goldberg, and J. P. Newhouse. "Effect of a Health Maintenance Organization on Physiologic Health." *Annals of Internal Medicine* 106, no. 1 (1987): 130–38.

Stuart, M. E., M. A. Handley, R. S. Thompson, et al. "Clinical Practice and New Technology: Prostate-Specific Antigen (PSA)." *HMO Practice* 6, no. 1 (1992): 5–11.

Wagner, E. H., and T. Bledsoe. "The Rand Health Insurance Experiment and HMOs." *Medical Care* 28, no. 3 (1990): 191–200.

Ware, J. E., R. H. Brook, W. H. Rogers, E. B. Keeler, A. R. Davies, C. D. Sherbourne, G. A. Goldberg, P. Camp, and J. P. Newhouse. Comparison of Health Outcomes at a Health Maintenance Organization with Those of Fee-For-Service Care." *The Lancet* 1 (1986): 1017–22.

General Discussion

Jon Christianson opened the discussion saying that he does not believe these studies settle all of the questions with respect to quality. He said that he was not convinced that Retchin, Brown, and Clement were able, with their data set, to really measure outcomes in the way that they wanted to. They were constrained to a readmission variable, and yet the outcome that they focused on showed a difference in the proportion of patients who were discharged with a neurological deficit. It appears that what the authors truly would have preferred was to have gotten to these people in ten months after discharge to see what had happened to that deficit. If people are discharged early and they have deficits, over time do the deficits disappear? Does it make sense to discharge people early? Should there be a plan for follow-up postdischarge? It is difficult for a nonclinician to know if readmission is too crude a measure, given that these deficits have been identified at discharge. In the concluding part of the paper, this could have been addressed, and the authors could have talked from the clinical standpoint about readmissions as a crude or sensitive measure of how patients of this kind are doing.

Sheldon Retchin commented on the remarks by Jon Christianson and Edward Wagner. He said that the technology of health status measurement sets the stage for doing more such research in the future, not just for stroke patients but in general. Health status measurements are going to have to be a part of whatever health care system might be imposed in the future. We have mortality figures but no systematic way of collecting health status data in the Medicare system except for the Medicare health status registry. There may be some opportunities in the registry, if the sample is large enough, to be able to follow up groups of patients like this to see if there are differences in outcomes.

Dr. Retchin said he wanted to take issue with some of Ed Wagner's remarks. In his opinion, investigators are going to have to continue to look at outcomes and many of those are going to be adverse outcomes. We are ratcheting back on expenditures. While one might be able to speculate that utilization falls in the elderly, one can expect to see some modest improvement in outcomes because of iatrogenesis. But those gains are going to be pretty small. In the long term, one would like to maintain outcomes. One still has to think about adverse outcomes, regardless of whether it is HMO care, reducing fees, or whatever action is taken. It is possible that reducing utilization will lead to improvements, but if reducing utilization does not lead to an increase in adverse outcomes, that is a terrific finding. There is no evidence in the literature to suggest the usefulness of rehabilitative care. Similarly, we looked at echocardiography in the literature, tying process to outcomes. We were trying to see if clinical judgment is active in HMOs. You would expect it to be if you have found at least some evidence of it. We do not know how physicians act on this kind of information. Early in the mid-1970s a study was made of the effects on utilization of reducing intensive care beds. They showed that the mortality rate after myocardial infarctions did not change, and that is the sort of effect we are looking for—that there are no worse outcomes.

Hal Luft commented that he thinks we need to go a step beyond that to look at what the patients want if HMOs become more sensitive to patient preferences. In essence, patients might say they do not want aggressive intervention. They may be interested in quality of life, and if that is impossible they may not want to live. If we focus only on mortality, we may not know that these are people who have chosen less intervention—to live a shorter but happier life with a lot more control. We may inappropriately blame a system for, in effect, giving people what they want. This may not be something that just shows up in "no code" variables; it may be a lot more subtle. Dr. Retchin responded that he thinks this is a fruitful area for study, not only in terms of an evaluative study but also to see what the different interventions in HMO settings are that actually will change the decision making.

Sheila Leatherman said that she wanted to pick up on something Sheldon Retchin said earlier. She said that it is important that we refine the units of analysis, to select more explicitly and realistically the various health care delivery systems and not to function in a polarity between the HMOs versus fee-for-service.

Dr. Retchin responded that he subscribes to that. Early on, he was involved in studies of the effects of different model types on ambulatory care and found that as you move along the continuum to the staff model with financial risk, those models further along are pretty good in terms of compliance with prevention, and so forth. As you look at those kinds of elements of care in the outpatient setting, and perhaps the inpatient setting as well, you are going to see some effects of the delivery system on process.

Louis Rossiter said that he would like to put on a health policy hat as opposed to a health services research hat. He reported on HCFA figures for Medicare contracts with prepaid organizations as of November 1, 1992. There were 95 plans that HCFA paid a total of $639 million in the month of November 1992. Enrollment is going up, and there are 15 pending applications from plans. He went on to say that the HMO program is not going away. HCFA has two ways to pay: fee-for-service and HMOs. HCFA needs to be vigilant in characterizing the whole program, both the fee-for-service and HMO sides of the program. We should stop asking if HMOs are better than FFS, and ask how we can make medical care better.

Part **IV**

Appropriate
Premium Levels

Chapter 10

HMO Market Share and Its Effect on Local Medicare Costs

W. Pete Welch

The payment received by an HMO for its Medicare enrollees is determined by the Medicare average adjusted per capita cost in the fee-for-service sector. The AAPCC is 95 percent of the U.S. average Medicare per capita cost (USPCC) in the fee-for-service sector, adjusted for the demographic characteristics of enrollees in the HMO (the demographic factor) and for local cost differences as measured by the ratio of Medicare costs in the county to costs nationally (the location factor). This formula was designed in the 1970s and has remained basically unchanged.

Since HMOs are only 3 percent of the national Medicare market, their presence currently does not affect costs in the fee-for-service sector in most areas, and, therefore, does not affect their reimbursement. As the HMO market share grows, however, the possibility increases that HMOs will, in fact, influence FFS costs. There are theoretical reasons why HMOs might either increase or decrease FFS costs. If they increase costs—by, for example, attracting lower-cost beneficiaries and leaving a smaller pool of higher-cost beneficiaries in the FFS sector—the current formula will increase HMO reimbursement, even though HMO costs are low relative to FFS costs.

This paper estimates the effect of HMO market share on total Medicare costs and indirectly on FFS costs. If new research should find that the HMO market share has a sizable effect on FFS costs, it would no longer be appropriate to base payments to HMOs on local FFS costs.[1] Alternative ways of calculating payments have been proposed by Rossiter, Adamache, and Faulknier (1990) and Welch (1989).

The Issue

High HMO penetration may affect costs in the fee-for-service sector through four mechanisms: selection, competition, spillover, and the 95 percent formula. The first way would probably increase costs, the second could either increase or decrease costs, and the last two would reduce costs.

Selection generally has been favorable to HMOs. To the extent that HMOs attract healthier clients who require less expensive care than nonenrollees, per capita cost in the FFS sector will increase as lower-cost individuals progressively join HMOs. The average costs of those individuals left in the FFS sector will increase because they are sicker, and HMOs, if paid on the basis of that average, increasingly will be overpaid. A simple numerical example illustrates the point. See Ellis and McGuire (1987) and Feldman and Dowd (1982) for extensive discussions. Suppose that average Medicare FFS costs are $100 per month in a county but that Medicare HMO enrollees would have cost only $80 on average in the FFS sector. As long as HMOs enroll a negligible proportion of the Medicare beneficiaries in the county, the FFS base of $100 will be unaffected and HMOs will be overpaid by 25 percent. Now suppose that half the Medicare beneficiaries in the county are enrolled in HMOs, still with an average cost in the FFS sector of $80. The average cost of those remaining in FFS is no longer $100, but rises to $120. HMOs are now being overpaid by 50 percent. The percentage of overpayment due to biased selection increases with HMO market share. Although much research has been done on selection bias at the individual level (e.g., Scheffler and Rossiter 1985), little is known about selection bias at a county or metropolitan level.

Previous research has shown that selection bias is greater for prepaid group practices than for individual practice associations (Brown 1988). The difference is that PGPs are HMOs in which physicians have only HMO patients, and IPAs are HMOs in which physicians have both HMO and FFS patients. IPAs have a majority of the Medicare beneficiaries enrolled in HMOs and half the enrollment in the general HMO market (Welch 1988).

The second way that HMO penetration may affect FFS costs is through competition between HMOs and fee-for-service physicians in the same health care market. Enthoven (1978) offers two alternative hypotheses. In one scenario, in the face of HMO competition, both conventional insurers and FFS providers might control costs in order to keep premiums and fees low and attract customers (as in the textbook case for any competitive market). In the other scenario, FFS providers, facing a loss of revenue due to loss of business to HMOs, might increase fees or utilization. In this latter scenario—as long as conventional insurers are passive, insurance coverage copayments are low, and consumers are influenced by physicians—higher fees will increase provider income and FFS costs, and competition would have a perverse effect.

In the case of Medicare, the conventional insurer is Medicare itself. Under Medicare regulations, providers have little opportunity to increase price per service, but they have considerable opportunity to increase utilization. And there is evidence that physicians respond to lower fees by increasing utilization (Gabel and Rice 1985). Because Medicare policy is implemented at the national rather than the local level, there is no mechanism for the conventional insurer to use to respond to HMO-induced increases in FFS utilization by containment activities in the local area. In addition, nonprice competition could entail greater accessibility, which might increase utilization. The perverse competitive effect might dominate.

A third way that HMO penetration may affect FFS costs relates to the IPA form of HMO, under which physicians have both HMO and FFS patients. IPAs encourage physicians to practice cost-effective medicine. The encouragements may take the form of capitating physicians for primary care services, sharing the surpluses from lower hospitalization, and utilization review.

In the case of IPAs, cost-effective practices might spill over onto FFS patients, thus reducing FFS expenditures.[2] Whether this happens, and how much, hinges on the extent to which IPA physicians have two very different styles of practice—one for HMO patients and one for FFS patients (Langwell and Hadley 1989, VII-9). It is plausible that each side of the practice influences the other. If so, the cost-controlling effect of HMO practice patterns spilling over onto FFS practice patterns would be attenuated by the reverse effect. However, it is not necessary that FFS patients be treated exactly like HMO patients for the net effects to be cost-reducing, only that the two sides affect each other.

Indirect corroborating evidence of this spillover effect comes from hospitals. Scheffler, Gibbs, and Gurnick (1988) found that Medicare's prospective payment system (PPS) encouraged hospitals to contain the costs of their FFS patients, in particular, those covered by Blue Cross. PPS was estimated to have lowered Blue Cross's inpatient payment by 4 percent in 1986. This spillover between prospectively paid cases and FFS cases in hospitals makes more plausible a spillover between HMO and FFS patients in IPAs.

In addition to the three substantive effects, there is one mechanical effect of HMO market share on Medicare costs in the current reimbursement formula. The current formula reduces Medicare expenditures by 1 percentage point for each 20 percentage points of HMO market share, simply because Medicare pays HMOs 95 percent of FFS costs.

The bulk of the literature so far suggests that the impact of HMO market share on the FFS sector may not be great. McLaughlin (1987), for example, found that PGP enrollment had no significant impact on hospital expenses per capita. In a careful review of the data from three areas with high HMO penetration—Hawaii, Rochester, and Minneapolis–St. Paul—Luft, Maerki and Trauner (1986) supported this finding; reported reductions in hospital use in these areas could not be plausibly attributed to HMO growth. Feldman et al. (1986) also found no impact on hospital costs per admission in the Twin Cities between 1979 and 1981. However, Dowd (1986) came to a somewhat different conclusion. Admission rates in the Twin Cities dropped sharply between 1978 and 1982 (2.8 percent per year compared to 0.3 percent for the nation). Half of this drop was attributed to consumers switching from FFS to HMOs and the other half to the drop in admission rates in the FFS sector, a spillover effect.

Only Rossiter (1989) has investigated the impact of HMO market share on Medicare costs. In his simultaneous equation model, the dependent variables were HMO market share in 1986 and the AAPCC rate in 1987, which is based on average Medicare expenditures in a county between 1980 and 1984. The county is the unit of analysis, and two-stage least squares were used. HMO market share in 1986 was found to have a positive effect on the AAPCC rate in 1987.

None of these studies used expenditure data more recent than 1984, however. The data used here may shed more light on the issue because they are for the 1984–1987 period, a period when Medicare HMO enrollment grew rapidly.

Methodology

The metropolitan statistical area (MSA) is used as the local area, rather than the county, as is used by Medicare, because the MSA is a better approximation of a market area ($N = 295$ in the data set). Patients often cross county lines to seek medical care but rarely leave their metropolitan area. All regression analyses are weighted by the population in the applicable MSA, and the data pertain to 1984–1987. The year 1984 is a good baseline, because it was the last year when Medicare HMO enrollment was restricted to the Medicare competition demonstration sites, and 1987 was the most recent year for which data were available. Finally, Medicare enrollment is defined as the enrollment of beneficiaries in HMOs with TEFRA-risk contracts, including enrollment under the Medicare competition demonstrations. Medicare HMO cost contracts are excluded because the incentives are quite different.

Dependent variable and functional form

The dependent variable is Medicare expenditures per beneficiary adjusted by a demographic factor. It was not possible to analyze FFS expenditures per FFS beneficiary, because FFS and HMO expenditures cannot reliably be separated in the data. (See the data section for further discussion.) To facilitate interpretation of the coefficients, the expenditure variable is defined in terms of percentage of the national mean. Each MSA's expenditures in 1987 (times 100) is divided by the national mean expenditure in 1987 (the weighted mean of all MSAs). That is,

$$E_m = (e_m/DF_m)/(e_{US}/DF_{US}) * 100 \qquad (1)$$

where e_m and e_{US} are the expenditures per beneficiary in metropolitan area m and in all metropolitan areas, respectively, and DF is a demographic factor that adjusts for age, sex, and mortality.[3] The expenditure variable for other years is defined the same way. Expenditure growth rates by state vary considerably from year to year (Congressional Research Service 1989, Table 6-1). This means that analyses of expenditure growth rates by state, MSA, or county are likely to be sensitive to the choice of base year and end year. This variance appears to be, in part, an artifact of the claims processing system.[4] Suppose, for instance, that in one state expenditures for an extra two months of 1986 were processed in 1987. Then the 1986 expenditures figure would reflect 10 months of experience, the 1987 expenditures figure would reflect 14 months of experience, and the 1987 growth rate would be incorrectly high.

To mitigate this problem (but not solve it), the dependent variable is the average expenditure over two years, 1986 and 1987. Although many variables traditionally are defined over a 12-month period, there is no institutional or theoretical reason why expenditures should be so defined in this paper. This variable is denoted E_{86-87}, and its summary statistics are presented in Table 10.1. The other key variable (market share) is also defined biennially. This approach corrects some situations—for instance, in which extra months of expenditures are shifted from 1986 to 1987, but not other situations—for instance, in which extra months of expenditures are shifted from 1987 to 1988.[5]

As a check on the robustness of the results, at one point expenditures for Parts A and B represent separate dependent variables. Part A claims are processed by intermediaries and Part B claims are mainly processed by carriers, so that claims-processing aberrations should be independent between Parts A and B. To presage the results, regressions of Parts A and B yield similar coefficients.

Table 10.1 Summary Statistics for Market Share and Expenditure Variables (For All MSAs, Weighted by MSA Population)

Variable	Mean	s.d.
HMO Market Share		
HMO 1986–1987	3.2	6.0
Expenditure per Beneficiary*		
1984–1985	2473	487.1
1984–1985, as percent of national mean for MSAs	100.0	19.7
1986–1987	2989	534.8
1986–1987, as percent of national mean for MSAs	100.0	17.9
$N = 313$		

*Adjusted for PPS policy changes and for age, sex, and mortality of Medicare beneficiaries (whether enrolled in HMOs or not).

I specify a partial adjustment model. The equilibrium level of expenditure in 1986–1987 (E_{86-87}^*) is a function of a vector of independent variables (M):

$$E_{86-87}^* = M\beta \tag{2}$$

where β is a vector of coefficients. The rate of adjustment is specified as

$$E_{86-87} - E_{84-85} = \alpha(E_{86-87}^* - E_{84-85}) + u_{86-87} \tag{3}$$

where α is the coefficient indicating the speed of adjustment. Inserting (2) into (3), and rearranging, yields

$$E_{86-87} = (1 - \alpha)E_{84-85} + M\beta\alpha \tag{4}$$

A simpler functional form would exclude E_{84-85} as an explanatory variable. The advantage of the partial adjustment model is its recognization that the expenditure level may not adjust completely and immediately to changes in market conditions and its other factors (M). Rather, the adjustment may take a number of years. Including E_{84-85} makes the functional form more general and allows for testing whether adjustment is instantaneous. The results below reject the hypothesis of instantaneous adjustment.[6]

Given this form, the market share coefficient can be readily interpreted. A market share coefficient of .5 indicates, for example, that a one percentage point increase in market share increases expenditures by .5 percentage points. The coefficient on expenditures in 1984–1985 is expected to be between 0 and 1, by the following logic: the higher expenditures are in 1984–1985, the higher expenditures will be in 1986–1987.

But the higher expenditures are in 1984–1985, the slower the growth in expenditures will be.

Independent variables

The choice of variables related to HMO market share involves two issues. First, one could measure either the proportion of Medicare beneficiaries enrolled in HMOs or the proportion of the general population enrolled. Whereas the HMO share of the Medicare market can be measured precisely using the Medicare data system, the HMO share of the general market cannot be reliably measured at the metropolitan area level. Individual HMOs, which have data available only at the plan level, often have enrollment in several MSAs (U.S. Office of Personnel Management 1986). Exploratory analysis with 1986 expenditure data found market share of Medicare to be significant but market share of the general population to be insignificant. Hence, the HMO share of the Medicare market is used.

Second, PGP enrollment and IPA enrollment might be included separately, because the hypothesized effects are different for the two types of HMO. However, the correlation between PGP and IPA market share is .91. Maddala (1977, p. 185) states that high multicollinearity can yield individual coefficients with incorrect signs or with magnitudes that are meaningless. Such was the case when both PGP and IPA market share variables were included. Given this, I chose to ignore the PGP-IPA distinction except for presenting market share by these components by MSA in Table 3 below. (Multicollinearity was also a problem when the HMO share of the general market was included.) Given that the expenditure variables are defined biennially, market share is also defined biennially.

Besides HMO market share, a number of variables might affect the change in Medicare expenditures between 1984 and 1987. (See Table 10.2 for the precise definitions of these variables.) This paper introduces two price variables, three demand variables, and five supply variables.[7] Demographic characteristics and beneficiary health status are also important, and their effects are captured by a composite variable that is used to deflate the dependent variable (see Equation 1).

The two largest components of Medicare spending are for hospitals and physicians. The price effect of the former is measured with the HCFA hospital wage index and of the latter with an index of prevailing charges for physicians.

The demand variables are intended to capture the effect on demand of the ability of beneficiaries to pay Medicare's out-of-pocket costs— either copayments or balance billing. The first variable is the proportion of the elderly with additional insurance coverage. The second is the assignment rate (the proportion of physician bills for which physicians

Table 10.2 Summary Statistics for Other Variables (For All MSAs, Weighted by MSA Population)

Variable	Definition	Mean	s.d.
Price			
Hospital wage	HCFA hospital wage index	1.11	0.15
Prevailing charge	Prevailing charge index (charges are weighted by frequency of service)	1.15	0.21
Demand			
Other insurance	Percent of the elderly with supplemental insurance (Medigap, Medicaid, VA, etc.)	58.2	7.1
Assignment rate	Assigned charges as a percent of total charges	65.4	15.0
Income	Per capita income of the elderly (in $1000s)	12.93	1.18
Supply			
Beds/1000	Hospital beds per 1000 population	5.10	1.61
Physicians/1000	Physicians per 1000 population	1.53	0.40
Primary care physicians	Primary care physicians (general practitioners, family practitioners, pediatricians, internists, and OB/GYNs) as a percent of all office-based physicians	44.8	3.1
Elderly population	Elderly as a percent of total population	10.4	2.9
Population size	MSA population (log)	7.1	1.2

Sources: Area Resource File, except as follows: income and other insurance are predicted from the Current Population Survey, and the prevailing charge index and the assignment rate were developed from Medicare administrative files (Holahan, Dor, and Zuckerman 1991).

do not charge beneficiaries anything beyond Medicare's allowed charge). The third is the per capita income of the elderly.

On the supply side, the specification includes three obvious variables: hospital beds per 1,000 population, physicians per 1,000 population, and the percentage of physicians who are primary care physicians. In addition, to reflect the fact that the elderly have higher utilization than the nonelderly, the percentage of the population that is elderly is entered. Finally, since utilization tends to be greatest in large metropolitan areas, the population of the metropolitan area is entered (in log form). (For convenience, the metropolitan area variable is classified here as a supply effect, but it could also be a demand effect.)

The issue of simultaneity bias

One methodological issue that needs to be addressed is simultaneity: that is, HMO market share affects expenditures, but expenditures also affect market share. Adamache and Rossiter (1986) found that HMOs were most likely to sign Medicare risk contracts in areas with high Medicare costs and high AAPCC payment. Although this may suggest the need for two-stage least square estimates of HMO Medicare market share and market costs, that technique is not necessary here because the independent variable is lagged and unrelated to the disturbance term. In other words, the equations constitute a recursive system, which can be estimated with ordinary least squares (OLS).

To illustrate this point simply, consider this model:

$$E_{86-87} = f(M_{86}, M_{87}, E_{84-85}) + u_{1,86-87} \tag{5}$$

where M is now HMO market share ($PGP + IPA$) and u's are the disturbance terms. (All variables are implicitly subscripted for MSA. The average for M_{86} and M_{87} is actually used.) This partial adjustment equation is derived from two equations that describe the equilibrium and the adjustment rate. The disturbance error is in the adjustment equation, and hence is year specific (Johnston 1972).

As demonstrated by Adamache and Rossiter,

$$M_{87} = f(AAPCC_{87}, X) + u_{2,87} \tag{6}$$

where X is a vector of independent variables. To simplify the formula, the $AAPCC$ can be written as:

$$AAPCC_{87} = (E_{80} + \ldots + E_{84})/5 \tag{7}$$

By substitution, we have

$$M_{87} = f[(E_{80} + \ldots + E_{84})/5, X] + u_{2,87} \tag{8}$$

OLS estimators of Equation 5 are unbiased *if* each independent variable is uncorrelated with the disturbance term ($u_{1,86-87}$). The key simultaneity bias issue is whether M_{87} and $u_{1,86-87}$ are correlated. What reason do we have to believe that they are correlated? By Equation 8, M_{87} is a function of E_{84-85}, but that is different from being a function of E_{86-87}. So the issue becomes one of whether $u_{1,86-87}$ is correlated with E_{84-85} (and hence M_{87}).

Although E_{84-85} and E_{86-87} are presumably correlated, there is no reason to believe that E_{84-85} is correlated with $u_{1,86-87}$, because $u_{1,86-87}$ is year-specific. Since these equations are recursive, OLS is the appropriate estimation technique.

It is instructive to compare this model with a related model that uses two-stage least squares: McLaughlin's (1987) simultaneous equation model of hospital costs and HMO market share. I use my notation for simplicity. She specified E_{87} (which represented hospital costs) as a function of M_{87} and other variables, and M_{87} was specified to be a function of E_{87} and other variables. Her specification differs from mine in two relevant ways: a lagged dependent variable was not entered as an explanatory variable, and market share was a function of hospital costs in the same year. In the general HMO market, which was her concern, the determination of HMO rates is not known, and McLaughlin could not safely assume that market share was affected by costs lagged by several years. But for Medicare HMOs, my concern, the formula is established by regulation.

Data

Expenditure data

The source of expenditure data was the AAPCC Master File, created by the Office of the Actuary (OACT) and the Bureau of Data Management and Strategy (BDMS) of the Health Care Financing Administration. This version (which was the basis of payment to HMOs in 1990) had expenditures for 1983 through 1987. The Office of the Actuary makes available raw expenditure data and expenditure data modeled for PPS. This latter file has the expenditures, say, in 1987, that would have occurred if 1990 PPS rules were in effect. For instance, if between 1987 and 1990 the transition to national rates will increase PPS expenditures in a county by 2 percent, the 1987 PPS expenditures are inflated by 2 percent. I used the modeled expenditure figures in order to factor out the effect of PPS changes between 1984 and 1987.

I had hoped to analyze expenditures in the fee-for-service sector, but OACT suggested that the data on HMO expenditures were not reliable. This is because, prior to April 1988, HMOs had the option of paying hospitals through Medicare's fiscal intermediaries, and Medicare's data systems have not distinguished between hospital payments on behalf of HMOs and those on behalf of FFS beneficiaries. To calculate the location factor, OACT first adds FFS and HMO expenditures, which include payments on behalf of HMOs and direct Medicare payments to HMOs. Then it subtracts projected direct and indirect payments to HMOs (Palsbo 1989). OACT apparently believes that the law gives it little choice but to subtract HMO payments, which are estimated as well as possible.

Therefore, I calculated an average expenditure per beneficiary as the ratio of "program reimbursement with pass-through" plus "direct GHP reimbursement" to "program enrollment." This was calculated for the aged for Part A and Part B separately, and the two figures were summed. The Medicare variables—HMO market share and expenditures—pertain to the aged beneficiaries.

Other variables

Per capita income of the elderly and the percentage of the elderly with additional insurance were derived from the current population survey (CPS). Because of small sample size, raw figures for small MSAs are subject to stochastic error. Therefore, a regression equation was used to predict such values (Holahan, Dor, and Zuckerman 1991).

Other variables were derived from Medicare administrative files and the Area Resource File.

Results

Tables 10.1 and 10.2, shown earlier, present the means and standard deviations of the variables used in the analysis. Table 10.3 has several key variables for the 35 MSAs in which the HMO share of Medicare exceeded 7.5 percent as of July 1, 1987. HMO market share was above 25 percent in only three MSAs, all in Minnesota: Duluth, Minneapolis–St. Paul, and St. Cloud.

Of the 35 MSAs in Table 10.3, 13 MSAs had faster expenditure growth than the national average for MSAs, but fully 22 MSAs had slower than average growth. Among the eight MSAs where HMO market share in 1987 exceeded 20 percent, two MSAs had faster than average growth but six had slower than average growth. These results suggest that HMOs may have slowed expenditure growth. Needless to say, this analysis does not control for other determinants of expenditures. Hence, I now turn to regression analysis.

As presented in Table 10.4, the coefficient of the HMO market share is negative and significant at 10 percent. (As noted further on, it is significant at 5 percent for Part B.) An increase of 10 percentage points lowers Medicare cost by 1.2 percent.[8]

This market share coefficient represents the short-run impact of HMO market share. To the extent that market share in 1986–1987 lowers expenditures in 1986–1987, in a partial adjustment model it will lower expenditures further in 1988–1989. Given that the lagged expenditures variable has a coefficient of .82, the long-term impact of market share is more than five times the short-run impact.[9] Of the coefficient of .12, .05 represents the impact of the 95 percent formula. By law this effect occurs immediately. Only the remaining .07 represents phenomena whose long-run effect may exceed their short-run impacts. Hence, an increase of ten percentage points in HMO market share decreases expenditures by 1.2 percent in the short run and by as much as 3.9 (i.e., .07/[1 − .82]) percent in the long run.[10]

Table 10.3   MSAs and Rural Areas with HMO Market Share Above 7.5 Percent

MSA or Rural Area*	HMO Market 1984 PGP	1984 IPA	1987 PGP	1987 IPA	Expenditure/ Beneficiary 1986–1987 (%)	Expenditure Growth 1984–1987 (%)
Albuquerque, NM	0.0	0.0	9.6	13.4	84	2.4
Anaheim–Santa Ana, CA	0.4	0.3	5.8	6.6	127	−0.5
Ann Arbor, MI	0.0	0.0	2.2	6.3	112	13.3
Colorado Springs, CO	0.0	0.0	4.7	5.2	87	11.6
Daytona Beach, FL	0.0	0.1	2.8	4.7	83	−0.8
Denver, CO	0.0	0.0	6.0	5.1	104	5.3
Duluth, MN	4.8	1.6	17.9	13.5	72	−7.1
Fargo-Moorhead, MN	0.0	0.0	2.8	6.7	81	−6.4
Flint, MI	0.7	4.5	2.6	7.8	129	1.2
Ft. Lauderdale–Hollywood– Pompano Beach, FL	1.8	9.1	7.3	11.9	123	−4.8
Honolulu, HI	0.0	0.0	4.2	17.9	90	−1.0
Indianapolis, IN	1.1	0.7	4.3	4.6	94	0.6
Lansing–E. Lansing, MI	1.9	1.6	2.8	6.3	98	4.5
Las Vegas, NV	0.0	0.0	7.1	8.4	104	−3.1
Lawrence, KS	0.0	0.0	3.7	10.3	80	−3.8
Los Angeles–Long Beach, CA	0.7	0.4	4.4	4.8	136	−3.3
Miami-Hialeah, FL	2.1	6.9	6.7	10.3	146	−4.3
Minneapolis–St. Paul, MN	13.9	2.9	23.2	21.9	96	−9.7
Oxnard-Ventura, CA	0.0	0.0	3.2	4.3	117	1.8
Pittsfield, MA	0.0	0.0	3.8	8.7	92	1.5
Portland, OR	3.9	0.6	9.7	7.7	91	−8.0
Pueblo, CO	0.0	0.0	16.2	5.6	81	3.8
Reno, NV	0.0	0.0	4.6	5.8	89	−10.2
Riverside–San Bernardino, CA	0.0	0.0	5.4	7.1	110	1.5
Rochester, NY	2.3	1.1	5.9	9.8	84	−0.8
St. Cloud, MN	1.2	0.2	15.5	32.8	74	−7.9
Salem, OR	0.1	0.0	4.3	3.4	73	−11.0
San Diego, CA	0.0	0.0	4.2	5.9	114	−0.4
San Francisco, CA	0.0	0.0	5.1	5.6	114	−2.1
Springfield, MA	1.0	0.5	6.2	2.3	85	−2.9
Tampa–St. Pete–Clearwater, FL	1.3	5.2	3.9	7.2	93	0.3
Vancouver, WA	5.2	0.9	12.0	8.1	75	−9.5
W. Palm Beach–Boca Raton– Delray, FL	2.1	9.3	5.0	8.7	104	−0.1

Continued

Table 10.3   Continued

MSA or Rural Area*	HMO Market				Expenditure/ Beneficiary	Expenditure Growth
	1984		1987			
	PGP	IPA	PGP	IPA	1986–1987 (%)	1984–1987 (%)
Wichita, KS	0.0	0.0	3.0	9.3	100	2.0
Worcester, MA	7.5	2.0	13.2	8.8	100	−2.6
Rural Hawaii	0.0	0.0	4.4	15.9	—	—
Rural Minnesota	0.1	0.0	5.8	9.4	—	—
Rural Nevada	0.0	0.0	3.5	4.4	—	—

*Rural areas are included here for background purposes and are excluded from all subsequent analyses. Expenditure per beneficiary and growth rate are adjusted for age, sex, and mortality. Expenditure per beneficiary is a percentage of the national mean for MSAs. The growth rate pertains to expenditure growth (relative to the national mean) between 1984–1985 and 1986–1987. Hence, a growth rate of 0 implies that expenditures grew at the national mean for MSAs.

Lagged expenditures have, as expected in partial adjustment models, a coefficient between 0 and 1. This indicates that MSAs with high expenditures in 1984–1985 tended to have slower growth rates in percentage terms. The other significant coefficients indicate that expenditures are higher: where the elderly commonly have other insurance, where few physicians are primary care physicians, and in MSAs with large populations.

Separate regressions for Part A and Part B expenditures were run with the same independent variables. The HMO market share had coefficients of −.13 (t = 1.79) and −.14 (t = 2.23) for Part A and Part B, respectively. Their coefficients are close to each other and to the coefficient for Parts A and B combined. These results suggest that HMOs encourage a lower admission rate, since Medicare pays a prospective price. It furthermore appears that HMOs encourage lower utilization in terms of physician and other Part B services.

Part A claims and Part B claims are processed through different fiscal intermediaries. If, in one state, extra Part A claims were shifted from one year to the next, there is no particular reason why Part B claims would be similarly shifted. The fact that HMO market share decreases both Part A and B expenditures lowers the likelihood that HMOs' negative impact is an artifact of the claims processing system.

Under the AAPCC formula, lower expenditures in an area with substantial HMO enrollment do not affect Medicare payments to HMO for several years. The expenditures in 1987 affect payment starting in 1990. The apparent lower expenditures due to HMO market share are just beginning to affect HMO payment.

Table 10.4   Expenditure Regression (Weighted by MSA Population)

Independent Variable	
HMO market share, 1986–1987	−0.12
	(1.94)
Expenditures per beneficiary, 1984–1985†	0.82*
	(21.48)
Price	
Hospital wage	1.30
	(0.33)
Prevailing charge	−3.81
	(1.34)
Demand	
Other insurance	0.24*
	(3.96)
Assignment rate	0.03
	(0.93)
Income	−0.06
	(0.17)
Supply	
Beds/1000	0.20
	(0.80)
Physicians/1000	−0.34
	(0.23)
Primary care physicians	−0.35*
	(2.82)
Elderly population	−0.20
	(1.47)
Population Size	1.91*
	(4.45)
Intercept	10.04
R-square 0.909	
F 234*	
N 295	

*Significant at $p < .05$.

†The dependent variable is the average of expenditures per beneficiary in 1986 and 1987, as a percent of the national mean for MSAs and adjusted for age, sex, and mortality of Medicare beneficiaries (whether enrolled in HMOs or not). Expenditures in 1984–1985 are similarly defined.

Conclusion

The paper predicts that an HMO Medicare market share of 10 percent will decrease Medicare expenditures per beneficiary in an MSA by 1.2 percent. (By itself, the 95 percent formula lowers expenditures by only 0.5 percent.) For the three MSAs that have HMO market shares exceeding 25 percent, this result suggests that expenditures will be decreased by at least 3.0 percent in the short run. In the long run expenditures could fall by as much as 9.7 percent. This result is consistent with the recent finding of Robinson (1991) that hospital costs in California grew more slowly in areas with a high HMO market share. The result parallels the finding of Scheffler, Gibbs, and Gurnick (1988) that PPS has had a spillover effect in terms of lowering the growth of Blue Cross costs. However, the result is apparently inconsistent with the literature on selection bias, the thrust of which is that HMOs attract healthier clients who require less expensive care than nonenrollees. As noted above, this is likely to increase total costs.

The two sets of findings are based on different methodologies. The unit of analysis is the market area in the spillover analyses, whereas it is the individual in the selection bias literature. Also, the spillover analyses compare the level of expenditures after HMO enrollment growth (controlling for expenditures prior to growth), whereas the selection bias literature compares the level of expenditures of two groups before possible HMO enrollment. The results are not necessarily inconsistent: in particular, HMOs may experience favorable selection, but their spillover effect may more than compensate. Selection may be less than pre-enrollment comparisons suggest, perhaps because of regression toward the mean (Welch 1985).

Not surprisingly, more work is needed on this topic. Within the general methodological approach taken here, several elaborations are possible. The most straightforward would be adding more years of data. The longer the time period, the more plausible any correlation between HMO market share and lower expenditures. Stochasticity, such as due to claims processing, has less effect in longer periods, and the idea that HMO styles of practice spill over into FFS medicine becomes more plausible as a mechanism. Another elaboration would be investigation of the impact by different HMO types. A problem here is that the PGP-IPA distinction is probably an inadequate classification scheme, but recognition of this in a regression model would increase probable multicollinearity.

A more important elaboration would be using HMO share of the general market, as distinct from the Medicare-only market, as the key independent variable. Just as it is plausible that practice patterns might spill over from the HMO to the FFS sides of a physician's practice, so might they spill over from the non-Medicare to the Medicare side. The difficulty here is obtaining data by market area for non-Medicare enrollment, particularly in a time-series.

Often new insights and results are best obtained by introducing a new unit of analysis rather than tinkering with the old one. Along these lines, the unit of analysis could be a physician's practice. The hypothesis of spillover would be strengthened by finding that as IPA enrollees increase, a physician's style of practice becomes more conservative for FFS patients.

The introduction raised the policy issue of how to pay HMOs in areas with high HMO market share. As the HMO market share in an area increases, using the FFS sector as the basis for HMO payment loses its straightforward appeal. Both HMO advocates and critics have had suspicions that large HMO market share affects FFS costs (albeit, often in opposite ways). The results here, although not definitive, tend to confirm those suspicions. If Medicare enrollment in HMOs ever threatens to increase rapidly, HCFA should consider moving away from basing HMO payments on local FFS costs.

Acknowledgments

Support for this research was provided by the Health Care Financing Administration to the Urban Institute through Grant no. 17-C-99223/3-01. Any opinions expressed are those of the author and not the Urban Institute or its sponsors. The author appreciates the assistance of Clifton Maze of OACT, Lynn Rabey and Bob Fortenbaugh of BDMS, Bob Bryant, Thy Dao, John Holahan, Steve Zuckerman, Marianna Diggs, Brian Dowd, Will Manning, Karen Mitchell, Ranjit Dighe, Stephen Norton, Al Peden, James Beebe, Felicity Skidmore, and Kathy Langwell.

Notes

1. Even a desirable effect on FFS costs could have an undesirable effect on HMO payments. For instance, suppose the HMO market share caused the fee-for-service sector to lower its costs to some efficient level. This impact, although desirable, would result in Medicare paying HMOs 95 percent of efficient costs, which would be neither fair nor sustainable.
2. PGPs may also have a spillover effect if the conservative style of practice of PGPs has an impact on local medical norms in the FFS sector.
3. Methodologically, this adjustment factor differs from the one used by HCFA's Office of the Actuary only by the addition of mortality as a predictor of expenditures.

4. Claims are attributed to a year according to their process date (that is, approval for payment), not when the service was rendered or when payment was made (Palsbo 1989).
5. This problem is a major reason why the adjustment of HMO payment for local cost differences is based on five years of data rather than on data for a shorter period. Because of interest in the impact of increased HMO market share on expenditures, I must calculate expenditures based on fewer years. Note also that expenditures for a year are first defined as a percentage of the national mean and are then averaged over years.
6. Because of the lagged dependent variable, the estimator is consistent only if there is no autocorrelation. As noted below, the estimate of the key coefficient changes slightly when instrumental variables are used.
7. I am indebted to John Holahan for supplying these data.
8. Using instrumental variables, the estimated coefficient is $-.10$ ($t = 1.57$). Hence, the finding of a negative impact appears robust with respect to econometric assumptions.
9. Let β_i represent the coefficient estimates in Equation 6:

$$E_{86-87} = \beta_0 + \beta_1 E_{84-85} = \beta_2 M$$

β_2 represents the short-run impact of HMO market share and $\beta_2/(1 - \beta_1)$ represents the long-term effect.
10. The coefficient of the lagged expenditure variable captures MSA-specific factors that are not controlled by other explanatory variables. Hence, the speed of adjustment is understated and the long-term effect is overstated. The estimate of 3.9 must be treated as an upper bound on the long-term effect of market share.

References

Adamache, K. W., and L. F. Rossiter. 1986. "The Entry of HMOs into the Medicare Market: Implications for TEFRA's Mandate." *Inquiry* 23 (Winter 1986): 239–364.

Brown, R. S. "Biased Selection in the Medicare Competition Demonstrations." Report to HCFA under contract #500-83-0047. Princeton, NJ: Mathematica Policy Research, Inc., 1988.

Congressional Research Service. "Prospective Budgeting for Medicare's Physician Service." Washington, DC: CRS, 1989.

Dowd, B. E. "HMOs and Twin Cities Admission Rates." *Health Services Research* 21 (June 1986, Part I): 177–88.

Ellis, R. P., and T. G. McGuire. "Setting Capitation Payments in Markets for Health Services." *Health Care Financing Review* 8 (Summer 1987): 55–64.

Enthoven, A. "Competition of Alternative Delivery Systems." In *Competition in the Health Care Sector*, edited by W. Greenberg. Germantown, MD: Aspen Systems, 1978.

Feldman, R. D., and B. E. Dowd. "Simulation of a Health Insurance Market with Adverse Selection." *Operations Research* 30 (November–December 1982): 1027–42.

Feldman, R., B. Dowd, D. McCann, and A. Johnson. "The Competitive Impact of Health Maintenance Organizations on Hospital Finances: An Exploratory Study." *Journal of Health Politics, Policy and Law* 10, no. 4 (Winter 1986): 675–98.

Gabel, J., and T. Rice. "Reducing Public Expenditures for Physician Services: The Price of Paying Less." *Journal of Health Politics, Policy and Law* 9, no. 4 (Winter 1985): 595–609.

Health Care Financing Administration, Bureau of Data Management and Strategy. *1987 HCFA Statistics*. HCFA Publication No. 03252, Washington, DC, September 1987.

Holahan, J., A. Dor, and S. Zuckerman. "Medicare Physician Expenditures: Sorting Out the Reasons for Growth." Washington, DC: Urban Institute working paper #3650-06, January 1991.

Johnston, J. *Econometric Methods*. New York: McGraw-Hill, 1972.

Langwell, K. and J. Hadley. "National Evaluation of the Medicare Competition Demonstrations, Summary Report." Report to HCFA under contract #500-83-0047. Princeton, NJ: Mathematica Policy Research, Inc., 1989.

Luft, H. S., S. C. Maerki, and J. B. Trauner. "The Competitive Effects of Health Maintenance Organizations: Another Look at the Evidence from Hawaii, Rochester, and Minneapolis/St. Paul." *Journal of Health Politics, Policy and Law* 10 (Winter 1986): 625–58.

Maddala, G. S. *Econometrics*. New York: McGraw-Hill, 1977.

McLaughlin, C. G. "HMO Growth and Hospital Expenses and Use: Simultaneous-Equation Approach." *Health Services Research* 22 (June 1987): 183–205.

Palsbo, S. J. "The AAPCC Explained." Group Health Association of America, Inc., Research Brief No. 8, February, 1989.

Robinson, J. C. "HMO Market Penetration and Hospital Cost Inflation in California," *Journal of the American Medical Association* 266 (20 November 1991): 2719–23.

Rossiter, L. F. "An Analysis of Long-Run Rate Setting Strategies for Risk-Based Contracting under Medicare." Report to HCFA. Williamson Institute for Health Studies, Richmond, VA, 9 March 1989.

Rossiter, L. F., K. W. Adamache, and T. Faulknier. "A Blended Sector Rate Adjustment for the Medicare AAPCC When Risk-Based Market Penetration Is High." *Journal of Risk and Insurance* 57 (June 1990): 220–39.

Scheffler, R. M., J. O. Gibbs, and D. A. Gurnick. "The Impact of Medicare's Prospective Payment System and Private Sector Initiatives: Blue Cross Experience, 1980–1986." School of Public Health, University of California, Berkeley. Report under HCFA Grant No. 15-C-98757/5-01, July 1988.

Scheffler, R. M., and L. F. Rossiter. 1985. *Advances in Health Economics and Health Services Research*. Vol. 6. Greenwich, CT: JAI Press, 1985.

U.S Office of Personnel Management. "1987 Enrollment Information Guide and Plan Comparison Chart." Washington, DC (pamphlet), 1986.

Welch, W. P. "Regression Toward the Mean in Medical Care Costs: Implications for Biased Selection in Health Maintenance Organizations," *Medical Care* 23 (November 1985): 1234–41.

———. "Individual Practice Associations: The Dominant Form of HMO." *Business and Health* 5 (February 1988): 14–16.

———. "Improving Medicare Payments to HMOs: Urban Core Versus Suburban Ring." *Inquiry* 26 (Spring 1989): 62–71.

Chapter 11

Strengths and Weaknesses of the AAPCC: When Does Risk Adjustment Become Cost Reimbursement?

Louis F. Rossiter, Herng-Chia Chiu, and Sheau-Hwa Chen

There are two significant conflicting facts about the nearly decade-long experience with the Medicare HMO risk contract program. On one hand, since the early demonstrations in 1981–1982, research on biased selection for Medicare risk contracts has consistently shown that a disproportionate number of plans experience favorable selection. By implication, the favorable selection has led to excess profits. On the other hand, only about 142 risk contract HMOs participated in the program at the beginning of 1991, enrolling 1.6 million beneficiaries. This enrollment represents about 4 percent of the total number of beneficiaries, or about 9 percent of those with the HMO option available in their area, and fewer than 25 percent of the number of federally qualified HMOs.

No one has satisfactorily answered the most conspicuous policy question about the Medicare risk program. If profits can be so easily made by risk contractors because of biased selection without even changing inefficient fee-for-service practices, why are only a fraction of the eligible HMOs participating in the program? The research studies show favorable selection, while the HMOs complain that the payment rate is too low given the risk they are expected to bear. What logic or data reconcile these two conflicting, longstanding facts about the program?

The purpose of this paper is to try to square the research on biased selection with the behavior in the market. The path to reconciliation yields the conclusion that some sort of risk adjustments beyond those used in the current AAPCC formula are required. But the risks should be for the health risks of the enrollees, not the business risks of the plans. Thus, while appropriate adjustments are required, that in no way means that HMOs should be guaranteed their costs.

Most research in the area of risk adjustments has been in vain because investigators have focused on individual data, not group data. Too often, we have slavishly adhered to simple statistical measures, like the R-square, to identify the best predictor models. A reorientation toward predictions of group means and distributions is required in the field. New approaches, such as the most promising new risk adjustment technique, the six-equation group adjustment model (SEGA model), should be studied and properly evaluated as the modifier for the AAPCC.

We begin the discussion with a review of the measurement and policy issues surrounding biased selection and then develop an example from actual Medicare risk contract data to illustrate how the SEGA model can be used to modify the AAPCC formula. A proposed plan of action in the near term and the long term is included in the last section.

The TEFRA HMO Conundrum

The conundrum. Why does research show that the plans should make excess profits through biased selection alone, yet the plans assert that payments are too low, and many HMOs avoid the market entirely?

By law, HCFA must pay HMOs 95 percent of what would have been paid had the HMO enrollees remained in the fee-for-service sector (Palsbo 1989). Thus the goal of the risk-based payment system is *not* to pay the HMOs their costs. It is *not* to make the HMOs whole in an actuarial sense for their costs (Cookson 1983). The system is inherently designed to create competition between the fee-for-service and risk-based sectors. HMOs that can deliver services more efficiently than the fee-for-service sector should thrive. Inefficient plans should fail or will not enter the market.

Some say that, if the AAPCC calculation is accurate, and HMOs do not enter the market or quit the market after trying it for a few years (Tompkins and Porell 1988), this demonstrates that HMOs are not economically competitive. Because most studies show that HMOs have lower costs, especially for hospital care, the notion that they are not competitive is difficult to accept in a market where hospital services predominate (Gold and Hodges 1989). Nevertheless, one explanation for the TEFRA HMO conundrum is:

Explanation 1. Most HMOs are not as efficient as the fee-for-service sector for elderly enrollees.

Most HMOs take their knowledge of patient care from enrolling relatively healthy employed individuals and families. The elderly and disabled Medicare beneficiary represents a far different set of medical conditions and multiple medical conditions. The economist would say that the production function for delivery of care to the elderly differs from that function for the normal population served by HMOs. It is entirely possible that most HMOs have not made the necessary investment in learning how to care efficiently for the elderly. Thus the payment system is accurate and adequate; it is just that HMOs cannot meet market expectations.

Another explanation for the conflict between the research and market experience is:

Explanation 2. The research on biased selection has not measured what really needs to be measured.

Not that the research itself is flawed, but the techniques for measuring biased selection only give indirect evidence of what fundamentally cannot be measured. Despite the best uses of statistical techniques, the counterfactual (what would enrollees have cost in fee-for-service) is impossible to determine conclusively (Porell et al. 1987; Gruenberg et al. 1988).

The best and latest results are reported by Hill and Brown (1990). They used two measures of biased selection for each of 98 different TEFRA HMOs. The first measure compared fee-for-service Medicare costs of enrollees in HMOs *prior* to enrollment to the same measure for nonenrolled beneficiaries in the same market area across AAPCC risk categories. The second measure compared enrollee-nonenrollee differences in prior hospitalization for diagnoses associated with high future Medicare costs. The validity of these measures of biased selection is in question because they assume pre-enrollment costs and service use to be valid indicators of Medicare costs after enrollment, as the authors point out.

Most observers feel that the selection process attracts low utilizers to the HMO and leaves high utilizers in the fee-for-service sector. Given the role of attachment to ongoing providers, this is a plausible scenario (Luft 1983). But measuring the magnitude of the supposed differences is fraught with difficulty.

Hill and Brown provide an excellent critique of the biased selection measures we have available. Most importantly, observed fee-for-service costs prior to enrollment could stem from a short-term difference in health care needs rather than from a major inherent enrollee-nonenrollee difference in health status. Moreover, if enrollee costs over time regress to the mean, as others have shown them to do (Beebe 1981), any pre-enrollment differences are overstated. Another valid criticism is that, inasmuch as Medicare HMO enrollees tend to be lower income than nonenrollees and less likely to have Medigap insurance, they may have faced barriers to care in the fee-for-service sector. Thus prior service use measures merely indicate the lower level of access experienced prior to joining an HMO (Rossiter 1988). By giving beneficiaries a structured source of care and perhaps enhanced access to care, HMOs increase costs by providing what amounts to a different, accessible product compared to fee-for-service Medicare—and one that cannot be delivered at Medicare costs for those most prone to enroll.

If a cross-section of beneficiaries is required to enroll, the AAPCC might adequately account for a prevailing level of access to care under fee-for-service medicine. On the other hand, people with Medigap tend to use more Medicare services, thus implicitly boosting the AAPCC.

In sum, as a counterfactual, biased selection is a concept that cannot be observed directly. Furthermore, we cannot be sure we are measuring it correctly. But even if we could measure it accurately, it would be difficult to interpret the results. This leads to the third explanation for the TEFRA HMO conundrum:

Explanation 3. The research and policy communities expect no biased selection to exist, which is unrealistic given the inherent stochastic nature of the contracts.

From a random assignment of beneficiaries to plans we would expect half of all plans to have favorable or neutral selection and half to have unfavorable or neutral selection. But assignment is not random. Plans are free to exit the market. Thus, in a practical setting we would expect the plans with adverse selection to leave the market and only plans with favorable or neutral selection to remain. Truly random selection differences will average out over time, in principal. However, marketing costs, inertia, and short profit horizons lead us to expect a disproportionate number of health plans with favorable selection at any point in time.

In fact, this is what we find. In the first study of the early demonstration experience, Eggers and Prihoda (1982) found evidence of favorable selection in two of three plans under study. These findings were confirmed by Kasper et al. (1988) and Eggers and Prihoda (1982). Brown (1988) found favorable selection for 13 of the 17 plans studied in the Medicare Competition Demonstrations, neutral selection for three plans, and adverse selection for one plan. In the most recent study, Hill and Brown (1990) found consistently favorable selection across the measures studied for 54 to 62 percent of the plans; the remainder had neutral selection, and none had adverse selection.

The proportion of plans with favorable, neutral, or adverse selection depends on one's definition of neutral selection and the size of the sample. But a look at the available studies is instructive. In summary, in the first study with three HMOs we would expect to find one with favorable selection, one with neutral selection, and one with adverse selection. Instead, we found two favorable, zero neutral, and one adverse. In the second study we would expect to find 5.6 plans with favorable selection, 5.6 plans with neutral selection, and 5.6 plans with adverse selection, with spillover from the neutral category in either direction. Instead we found 13 favorable, 3 neutral, and 1 adverse. Perhaps there were plans that had adverse selection and dropped out of the market, which would make the result closer to expectations. In the third study we expect about 33 plans in each category of biased selection, with spillover from the neutral category. The study found about 60 plans with favorable selection and 38 plans with neutral selection. At the same time, 33 plans did not renew their contracts. While there would appear to be a clear tendency toward plans with favorable selection, the number of plans by category is not especially different from what we would expect when the nonrenewing plans are factored in by category. Given market forces, we would expect plans with adverse selection to drop out, and only favorable or neutral selection plans to remain.

The final issue concerns the very nature of the measures used to indicate biased selection:

Explanation 4. Service use before joining the plan is an especially poor measure of biased selection.

Yet another important point is that *all* of the studies have relied on a one-time snapshot of the biased-selection issue. Normally, indications of prior use of services before joining an HMO are used to imply biased selection after enrollment. It is particularly unrealistic to expect plans always to have neutral selection, especially at start-up. The selection issue needs to be examined from a longitudinal standpoint, which of course is difficult to do. But the nature of risk contracting typically involves favorable selection one year and adverse another. Over several years plans should be made whole, and in fact must be, or they will leave the market.

To look only at new-enrollee prior service use, even for plans that are in the market several years, is not appropriate. The Hill and Brown study, for example, took samples of 1,000 new enrollees from 98 plans for a total of 98,000 beneficiaries. This is a snapshot of about 7 percent of one extreme portion of the total enrollment of 1.3 million beneficiaries. An additional 1.2 million beneficiaries were essentially excluded from the analysis because they had not recently enrolled. There are two problems here. One is the exclusion criteria, necessitated by the use of prior service use as the indicator of biased selection. The second issue is the size of the sample required to capture the very high-cost cases that have a large impact on a plan's cost experience.

Researchers have used a tiny segment of the total to describe the entire enrollment. This is not the problem of the research, since prior service use and costs are all that can be measured accurately for estimating a fee-for-service concept that is unobserved when enrolled in an HMO. But the problem with using prior service use and costs as measures of biased selection for only new enrollees is that the market experience for *all* enrollees may be quite different.

Hill and Brown found an average level of favorable selection for new enrollees equal to 23 percent of payments. If that is an accurate estimate of favorable selection today in the program, 5 percent of the 23 percent is removed by the payment formula because it pays 95 percent of the adjusted average cost. Thus the level of favorable selection for payment purposes is 17 percent. One has to wonder if biased selection among the other 97 percent of enrollees, unmeasured in dollar terms with conventional techniques, could somehow be measured. One goal would be to incorporate changing health status as beneficiaries remain in the HMO more than two years (the cutoff for the sample design in the HCFA evaluation). If this could be done, would the estimated level of 17 percent favorable selection be lower?

Changing health status and service use after enrollment may be the explanation for the conflict between the research and the market experience, and the answer for the TEFRA HMO conundrum.

Tyranny of the *R*-Square

The research indicates favorable selection for Medicare HMOs. The market experience of HMOs indicates adverse selection. The AAPCC formula, just as the research, makes no allowances for changing health risks over time, using only age, sex, institutional status, and welfare status as payments adjusters. One way to reconcile the conflict between the research and the experience of the market might be to incorporate further risk adjustments that capture the changing health risk of an enrolled population.

Prior research on prior service use

Many studies in the Medicare market measure prior service use, including those just summarized. There have been other attempts to incorporate health risk adjustments in the formula as well. One more notable risk adjustment technique is the diagnostic cost groups approach (Ellis and Ash 1988). Eight classifications of beneficiaries are created. *Individuals* are classified into the highest-reimbursement DCG on the basis of the principal diagnosis if they have more than one hospitalization in a year. Individuals with no hospitalizations in the prior year are classified as DCG 0. Other classifications follow according to principal diagnoses defining each diagnostic cost group. A DCG rate book defines the cost weights, much like the demographic factors for the AAPCC system, for payment purposes. In their paper outlining DCGs, Ellis and Ash showed that future Medicare costs were predicted better by DCGs than by current demographic factors alone.

Hornbrook, Bennett, and Greenlick (1988) present four major problems with DCGs. First, DCGs rely on prior hospitalization experience for HMO enrollees. Because it is well known that HMOs lower hospitalization, the HMOs would not be made whole with respect to the level of hospitalization expected under fee-for-service, which is the goal. This, despite the fact that discretionary and nondiscretionary hospitalizations are identified in the DCG system. Second, they are based on hospitalization only. Hospitalization rates can be unstable for smaller groups and could lead to swings in payments. Third, multiple episodes of hospitalization are not readily accounted for in the system. Fourth, there is an inherent aspect of the system that brings us back to cost reimbursement and could dramatically change the incentives for HMOs. Instead of avoiding hospitalizations, HMOs could be rewarded for hospitalizing individuals, knowing the clinical categories of DCGs that would produce higher payments. The fact that the system works at the individual level in determining payments—that certain types of hospitalizations in the previous time period produce higher payments—makes the system a version of individual experience rating.

What is perhaps most troubling about the DCG model is the methodological reliance on the R-square for determining its usefulness. A well-known and often quoted fact regarding the AAPCC is that the demographic factors explain less than 1 percent of the variance in per capita Medicare costs for aged beneficiaries (Lubitz 1987; Howland et al. 1987; Schauffler, Howland, and Cobb 1993). Hornbrook (1991) has extensively developed new methods for evaluating payment systems using simulations for individual data. Likewise, Robinson et al. (1991) appropriately employ simulation analyses.

The field seems to have recognized that individual level R-square analysis, while not exactly incorrect, nevertheless does not answer the question that needs to be answered. HMO payments need not, and arguably perhaps should not, be good predictors of individual enrollee expenses. The question is whether they adequately predict the expenses for groups.

Past reliance on the individual R-square may be explained by the following three propositions:

Proposition 1. A higher R-square from analysis of demographic factors and their effect on service use and costs using data on individuals should lead to better risk adjustment for groups.

Proposition 2. A low R-square using individual data does not necessarily imply poor risk adjustment for groups.

Proposition 3. R-square using individual data is not the best validation measure for payment models. Rather, simulations of predicted group means and the reliability of such estimates should be the standard for validation.

Proposition 3 is an argument against using R-square. People have tended to rely on the simple R-square for individual data because it is easy to understand and it makes sense intuitively that a model that predicts well at the individual level will predict well at the group level. While this is true, it is also true that a model that predicts poorly at the individual level can, nonetheless, predict well at the group level.

An epilogue for prior use measures

With the recent flurry of new papers on risk adjustment in the early 1990s, notably Hornbrook (1991) and Robinson et al. (1991), it may be possible to progress beyond the early attempts of the 1980s to develop individual level risk adjustments. By recognizing that the goal is risk adjustments for enrolled groups, we can view the analysis and assessment of R-squares based on individual data as early attempts.

We can see also that group adjustments eliminate the perverse incentives of individual adjustments. An individual adjustment encourages gaming of the system. Individual adjustments based on service use can even encourage higher service use because reimbursement for that individual will increase as a result.

One of the most promising new approaches to risk adjustment is the model developed by Robinson, Luft, Gardner, and Morrison in 1991.

We suggest that this type of model and the techniques used to validate are the yardstick of the 1990s for risk adjustment models.

The SEGA Model Applied to Medicare

The six equation group adjustment (SEGA) model a.k.a. the RLGM (Robinson, Luft, Gardner, Morrison) model, was developed in 1991 by the originators to predict medical care service use and expenditures for groups of fee-for-service plan and HMO enrollees, using characteristics commonly available in the personnel files of large employers. Simulation of the methodology showed that the six-equation, maximum likelihood model predicted quite well for groups of 1,000 or more. We have used the same six-equation group adjustment model to apply to data we had available from Medicare. In addition to using the traditional demographic factors, age and sex, we used beneficiary-reported data on health status and chronic conditions to show how the SEGA model might be used to modify the AAPCC.

Model development

The multi-equation model developed by the RAND Health Insurance Experiment (Duan et al. 1982) and then expanded by Robinson et al. (1991) forms the basis for the analysis. The SEGA model consists of six regression equations to estimate medical expense based on patient characteristics. Predicted values generated by each equation are then compiled in one formula to generate a single estimate of predicted medical expenditures.

The six equations adopted from the SEGA model are:

$$Pr(MED > 0) = L(XA_1) \tag{1}$$

$$Pr(INP > 0, \; if \; MED > 0) = L(XA_2) \tag{2}$$

$$Pr(MED \geq \$10,000, \; if \; INP > 0) = L(XA_3) \tag{3}$$

$$\log(MED, \; if \; INP = 0 \; and \; MED > 0) = XB_1 + U_1 \tag{4}$$

$$\log(MED, \; if \; INP > 0 \; and \; MED < \$10,000) = XB_2 + U_2 \tag{5}$$

$$\log(MED, \; if \; INP > 0 \; and \; MED \geq \$10,000) = XB_3 + U_3 \tag{6}$$

where *MED* is Medicare costs, X includes variables describing the individuals, and *INP* is any hospital inpatient expense. Thus hospital and ambulatory expenses are recognized in the model. The *A*s and *B*s are parameters to be estimated, and the *U*s are error terms. The function L is the logit function.

When Robinson et al. used the SEGA model, they had age, sex, type of plan, marital status, length of employment, education attainment, occupational level, salary level, and eligibility as independent (X) variables. We tried a number of measures from the data we had available, but found only a few variables appropriate (non-gameable) and significant in preliminary estimates.

We have chosen age (three categories), gender, marital status (two categories), educational level (two categories), income level (two categories), functional ADL level (two categories), and chronic problems (two categories). We hope to receive funding at some point to explore more fully the variables that would be best for predicting Medicare costs using the SEGA model. But we consider this empirical work a preliminary investigation enabling us to understand the potential of the SEGA model for Medicare risk contracting.

The data, taken from the 1983–1987 National Medicare Competition Demonstration Evaluation household-reported data, were drawn from records on 1,059 comparison group Medicare beneficiaries. They were sampled from cities that did not have Medicare HMOs, but they were similar in a number of characteristics to the cities with Medicare HMOs at the time. We used their household-reported data of independent variables in conjunction with Medicare claims file data on dependent variables to estimate the parameters of the SEGA model. These results were then used to predict the Medicare costs of 3,097 Medicare beneficiaries who joined one of the demonstration HMOs and who were interviewed with the same set of questions as that posed to the comparison group. The Medicare cost data represent the claims experience of the enrollees one year before joining the HMO. So we use their characteristics to predict their prior year fee-for-service cost experience, as though they had joined the HMO one year earlier.

Table 11.1 and Table 11.2 simply indicate the distribution of the subsamples used in each equation.

Returning then to the equations, Equation 1 calculates the probability of any medical services utilized: $Pr(MED > 0)$. The full sample of the comparison group is included ($N = 1,059$). Equation 2 uses individuals who ever incurred any medical costs ($MED > 0$, $n = 832$), to compute the probability of using any inpatient services: $Pr(INP > 0)$. Equation 3 includes 307 individuals who used any inpatient services ($INP > 0$) and obtains the probability of incurring medical expenditure of $10,000 or more: $Pr(MED \geq 10,000)$. Logistic regression is performed on Equation 1 through Equation 3.

Equation 4 through Equation 6 calculate the logarithm of medical expenditure using an ordinary least square model. For Equation 4, individuals who had medical expenditures but no inpatient services (*INP*

Table 11.1   Frequency Table of Medical Care Utilization by Inpatient
Service Use

		Medical Care Utilization		
		1 (Yes)	2 (No)	
Inpatient Service Use	1 (Yes)	307	0	307
	0 (No)	525	227	752
		832	227	1059

Table 11.2   Frequency Table of High-Cost Medical Utilization
(≥ $10,000) by Inpatient Service Use

		High-Cost Medical Utilization		
		1 (Yes)	2 (No)	
Inpatient Service Use	1 (Yes)	72	235	307
	0 (No)	0	752	752
		72	987	1059

= 0 and *MED* > 0) are included (*n* = 525). Equation 5 examines 235
individuals who utilized inpatient care but incurred medical expenditure
of less than $10,000. Finally, Equation 6 includes only 72 individuals who
used inpatient services and incurred medical costs of over $10,000.

Ideally, we would want to estimate these equations with a much
larger sample. Such data are available at the Williamson Institute from the
various studies conducted in the 1980s on the Medicare HMO experience
in the 1980s. We hope to seek funding to investigate further the most
appropriate independent variables in the Medicare context for the SEGA
model.

The predicted probability estimated by Equation 1 through Equation 3 is obtained, denoted as P_i, Q_i, and R_i, respectively. Logarithmic
medical expenditures predicted by Equation 4 through 6 are denoted
as X_4B_4, X_5B_5, and X_6B_6, respectively. Z, a nonparametric adjustment

developed by Duan et al. (1983) is calculated for each of Equation 4 through Equation 6 to modify the predicted dollar values, denoted as Z_1, Z_2, and Z_3, respectively.

All of these values are then compiled into a unique value of predicted medical costs using the formula:

$$P_i * \{[(1 - Q_i) * \text{EXP}(X_4 B_4) * Z_1]$$
$$+ [Q_i * [[(1 - R_i) * \text{EXP}(X_5 B_5) * Z_2]$$
$$+ [R_i * \text{EXP}(X_6 B_6) * Z_3]]\}$$

We first validated the model in our pilot examination by applying the parameters to the comparison group to estimate the medical expenditure for the very same observations used to generate the parameter estimates. Mean estimated medical expenditures were then compared to mean actual medical expenditures. The prediction error is calculated by subtracting the predicted from actual expenditures, dividing by actual expenditures, and then multiplying by 100.

The estimated parameters from the comparison group were then applied to the HMO enrollee group. Predicted medical expenditures were obtained and compared to actual medical expenditures. The prediction error is also calculated.

Results

The results of the simulations are shown in Table 11.3. Generally, the composition of the comparison group and the HMO enrollee group is not much different. That does not matter, however, because the purpose is to impute fee-for-service Medicare costs to a group of enrollees no matter what their characteristics. Both groups include a similar distribution of women and more highly educated individuals. In both groups, over 90 percent of the individuals could perform over two IADLs, and 66.6 percent had chronic problems. The comparison group is older, with 11.8 percent over the age of 85, as opposed to 5.6 percent for the HMO enrolled group. The comparison group is better in physical function measured by IADL. The other difference is that the comparison group has higher income than the HMO enrollee group.

The average predicted medical expenditure for the comparison group was \$2144.47 ± 2095.82 (s.e.), while the actual medical expenditure was \$2510.20 ± 5365.41 (s.e.). The prediction error is −14.5 percent. We did not determine why the model does not predict better for the very observations used to generate the parameter estimates, but we are continuing to explore this. Robinson, Luft, Gardner, and Morrison found

Table 11.3 Frequency Summary of Study Variables

Variable	Category	Total (N = 3157)	Comparison Group (n = 1059)	HMO Enrollee Group (n = 2098)
Age	1:65–74	1701(53.9%)	518(48.8%)	1183(56.4%)
	2:75–84	1221(38.7%)	423(39.9%)	798(38.0%)
	3:85+	235 (7.4%)	118(11.8%)	117 (5.6%)
Gender	1:Male	1293(41.0%)	416(39.3%)	877(41.8%)
	0:Female	1864(59.0%)	643(60.7%)	1221(58.2%)
Marital Status	1:Married	1527(48.4%)	484(45.7%)	1043(49.7%)
	0:Others	1630(51.6%)	575(54.3%)	1055(50.3%)
Education	1:>9th grade	2063(67.9%)	707(69.2%)	1356(67.2%)
	0:≤9th grade	976(32.1%)	314(30.8%)	662(32.8%)
Income	1:≥$10,000	1603(50.8%)	591(55.8%)	1012(48.2%)
	0:<$10,000	1554(49.2%)	468(44.2%)	1086(51.8%)
Function	1:can perform over two IADLs	3013(95.4%)	981(92.6%)	2032(96.9%)
	0:can perform fewer than two IADLs	144 (4.6%)	78 (7.4%)	66 (3.1%)
Chronic Problems	1:have any chronic problem	1942(61.5%)	660(62.3%)	1282(61.1%)
	0:have no chronic problem	1215(38.5%)	399(37.7%)	816(38.9%)

that the SEGA method did less well at predicting for groups smaller than 1,000. Thus we hope that using larger databases at a later time will improve our estimates.

The average predicted medical expenditure for the HMO enrolled group is $1903.32 ± 1780.12. Since the actual medical expenditure is $1967.95 ± 4355.14, the prediction error is only as small as 3.2 percent. We were particularly pleased to see the model predict this well for a relatively small group of enrollees, and are optimistic it could predict even better given a larger sample to generate the parameters and a greater number of HMO enrollees requiring predicted expenditures.

It should be noted that the measures of physical functioning we included in the model consistently performed well in the equations in terms of significance. The other variables were less reliable as predictors of Medicare costs. Again, larger datasets would be helpful in seeing which variables are best for SEGA modeling in the Medicare context.

The SEGA approach could be used to modify payments for HMOs. Each HMO would be required to submit data on the characteristics (X variables) of their enrollees, based either on sample data or on a census. These characteristics would be used to generate a case-mix factor for each plan (not unlike the Medicare hospital case-mix indicator) and published in the *Federal Register* each year along with the new AAPCC rates published each September 7. The characteristics would pertain to enrollees in the previous year, but we would not expect massive shifts in enrollment from year to year, just as we do not expect massive shifts in case mix for PPS hospitals. The group level modifier would be based on fee-for-service estimating parameters for the characteristics of the HMOs. SEGA modeling would be administratively simple, and it would not require detailed data on hospitalizations and ongoing service use. We recommend, however, that it incorporate some sort of measure of chronic conditions in the enrollee group.

More data would be required from HMOs than are now collected, and there would be some potential for manipulation of the reported data. But the demands from the data are no more onerous than those for hospitals, and the process could be audited just as it is for hospitals.

What Should Be Done with the Medicare Risk-Based Payment System?

Fundamental philosophy

One critical area of philosophical agreement must be reached by those involved with the Medicare risk-based payment system. The current system is clearly based on the principle that the fee-for-service and risk-based sectors should be connected. The risk-based payment is drawn from the fee-for-service experience by design. Risk-based contractors who can better organize the delivery system and provide higher quality, more efficient care should thrive under such a competitive system. As a prudent purchasing model, the approach makes sense (Gruenberg, Pomeranz, and Porell 1988).

On the other hand, we must be concerned with a shrinking fee-for-service sector and the appropriateness of basing payments in a small area on a relatively few individuals and perhaps a biased set of individuals (Rossiter, Adamache, and Faulknier 1990). By the same token, if one believes the fee-for-service sector is not a part of the long-term future of health care in this country, including Medicare, we must begin now to develop a payment system that can establish payment rates separately from fee-for-service medicine (Lewin/ICF 1991).

For now, the law requires a linkage, and there is some sense to that so long as risk contracts comprise only 4 percent of all enrollment. A managed competition approach, with bids submitted by competing health plans might be a reasonable alternative and should be tested (Roper et al. 1988). Rather than HCFA posting take-it-or-leave-it prices, as it does today, the risk contract would be organized much like a private employer organizes procurement of health benefits. Plans would be invited annually to submit bids. HCFA would establish its payment level in an area based on those bids, and people would be free to supplement the payment to join a plan. Ideally, Medigap policies should be included in the process as well (Florida Department of Insurance 1983).

What should be done now?

The search must continue for appropriate, adequate, and stable payment rates in Medicare for risk-based contractors. Two things should be done for the next set of rates to be published. First, a working aged adjustment should be created (Office of Research and Demonstrations 1987; Porell et al. 1987). This would amount to a new demographic factor to account for the difference in expected Medicare payments for the working aged, who have their employer's private insurance as the primary payer. HMOs that disproportionately enroll the working aged are overpaid, and those who disproportionately do not enroll the working aged are underpaid. The overpaid problem is a larger one, because some plans could be targeting marketing efforts to enroll working aged, but plans that are not enrolling the working aged are receiving an underpayment estimated at about 2 percent of the AAPCC. The HCFA actuary has committed to doing this adjustment when the data are available, which should be for the 1994 rates.

The second thing that could be done right away is to change the definition of the geographic factor (Beebe 1982; Rossiter and Adamache 1990; Welch 1991). The current configuration leaves most counties with too few beneficiaries to make reliable predictions of future expenses and is a source of variability, year to year, in the AAPCC for an area. The GHAA has proposed a geographic configuration that is acceptable to most current risk contractors. It consists of collapsing most counties in metropolitan statistical areas to define a larger geographic area than the current county-based system. Some so-called ring counties around large MSAs would form other geographic areas when it made sense to do so. Rural non-MSA counties would have their own separate reimbursement. The GHAA approach would be easy to implement and would greatly improve the year-to-year reliability of the AAPCC, which has been a source of concern for risk contractors. Because marketing is often done on a wide geographic basis, this approach also reduces the chances of selective marketing and enrollment as well.

The two actions just discussed require no legislative action. Another action that would require legislation, but could be done now, is the development of an outlier pool. The Bush administration proposed one easy step that would greatly reduce the riskiness of contractor participation in Medicare (Wilensky and Rossiter 1991). Twenty-seven states have established this approach for their own private insurance market. It is well tested and easily implemented (Congressional Budget Office 1982). The proposal would pay HMOs an outlier payment above the 95 percent payment that they currently receive with respect to the AAPCC. The current formula does not adjust for the health status of the beneficiary enrolled, nor are there adjustments if a disproportionate number of high-cost Medicare beneficiaries are enrolled in an HMO in any year.

Hospitals now receive an outlier adjustment. Many HMOs are no more prepared to accept full risk for high-cost Medicare beneficiaries than many hospitals. Case studies done by HCFA evaluators of the risk contract experience and HMOs that dropped their contract bear out the concern that a few high risks can be an excessive financial burden. Further, the cost of reinsurance in the market may be higher than what could be guaranteed through a Medicare outlier policy. Economies of scale from a Medicare-provided program could greatly reduce the costs of reinsurance while providing greater risk protection.

This proposal would change the current payment policy by creating an outlier pool to pay HMOs for a portion of the costs of very high cost cases. The outlier pool would be funded from the Medicare Trust Funds by setting aside 2 percent more of the AAPCC above the current 95 percent limit. Payments would be made to plans from the outlier pool for a portion of costs above some threshold (for example, Medicare costs above $50,000). HMOs would be responsible for identifying cases that exceed the threshold and reporting them to a Medicare fiscal agent that would process the outlier payments.

Beebe (1992) used Medicare data for 27,326 Medicare beneficiaries to simulate the impact of an outlier pool with a $50,000 deductible. Of the persons in the sample, 20.1 percent had at least one hospital stay, and 216 people had Medicare expenses in excess of $50,000. Paying separately for such high-cost persons would improve the AAPCC by protecting HMOs against risk they cannot readily control.

Half of Medicare benefit costs are spent on beneficiaries who are in their last two years of life (McCall 1984; Wagner et al. 1983). As much as 10.2 percent of all Medicare spending is for less than 0.5 percent of beneficiaries with costs above $50,000 per year. The outlier pool would afford protection against very high cost cases that make the Medicare population so risky for many plans.

What should be done in one to three years?

The next thing to do is to begin to develop the SEGA model for the Medicare market. It would take less than one year to develop the parameter estimates with larger sample sizes. The data are in hand from the TEFRA HMO evaluation. Simulations could be performed for the 98 HMOs in that study. Each plan would receive a SEGA adjustment factor and could simulate payments for its entire population. Procedures would need to be developed to report the necessary independent (x) variables on an ongoing basis through the current enrollment-disenrollment system, or to develop beneficiary surveys to collect the self-reported data, if they are required for the independent variables. Legislative action might not be required to implement the system. The HCFA actuary is free to use the most appropriate actuarial values to estimate HMO payments, according to the law. Thus the development and testing could and should be done within three years, just in time for the tenth anniversary of the Medicare risk contracting program.

References

Adamache, K., and L. Rossiter. "The Entry of HMOs Into the Medicare Market: Implications for TEFRA's Mandate." *Inquiry* 23, no. 4 (Winter 1987): 1314–1418.

Anderson, G. F., E. P. Steinberg, M. R. Powe, S. Antebi, J. Whittle, S. Horn, and R. Herbert. "Setting Payment Rates for Capitated Systems: A Comparison of Various Alternatives." *Inquiry* 27, no. 3 (19 February 1990): 225–33.

Beebe, J.C. "An Examination of the Geographic Factor Used in the AAPCC." Baltimore, MD: HCFA, Office of Research, 29 April 1982.

———. "An Outlier Pool for Medicare HMO Payments." *Health Care Financing Review* 14, no. 1 (Fall 1992): 59–65.

———. "Two Studies in the Evaluation of the AAPCC." Baltimore, MD: HCFA, Office of Research, 21 September 1981.

Brown, R. "Biased Selection in the Medicare Competition Demonstrations." Princeton, NJ: Matehematica Policy Research, Inc., 1988.

Congressional Budget Office. "Catastrophic Medical Expenses: Patterns in the Non-Elderly, Non-Poor Population." Washington, DC, December 1982.

Cookson, J. "Review of AAPCC Methodology for Implementing Prospective Contracts with HMOs." Prepared under HCFA contract no. 500-38-0018. Washington DC: Health Care Financing Administration, August 1983.

Duan, N., W. G. Manning, C. N. Morris, and J. P. Newhouse. "A Comparison of Alternative Models for the Demand for Medical Care." RAND Publication no. R-2754-HHS. Santa Monica, CA, January 1982.

Ellis, R. P., and A. Ash. "Refining the Diagnostic Cost Group Model: A Proposed Modification to the AAPCC for HMO Reimbursement." Boston: Boston University, February 1988.

Eggers, P., and R. Prihoda. "Pre-Enrollment Reimbursement Patterns of Medicare Beneficiaries Enrolled in 'At Risk' HMOs." *Health Care Financing Review* 4, no. 1 (September 1982): 55–73.

Florida Department of Insurance. "Medicare Supplement Insurance Shopper's Guide." *Florida Department of Insurance* (Pamphlet) March 1983.

Gold, M., and D. Hodges. "Health Maintenance Organizations in 1988." *Health Affairs* 8, no. 4 (Winter 1989): 125–38.

Gruenberg, L., D. Pomeranz, and F. Porell. "Evaluation of the Accuracy of the AAPCC." Prepared under HCFA Cooperative Agreement no. 18-C-98526/1-03. Washington DC: Health Care Financing Administration, August 1988.

Hill, J. W., and R. S. Brown. "Biased Selection in the TEFRA HMO/CMP Program." Prepared under HCFA contract no. 500-88-0006. Washington DC: Health Care Financing Administration, March 1990.

Hornbrook, M. C. (Volume Editor) "Risk-Based Contributions to Private Health Insurance." In *Advances in Health Economics and Health Services Research*, edited by R. M. Scheffler and L. F. Rossiter. Greenwich, CT: JAI Press, 1991.

Hornbrook, M., M. Bennett, and M. Greenlick. "Diagnostic Cost Groups: Validation from an HMO's Experience." Prepared under HCFA Cooperative Agreement no. 18-C-988804-1/04. Baltimore, MD: Health Care Financing Administration, October 1988.

Howland, J., J. Stokes, S. Crane, and A. Belanger. "Adjusting Capitation Using Chronic Disease Factors: A Preliminary Study." *Health Care Financing Review* 9, no. 2 (Winter 1987): 15–23.

Kasper, J. D., G. F. Riley, J. S. McCombs, and M. A. Stevenson. "Beneficiary Selection, Use and Charges in Two Medicare Capitation Demonstration." *Health Care Financing Review* 10, no. 1 (Fall 1988): 37–49.

Lewin/ICF. "A Research and Demonstration Agenda on Health Services Delivery to Older Persons in HMOs." Washington DC: Lewin/ICF, 1991.

Luft, H. "Competition and Regulation: The Selection and Competitive Effects of Health Maintenance Organizations." Prepared under HCFA Grant no. 8P-975569/901. Washington DC: Health Care Financing Administration, September 1983.

Manton, K. G., and E. Stallard. "Analysis of Underwriting Factors for AAPCC." *Health Care Financing Review* 14, no. 1 (Fall 1992): 117–32.

McCall, N. "Utilization and Costs of Medicare Services by Beneficiaries in Their Last Year of Life." *Medical Care* 22, no. 4 (April 1984): 329–42.

Office of Research and Demonstrations. "Technical Study and Recommendations for Refining the AAPCC, 1987." Baltimore, MD: Health Care Financing Administration, September 1987.

Palsbo, S. J. "Analysis of 1989 USPCCs and AAPCCs." *Research Briefs*. Group Health Association of America, Inc., September 1988.

Palsbo, S. J. "The AAPCC Explained." *Research Briefs*. Group Health Association of America, Inc., February 1989.

Porell, F., C. Tompkins, D. Pomeranz, and L. Gruenberg. "Medicare TEFRA Risk Contracting: A Study of the Adjusted Community Rate." Report supported by HCFA Cooperative Agreement no. 99-6-98526/0-04. Washington DC: Health Care Financing Administration, September 1987.

Robinson, J. C., H. S. Luft, L. B. Gardner, and E. M. Morrison. "A Method for Risk-Adjusting Employer Contributions to Competing Health Insurance Plans." *Inquiry* 28 (Summer 1991): 107–16.

Roper, W. L., W. Winkenwerder, G. Hackbarth, and H. Krakauer. "Effectiveness in Health Care, An Initiative to Evaluate and Improve Medical Practice." *The New England Journal of Medicine* 319, no. 18 (3 November 1988): 1197–1202.

Rossiter, L. F., L. M. Nelson, and K. W. Adamache. "Service Use and Costs for Medicare Beneficiaries in Risk-based HMOs and CMPs: Some Interim Results from the National Medicare Competition Evaluation." *American Journal of Public Health* 78, no. 8 (August 1988): 937–43.

Rossiter, L. F., and K. Adamache. "Payment to Health Maintenance Organizations and the Geographic Factor." *Health Care Financing Review* 21, no. 1 (Fall 1990): 19–30.

Rossiter, L. F., K. W. Adamache, and T. Faulknier. "A Blended Sector Rate Adjustment for the Medicare AAPCC When Risk-Based Market Penetration is High." *The Journal of Risk and Insurance* 47, no. 2 (June 1990): 220–39.

Schauffler, H. H., J. Howland, and J. Cobb. "Using Chrinoic Disease Risk Factors to Adjust Medicare Capitation Payments." *Health Care Financing Review* 14, no. 1 (Fall 1992): 79–90.

Tompkins, C., and F. Porell. "An Empirical Study of HMOs That Did Not Renew Their TEFRA Risk Contracts for 1988." In *Medicare: Issues Concerning the HealthChoice Demonstration Project*. Washington, DC: U.S. Accounting Office, 1988.

Wagner, D. P., W. A. Knaus, E. A. Draper, and J. Zimmerman. "Identification of Low-Risk Monitor Patients Within a Medical-Surgical Intensive Care Unit." *Medical Care* 21, no. 4 (April 1983): 425–34.

Wilensky, G. R., and L. F. Rossiter. "Coordinated Care and Public Programs." *Health Affairs* 10, no. 4 (Winter 1991): 62–77.

Welch, W. P. "Defining Geographic Areas to Adjust Payments to Physicians, Hospitals, and HMOs." *Inquiry* 28, no. 2 (Summer 1991): 151–60.

———. "Medicare Capitation Payments to HMOs in Light of Regression Toward the Mean in Health Care Costs." In *Advances in Health Economics and Health Services Research*, Vol. 10, edited by R. M. Scheffler and L. F. Rossiter. Greenwich, CT: JAI Press, 1989.

Chapter 12

Responses and Discussion

Susan E. Palsbo

Both of these papers address reimbursement issues under the Medicare risk contracting program and have implications for government-capitated plans in national health care reform proposals.

I would like to spend a few moments elaborating on the TEFRA HMO conundrum raised by Rossiter and associates. The program is much more concentrated than most policymakers realize.

Patterns in risk contracting

GHAA data show that year-end 1991 enrollment stood at 18 percent of the national population, and nearly 20 percent of covered lives. At 2.5 million members, HMO penetration is 28 percent of the Federal Employees Health Benefits Program. In stark contrast is the penetration of the Medicaid market, at only 4 percent (1 million recipients), and the Medicare market at only 7 percent (2.3 million beneficiaries). The low penetration rate of the Medicare market is disappointing, given the high hopes we had for risk contracting a half-dozen years ago. GHAA estimates that another 500,000 beneficiaries are enrolled in HMO prepaid Medigap plans, in which the HMO bills HCFA on a fee-for-service basis. These plans are regulated by state governments rather than the federal government.

Table 12.1 shows the October 1992 Medicare enrollment by contract type. Many people are not aware that one-third of Medicare beneficiaries in HMOs are *not* enrolled in risk contracts, but instead are enrolled in HMOs that have cost-based reimbursement contracts. In fact, nearly one-quarter of all Medicare beneficiaries in HMOs are enrolled in health care prepayment plans (HCPP), under which HMOs are paid their actual costs rather than being held financially at risk.

The risk contracting is very concentrated geographically, with half of the risk enrollees residing in only two areas—southern California and southern Florida. About 80 percent of risk enrollees reside in only 50 of the over 3,000 counties in the country. This concentrated geographic enrollment leads to market penetration rates equivalent to, or some times exceeding, the total HMO penetration rate (Table 12.2). My informal observation is that risk contract penetration is highest where the out-of-pocket premiums are lowest. Clearly, if an HMO can offer a risk contract at a nominal out-of-pocket premium, beneficiaries will enroll in large numbers. Thus, we can hypothesize that the main reason for Rossiter's conundrum lies not in beneficiary concerns about enrolling in a managed care system, but in HMOs being encouraged to sign contracts with the Health Care Financing Administration.

Table 12.1   Medicare Enrollment by Contract Type

October 1992	Number of Plans	Number of Enrollees	Percentage
Total	190	2,311,022	
Risk	94	1,524,761	66%
Cost	26	131,361	6
Risk with Cost	4	4,262	0.2
Health Care Prepayment Plan (HCPP)	52	534,980	23
Risk with HCPP	10	93,903	4
S/HMO	4	21,755	1

Table 12.2   Penetration in Specific Markets: Total versus Medicare Risk, 1991

Metropolitan Area	Total	Risk
Seattle	24%	17%
Portland, OR	34	39
San Francisco	46	4
Los Angeles	32	30
Washington, DC	22	0.4
Miami	21	27
Minneapolis	44	20

Source: Group Health Association of America and the Health Care Financing Administration.

Risk enrollment is concentrated in a few large plans. Most plans have fewer than 25,000 enrollees, but some have 150,000 enrollees or more. Risk enrollment is also very concentrated by HMO owner (Figure 12.1). About 75 percent of risk enrollment is concentrated in plans operated by only eight owners. All of these operate HMOs in more than one state. Some are regional; some are national.

Note that indemnity insurer–owned HMOs are noticeably absent from the playing field. This is an even more dramatic observation when one realizes that insurer–owned HMOs enroll 15.4 percent of all HMO enrollees, and CIGNA enrolls the second-largest number of members (1.9 million, versus Kaiser's 6.8 million). The small enrollment in Aetna plans resulted when Aetna acquired the "Partners" chain, rather than making a corporate decision to participate in the risk contracting program.

The one national insurer that did decide to enroll in TEFRA, Prudential, made a corporate decision to pull out a year later. This accounts for the large number of contract terminations in 1989, shown in Figure 12.2. This figure may illustrate that the kind of competitive activity in the early years of the TEFRA program, as hypothesized by Rossiter et al., did in fact occur. The plans that terminated operations in 1987 through 1989

Figure 12.1   Percent of Total Risk Enrollment by Ownership, February 1992

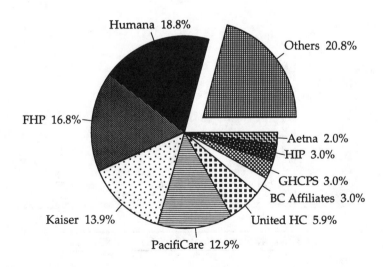

Source: Group Health Association of America analysis of data from the Health Care Financing Administration.

tended to be small, enrolling fewer than 5,000 Medicare members despite having, in some cases, a substantial number of private sector enrollees.

Figure 12.3 shows the number of Medicare contracts from 1986 through HCFA's estimates for January 1993. It appears that the TEFRA program has stabilized, and 1993 will see the greatest number of contractors since 1989: yet this is fewer than one-fifth of all HMOs in the country.

Finally, Figure 12.4 shows that, despite contractors leaving TEFRA risk contracts and either switching to a cost contract or an HCPP contract, or dropping out altogether, the total number of Medicare beneficiaries enrolled in risk HMOs has continued to offset the losses and has shown a fairly steady growth rate.

To recapitulate, the TEFRA HMO program is a phenomenal success in some parts of the country for some HMOs, but a disappointing failure in most of the country. The obvious questions are:

Figure 12.2   Contract Terminations/Service Reductions December 31, 1987–1992

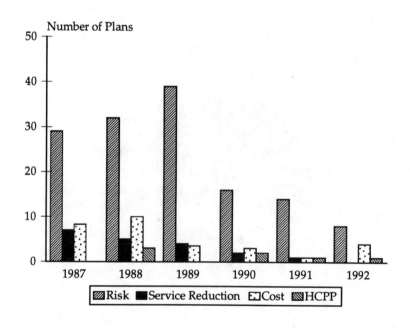

Source: Group Health Association of America analysis of data from the Health Care Financing Administration.

1. Why do HMOs not sign contracts? or after they do sign one, why do they drop it?
2. Can the government take action that will encourage more HMOs to participate?

The rest of my remarks will address these two questions.

Why do HMOs drop risk contracts?

HMOs cite many reasons for dropping risk contracts or not signing one in the first place: the peer review organization (PRO) process, HCFA's procedures for reviewing marketing materials, and the beneficiary appeals process for reconsideration of medical care coverage. But the primary reason is concern about financial performance.

On the revenue side of the financial equation, HMOs have many concerns about the level of payment. On its face, the adjusted average

Figure 12.3 Number of Plans by Contract Type January 1, 1985–1993

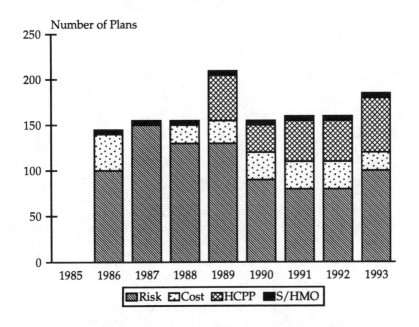

Source: Group Health Association of America analysis of data from the Health Care Financing Administration. Data for some contract types before 1989 are unavailable.

Figure 12.4   January 1 Enrollment by Contract Type 1987–1993

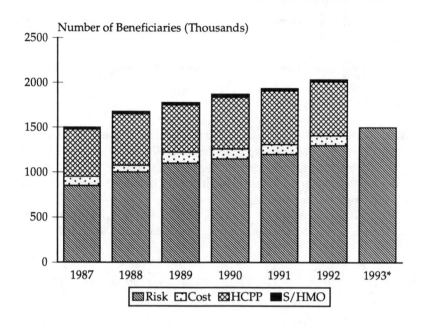

Source: Group Health Association of America analysis of data from the Health Care Financing Administration.
*HCFA estimate.

per capita cost (AAPCC) is geographically inequitable. For example, risk contractors in southern California charge a nominal premium, but risk contractors in New England charge beneficiaries a $90–$100 premium— for essentially the same benefit package. It is difficult to believe that regional differences in utilization solely account for this disparity in risk contract premiums.

The root of the problem apparently lies in TEFRA itself, which requires HCFA to develop an actuarially equivalent rate. Risk contractors are capitated at 95 percent of what would be paid by HCFA, at HCFA's rates. In many markets, HCFA is the 500-pound gorilla that can pay hospitals any rate it wants. This requires hospitals to shift their costs to other purchasers, such as HMOs.

A second difficulty of tying capitation to fee-for-service sector payments is that the TEFRA program perpetuates overpayments in geographic areas with overutilization and results in underpayments in areas with low utilization. The utilization may be low because of access problems of Medicare beneficiaries rather than because of any higher relative health of the beneficiary population.

A third difficulty is the one raised by Welch: the impact of the spillover effect and competitive markets on what Medicare pays. Additional research might help distinguish the relative importance of spillover practice patterns versus the constraint of medical costs that occurs as a result of competitive market forces. Also, there are some anecdotes about physicians modifying their treatment depending on the patient's insurer; additional research might be able to quantify this.

I suggest three additional lines of investigation to continue Welch's work on HMO market share and its effect on Medicare costs. The first is to look at the five years of geographic adjusters (GAs) HCFA uses to calculate the AAPCCs. The geographic adjuster is the ratio of county per capita payments to national per capita payments. I've been tracking these for several years for the counties with the largest risk enrollment, and it is clear that the geographic adjuster is dropping from values well above one (1.0) to a value closer to one in areas with a high overall HMO market penetration. This has implications for the AAPCC itself, because when a high GA is dropped off the rolling five-year average and is replaced with a lower GA, the AAPCC is lower than it would otherwise be.

The second is to look at the role of increasing physician participation in HMOs, not only in terms of numbers, but in terms of the percentage of the physician's practice that is HMO-enrolled. Some of this information is available by medical specialty.

The third is to see if including the market share of HMOs with health care prepayment plan contracts in Table 10.3 of Welch's paper has an impact on the Part A and Part B coefficients. For example, HMO penetration of the Twin Cities Medicare market is probably twice as great if HCPP enrollees are included.

If Welch's hypothesis is correct, risk contractors become the victims of their own success. The HMO industry cannot be expected to be paid 95 percent of a fee-for-service system that is all muscle and no fat. Furthermore, merely raising the capitation rate to 100 percent of the AAPCC may not be enough to get more HMOs to sign TEFRA contracts, especially in markets where HCFA payments are lower than HMO costs.

For these reasons and others, GHAA has proposed development of an economically based or administered capitation rate, rather than an actuarially based rate. Conceptually, risk contractors would be capitated at a rate that reflects the input costs for an efficient HMO in their geographic location, allowing for some amount of conformance to local practice patterns and expectations. Some standard of comparison will still be needed to assure taxpayers and beneficiaries that they are getting a good value for their money. But these standards should include quality and comprehensiveness of care, access to Medicare benefits, and enrollee satisfaction, not just payment savings to the government.

Controlling costs

The other side of the financial performance equation is for HMOs to control their costs. My perception is that the most successful risk contractors, and those that are expanding their service area and keeping premiums low, are those that treat Medicare as a separate line of business. Many of these HMOs have established a "duplicate" HMO, or an HMO within their HMO, that administers Medicare beneficiaries, exclusively. They have separate member services and marketing departments, board-certified geriatricians, and more integrated case management teams, and the plans go to a great deal of effort to identify the small percentage of beneficiaries who account for the bulk of the services. These HMOs often have an individual, visionary clinician who is innovative in providing care to the elderly and who has the full support of the HMO management.

Areas for future research

HCFA has contracted with researchers at least twice to find out why HMOs drop out of the risk contracting program. I propose that HCFA instead identify the best practices of the successful risk contractors and perhaps fund training programs for risk contract administrators. For example, I'm sure many risk contractors could learn a lot from the Social/HMO (S/HMO) program about managing the care of the frail elderly.

Study after study of the risk contracting program addresses selection bias. As Rossiter noted, the preponderance of evidence is that relatively healthy beneficiaries are more likely to choose an HMO delivery system. What is the best way to adjust the capitation payment to correct for this patient self-selection?

This is an important question because current measures are inadequate. The four AAPCC adjusters—age, sex, institutional status, and Medicaid status—result in HMOs being overpaid for relatively healthy beneficiaries and underpaid for sick beneficiaries, with a net loss to the Medicare program. It is important, however, not to view these findings as a condemnation of the risk contracting program. Rather, it adds urgency to the need to further the state of the art of assessing a beneficiary's likelihood of consuming health care resources in the upcoming year.

Rossiter's paper suggests the six equation group adjustment (SEGA) model. One difficulty is that the model is complex and somewhat difficult to understand. However, this obstacle is not insurmountable. As

Rossiter and his colleagues move beyond the preliminary stage, I advise them to concentrate on measures that the government and HMOs are likely to have in their computerized files. The government will need this information to determine the case-mix factor for each risk contractor, as well as for the fee-for-service sector, in HCFA's AAPCC calculations. Rossiter's suggestion to have independent data collection to sample non-HMO beneficiaries may be feasible, since as a practical matter we're talking about surveying non-HMO beneficiaries only in those counties with risk contracting HMOs (100 out of the over 3,000 counties in the country).

Other researchers have suggested alternative risk adjusters, such as the Ambulatory Care Groups (ACGs) developed by Weiner, Starfield, and colleagues at Johns Hopkins. In terms of conceptual simplicity, I consider the ACG model to be superior to the SEGA model. However, the requirement for ambulatory diagnostic data may preclude its widespread use, even among HMOs. GHAA is currently developing a research proposal to evaluate the use of ACGs as capitation adjusters.

Summary

I think the way to get more HMOs, especially the efficient ones, interested in signing new contracts and expanding existing ones, is to increase reimbursement in geographic areas with low AAPCCs and decrease the variability in net income. While reinsurance for catastrophic cases can help to decrease the variability of net income, it does not address the problem of adequate and appropriate reimbursement for the bulk of enrollees. To do this, HCFA should devote its efforts to:

1. develop an economically based rate;
2. develop alternative measures of value, quality of care, and satisfaction of beneficiaries in TEFRA risk contracts;
3. identify the characteristic success of the most efficient risk contractors and disseminate that information;
4. develop a managed competition reimbursement scheme for markets with multiple Medicare and Medigap offerings; and
5. coordinate open enrollment of individual Medicare beneficiaries, accommodate the needs of group retirees who may be on a noncalendar year benefit cycle, and require a one-year lock-in to the HMO after a three-month trial period.

Perhaps, in this way, we will no longer have a conundrum, but a success story.

Jon B. Christianson

Imagine that you have been summoned to the corporate offices of a large, private sector employer to provide consultation on the firm's health benefit options. The firm is a staunch advocate of offering multiple HMOs to its employees, along with a fee-for-service alternative. However, corporate management is unhappy with the results. Relatively few employees have enrolled in the HMOs, and the managers are not sure if offering the HMOs helps to contain health benefit costs. You learn that the firm bases its premium contribution to the HMOs on the costs of the fee-for-service plan, has no systematic process for distributing information about the HMO options to employees, and allows HMOs to disenroll employees continuously to the fee-for-service insurance plan. You are told that all of these practices must be continued as long as the HMOs remain as part of the employer's health benefit plan. What advice would you give this employer?

My advice would be to drop the HMOs from the firm's health benefit offering. The firm could probably reduce the total premiums paid for health insurance (combined employer and employee contributions) by offering only the fee-for-service plan. However, I would offer two qualifications to this recommendation. Offering the HMOs in addition to the fee-for-service plan might somehow hold premium increases in the fee-for-service plan in check or possibly reduce overall costs to the firm if the HMOs experienced adverse selection (and, for some reason, did not respond by dropping the firm).

Medicare as it is now structured is, of course, the health benefits program in question. If it does not have the political will or imagination to carry out fundamental reforms in the way in which reimbursement rates are set for HMO risk contractors and in which enrollment of beneficiaries is carried out, HCFA should consider terminating its program of contracting with HMOs. The reason that the papers by Welch and Rossiter et al. are so interesting is that they address important issues relating to the qualifications I noted.

Using data from 1984–1987, Welch concludes that "every 10 percentage points of HMO market share decreases Medicare expenditures by 1.2 percent in the short run and as much as 3.9 percent in the long run" and that this is a far bigger impact on expenditures than is generated by the 5 percent discount in the AAPCC formula alone. Thus, the Welsh findings appear to support the continuation of HCFA's risk-based contracts with HMOs. Despite the obvious flaws in the design of the existing program (which Welch readily acknowledges), the program has helped to contain overall Medicare spending. Or, at least it appears to have had that effect five to eight years ago.

Unfortunately, the conclusion seems less compelling when one considers that Welch did not, in fact, relate HMO market share to Medicare expenditures. Instead, the "market share" variable was the percentage of Medicare beneficiaries in a given geographical area enrolled in HMOs. In developing his model, Welch suggests that the HMO market share in a community could be inversely related to fee-for-service expenditures if it served as a proxy for the competitive pressures that HMOs brought to bear on fee-for-service providers. For example, in communities where the HMO market share was high, traditional insurers might attempt to more aggressively manage the care delivered by fee-for-service providers. As providers became accustomed to more conservative managed care practice styles, either through the efforts of traditional insurers or through providing services to HMO enrollees in their practices, their practice "norms" would gradually change. Over time, they would provide care more conservatively, in terms of resource use, to all patients, including Medicare beneficiaries. In effect, we have a "trickle down" theory of competitive pressure, where the degree of pressure is proxied by the overall HMO market share in the community.

Unfortunately, as Welch correctly notes, measuring overall HMO market share is a difficult and imprecise undertaking. While it is possible to collect data on HMO enrollment and on counties served by the HMO, enrollment by county is not available. The analyst has three choices in this situation, and all are less than satisfactory: abandon the analysis, choose a variable that can be measured precisely but doesn't represent the underlying construct as well, or accept some imprecision in the measured value and attempt to determine how sensitive the results are to that measurement error. Welch chooses the second approach. He uses the percentage of the Medicare beneficiaries enrolled in HMOs as his market share measure. It may be argued that this is an appropriate measure of competitive pressure due to HMOs, if one views the Medicare beneficiary market as self-contained. However, even if one accepts this assumption, there remains a serious problem of face validity associated with this measure. There simply were not many markets in which the share of Medicare beneficiaries in HMOs was significant during the 1985–1987 study period. As Welch points out, HMO Medicare market share exceeded 25 percent in only three communities, all in Minnesota. I think the Medicare market share measure is most usefully viewed as a proxy that may be correlated with the overall (but unobserved) market share measure.

I would have preferred the third approach. It is possible to construct overall market share measures by allocating HMO enrollment to the county, prorating by the population of the county served. For HMOs where major problems are obvious, additional information can be gathered through direct contacts with the plans. Also, the empirical analysis can include binary control variables for statewide IPAs or for plans where, based on the information collected through telephone conversations, the allocation scheme chosen seems most problematical. The sensitivity of the regression findings to the nature of the assignment algorithm chosen by the analyst could be explored. In my view, the research question is important enough to merit the expenditure of considerable effort in developing measures of market pressure imposed by HMOs. In this same vein, it might well be useful to introduce into the regression models other measures of HMO market structure as well. For example, the degree of competitive pressure felt by fee-for-service providers is likely to be different, for the same HMO market share, if all HMO enrollees are in a single IPA that includes all community physicians versus three group practice HMOs with physician panels that do not overlap versus a single staff model plan. Other measures of market structure that capture differences of this sort could be interacted with market share in the empirical analysis.

While I would be cautious about placing too much emphasis on the empirical results in the paper, given the problems encountered in model specification, I fully concur with Welch's concluding comment that "as the HMO market share in an area increases, using the FFS sector as a basis for HMO payment loses its straightforward appeal." I would go further, however, and suggest that there is little "straightforward appeal" in basing HMO rates on fee-for-service costs even when the HMO market share is low.

The paper by Rossiter and associates addresses the second qualification pertaining to adverse selection. He correctly notes that findings in the literature on this issue suggest that HMOs experience favorable selection in the Medicare market. In explaining why, he summarizes previous literature pointing out the shortcomings of the various approaches used to determine if adverse or favorable selection occur. He also notes that these studies have been done on beneficiaries in contracting HMOs, and for this reason alone it is not surprising that they find favorable selection for the HMOs. Those HMOs that had some reason to expect that they would experience adverse selection would be unlikely to contract with Medicare or would terminate existing contracts if they felt that adverse selection was likely to be chronic. As the program is now structured, if HMOs happen to enroll a disproportionate share of high utilizers, they can encourage them to disenroll or they can terminate their Medicare contract.

The primary focus of the paper by Rossiter et al. is on testing an approach for risk rating that could be used to "modify the AAPCC." This model is based on previous work done by Robinson et al. (1991)

for employed groups and uses six equations to predict the average medical expenses in a group. As implemented by Rossiter et al. the model requires individual level data on age, gender, marital status, education, income, functional ADL level, and presence of chronic health problems. The model was tested using data from the 1983–1987 National Medicare Competition Demonstration Evaluation and appears to work quite well. However, to be implemented, this approach would require each contracting HMO to provide HCFA with data on chronic conditions and functional status for all or a sample of its enrollees. Since the predictions appear to be influenced strongly by these measures, the potential for gaming on the part of HMOs is obvious. "Physical functioning creep" will become a new term in the health services researcher's vocabulary. Also, as Rossiter et al. point out, the rates for any given year will be based on data submitted by the HMO on enrollees in the previous year or (more likely) from two years previously. This is not a matter of concern to them as they do not "expect massive shifts in enrollment from year to year." However, while enrollment shifts may not be "massive," they could nevertheless be important, since disenrollment is continuous and HMOs have an incentive under this system to identify and encourage disenrollment on the part of high utilizers.

The Rossiter et al. paper adds to the already impressive amount of research attention that has been devoted to developing better methods of risk rating in HCFA contracts with HMOs. However, as Pauly (1984) points out, forcing health plans to charge the same premium within any preset actuarial category is the essential precondition for "cream skimming." Adverse selection will always occur to some degree. The essential issue is how to allocate scarce administrative and analytical resources in future efforts to improve the Medicare risk contracting program if, indeed, the program is to be continued in anything approaching its present form. In this respect it would seem worthwhile to at least consider the possibility that the concern over risk selection arises largely because of the nongroup nature of the Medicare market. Open enrollment periods with limited plan switching might be a more effective reform than experimentation with ever more complex systems for risk rating HMO payments. Individually risk-rated premiums (within a group) and risk-rated premium contributions are rare for group insurance in the nonelderly employed population. Introducing more complicated risk adjustments that involve the health status of the enrollee, treatment decisions, or similar variables that can be influenced by the health plan could easily backfire if new forms of gaming behavior on the part of health plans are rewarded.

Another reason to be concerned about further experimentation with risk rating systems is that it may well distract HCFA from undertaking more fundamental reform of Medicare's risk contracting process with HMOs. Both Welch and Rossiter et al. acknowledge that the present approach is fundamentally flawed, in that it provides HCFA with little information about the "right" price to pay contracting HMOs. Linking HMO payment to the fee-for-service sector could lead to under- or overpaying HMOs relative to the real cost of providing health care to Medicare beneficiaries using an efficiently organized and managed delivery system.

Rossiter et al. conclude their paper by proposing several useful changes that could be made in the present system. I would argue, in addition, that HCFA should devote most of its attention to developing alternatives to administrative pricing models that would break the link between fee-for-service and HMO payments. In particular, if HCFA wants to continue offering multiple HMOs to Medicare benificiaries in a given market area, it should give consideration to mounting a competitive pricing demonstration in selected market areas. At present, there are 57 metropolitan statistical areas with more than one active Medicare HMO, and these areas contain more than 40 percent of the U.S. elderly population. In such a demonstration, the government might consider setting its premium contribution equal to the lowest bid for Part A and Part B benefits by a qualified plan in a given area, paying all plans the same amount, including the fee-for-service Medicare "plan." The price of the fee-for-service alternative could be set based on the expected average cost of caring for beneficiaries in the contract year. Bids for basic Medicare coverage could be collected annually in the period prior to open enrollment. (Additional suggestions for reform can be found in Dowd et al. 1992.) In the demonstration, HCFA may wish to require bids by risk category. However, bids by health plans that vary by risk category are not common in private sector benefit offerings, including situations where firms have offered multiple plans to employees for years. Thus HCFA should not delay implementation of such a demonstration until the elusive "perfect" (or even "acceptable") risk-rating approach is developed.

General Discussion

Opening the discussion, Jon Christianson commented that the question is, who bears the risk? The government wants the HMOs to bear the risk, and the HMOs want the government to bear the risk. Ideally, from the HMOs' point of view, there would be an outlier pool that would take care of all the high-cost patients. There would be perfectly adjusted risk, so no risk would be borne by the HMO. They would provide their services, and they would be paid on the basis of the administrative fee plus the cost of services. In other words, cost-based reimbursement. What could be better than that? You would have no risk, and you would get your profits. Louis Rossiter responded that this relates to the subtitle of his paper, "when does risk adjustment become cost reimbursement?"

Christianson mentioned that insurance companies own a large number of HMOs, and that the insurance company way of thinking about risk or avoiding risk is becoming more and more common among HMOs. This is the point of view that if we could only structure this like we did in the past with insurance, HMOs would work perfectly. The government needs to be concerned about that perspective. One could make a good case for the government bearing the risk; the government might be much better at pooling risk than dividing it up. Maybe the government is risk neutral, and maybe the HMOs are risk averse, so one would have to pay them a premium. Maybe it makes sense just to do cost-based reimbursement with HMOs and terminate the risk contracts.

Another participant commented that there are many reasons for variations in cost. All we are trying to do is partition out that part of the variance that relates to the permanent health status. The government wants to spread the risk to everyone so that a person's choice of health plan is independent of the risk of a neighbor's choice. Now you are rewarded for finding a health plan that eliminates the sick. There will always be some variation in sickness, and a plan will always want to be compensated for the sick people who are treated. Over time, it should average out. We want the HMOs to be in the market long enough to complete the cycle.

Harold Luft commented that this seems to be one of the asymmetries in the market. He said, "If I were an HMO and I had a large employer with adverse selection from them, I might be concerned about it but I wouldn't drop the contract, because that would give a loud message to every one of my other contracts that they might also be dropped. This could drive me out of business. However, I could drop HCFA if I don't think they are paying me fairly because they are a separate market. Moreover, I don't have to drop the enrollees; I could just go over to a cost-based contract under which I keep the enrollees and I get paid better for them. Thus, there would be no risk and a lot of gain."

Bryan Dowd said that he has a paper coming out soon reporting on a study of the relationship between enrollment and supplementary premiums charged by Medicare HMOs. They found that they could calculate a markup for this supplementary coverage that HMOs offer in the range of 10 percent. The reason that an HMO might even get a high AAPCC payment but still complain about it being too low is that because even after receiving this government allocation they still find themselves in a competitive market on the supplementary premium side. Even if they are in a sense overpaid, they still have to spend away their profits offering supplementary benefits in a competitive market, usually against the fee-for-service Medigap plans.

Dowd continued with a second point. For its retirees, the state of Minnesota already offers a choice of health plans that includes three HCPPs, two TEFRA risk plans, and some others. They have annual open enrollment periods, and they have a level dollar premium contribution that is set at zero so they don't pay anything. Retirees have to pay the full premium out of their pocket, but they get the advantage of group purchasing. They run the whole thing based on the HCFA contract year. This is an example of a large employer that offers open enrollment and choices and a level dollar contribution. They do not risk adjust; that is the one ingredient they do not have, and Dowd believes that we can learn something from the fact that they do not do risk adjustment.

Susan Palsbo argued that risk adjustment is desirable because when a retiree is shopping on the basis of price, the price will be reflecting the HMO's efficiency in providing care, rather than reflecting the success of underwriting out risks.

Dowd responded that the severity of that problem is an empirical question. The empirical data suggest it may not be as important as one might expect. Furthermore, as Jon Christianson indicated, setting an annual open enrollment, rather than continuous plan switching throughout the whole year, may reduce some of the concern that we have about risk adjusters.

This preceded a comment that there is a risk to moving to cost reimbursement, which is one of the major reasons at least one plan was willing to keep a multimillion dollar loss in our risk contract. If we go that route we are undermining the whole conceptual basis of HMO care.

Part V

Integrative Overviews

Chapter 13

Research Perspectives on HMOs and the Elderly

Joseph R. Antos

Held on the eve of what promises to be sweeping national health care reform, the FHP Foundation–Institute of Health Policy Studies Conference on HMOs and the Elderly brought together some of the most significant findings from a decade of research. The conference focused on four major questions:

- How have health maintenance organizations influenced the utilization of medical services for the elderly?
- Can HMOs maintain quality of care equal to that provided in a fee-for-service setting, in the presence of incentives to reduce utilization and costs?
- How satisfied are HMO enrollees with their participation in managed care?
- Do HMOs increase or decrease the cost of health care for the elderly?

Conference participants representing research and business interests probed both the methodological rigor and the applicability of the research to the policy challenges facing HMOs.

This paper highlights some key findings from the conference on the effects of HMOs on health care utilization, quality of care, patient satisfaction, and cost. It then turns to what we need to know about HMOs, in order to improve their functioning and to inform policymakers as they grapple with the challenge of improving access to appropriate and affordable health care in America. This review, necessarily brief, is merely intended to outline current and future research directions in this important field.

Service Utilization

Do HMO physicians practice a less intensive style of medicine? Do enrollees avail themselves of the additional preventive services offered by HMOs? One recent study suggests that HMOs are fulfilling their promise of more conservative medicine, compared to fee-for-service.

Brown and Hill's analysis of 1989–1990 Medicare data finds that HMOs did not reduce hospitalization rates, but did reduce length of stay. This finding is remarkable in that it occurred well after the prospective payment system had squeezed excessive hospital days out of FFS. This reduced length of hospitalization is accompanied by evidence of more frequent, although less intensive, posthospital care. This is just what one would expect if HMO case managers are aggressively seeking the least intensive and least expensive site of care.

A similar pattern is seen for ambulatory care, with more HMO enrollees receiving physician care but fewer receiving extensive services than FFS beneficiaries. For example, enrollees were more likely to have received a physical examination but less likely to report 12 or more physician visits per year than FFS beneficiaries.

Quality of Care

Capitated payment arrangements, such as those existing in Medicare risk HMOs, are intended to contain health care costs. Cost containment is acceptable only if the quality of care provided remains at a high level. Assessing quality of care is, however, a challenging task. There are wide geographic variations in what is considered appropriate care for given conditions, relatively little research comparing the efficacy of alternative treatments, and an explosion of new techniques and variants on the course of treating scores of conditions.

Rather than attempting to assess HMO quality generally, it is only feasible to study a few key conditions for which the standards of care are reasonably well established and for which we have assurance that proper care is effective in ameliorating the conditions. This is the approach taken by Retchin, Clement, and Brown, and by Carlisle et al. These papers find that HMO care is at least equal to FFS care for stroke and acute myocardial infarction. There appears to be less reliance on some types of diagnostic testing by HMOs, although the contribution of those tests to favorable outcomes is not clear. HMO patients are discharged from the hospital "quicker" and somewhat "sicker." Recovery takes time, however, and condition at discharge may simply reflect the natural course of recovery and not differences in treatment. Posthospitalization experience differs between HMO and FFS patients, but again it is not clear that the differences affect patient outcomes.

Although these generally positive results for HMO quality are reassuring, the idea that managed care can mean high-quality care for the conditions studied should come as no surprise. The conditions selected are high-cost, involving substantial resources in the hospital and afterward. They are obvious candidates for case management. Even under less dramatic circumstances, however, there is evidence that HMO quality is appropriate. Under contract to HCFA (500-83-0047), Retchin et al. analyzed care for diabetes, hypertension, and routine care, such as physical examinations and immunizations, and found HMO care to be equal or superior to FFS care for these services.

Satisfaction

HMOs appear to have reduced utilization of some higher-cost services without sacrificing quality of care. To a policy analyst, these are very favorable results. But what do HMO enrollees think about HMOs? Unless HMOs can also satisfy their customers, they will not be successful in selling their services in the market.

In most cases, HMOs offer Medicare beneficiaries enhanced services at substantially lower cost than FFS Medicare (with or without supplementary insurance). Not surprisingly, HMO enrollees are very satisfied with their out-of-pocket expenses, but they are not as satisfied with the care they receive. Clement, Retchin, and Brown find that enrollees are less likely than FFS beneficiaries to be highly satisfied with the level of personal attention they receive and their access to desired services. Enrollees recognize a tradeoff between cost and other aspects of care.

In interpreting these results, one must weigh how much of the problem is poor customer service and how much is unreasonable expectations on the part of the customers. HMO enrollees have consciously chosen HMOs for their health care, and are likely to be more conscious of a tradeoff between service and cost than FFS beneficiaries. It may also be more informative to focus on recent HMO disenrollees' attitudes and experiences to ascertain what is, and is not, being managed well by HMOs.

Cost

The debate over whether HMOs save money for the Medicare program has raged for a decade, and shows no signs of abating. The major debating points:

- Risk HMOs are paid 95 percent of estimated FFS costs. If those costs are misestimated, payments are off.

- FFS costs do not reflect the cost of efficient practice. If HMOs are more efficient, the adjusted average per capita cost (AAPCC) can lead to overpayment.

- The AAPCC makes no allowance for the pent-up demand for services encountered when Medicare beneficiaries first enter HMOs offering broader benefits and lower copayments than FFS.

- HMOs may serve a less costly population than FFS providers, more than compensating for the 5 percent payment reduction mandated by law.

In the most thorough analysis to date of Medicare risk HMOs, Brown and Hill find that Medicare pays out 5.7 percent more for enrollees in capitation payments than the costs it would have incurred had these individuals remained in FFS.

Rossiter, Chiu, and Chen's paper points out that the voluntary nature of the Medicare risk program virtually assures that risk HMOs will have favorable selection. HMOs facing a sicker than average population will eventually drop out of the risk program in the face of repeated financial losses. Those with fewer sick enrollees will be profitable and remain with the program. If, however, the AAPCC could be adjusted to compensate properly HMOs with unfavorable enrollee selection (and reduce the overpayment to HMOs with favorable selection), the Medicare risk program could become more attractive to HMOs and Medicare beneficiaries.

Many are skeptical that an adequate risk adjuster can be found. Rossiter et al. criticize adjusters based on prior utilization, but their endorsement of the SEGA model hinges on the validity of enrollee-reported health status. It is arguable that individuals know more about their own health than physicians who treat them. Settling the choice of model is ultimately an empirical question: Which model better predicts health expenditures for a group of HMO enrollees?

It remains to be seen whether even the best possible risk adjuster can resolve the HMO biased selection problem. Other program modifications—such as the institution of long-term contracts between Medicare and risk HMOs to improve payment predictability, annual coordinated open enrollment periods, enrollee lock-in for 12-month periods, and use of Social Security district offices or other independent brokers for enrolling beneficiaries—may be needed to reduce the amount of selection bias that must be accounted for by the payment system.

Future Research

As this discussion suggests, a great deal is known about the impacts of HMOs on utilization of services, quality of care, patient satisfaction, and cost for the Medicare program. A good deal more can still be learned through future research projects. Several themes are evident:

- Analysis is needed on how to better manage care in general, and care of the elderly in particular. The elderly frequently have chronic, multiple conditions requiring different types of care management interventions than those for the under-65 population.
- Studies would be useful that closely examine HMO quality of care, as well as the systems by which HMOs manage and improve their quality. Studies that combine process, outcomes, and patient satisfaction measures of quality could provide a more complete view of these issues.
- The challenge of the frail elderly and the disabled is increasing. Research on the role of coordinated care in serving these special populations may lead to more efficient ways to handle their broader needs for clinical and social supports.
- Organizational and administrative innovations should be tested for their applicability to care for the elderly. The development of new models of care, and new ways to pay for that care, requires careful analysis.

Areas of Greatest Research Need

HMOs vary greatly in business organization, provider choice, coinsurance, access to services, incentive structures, and case management methods. Many existing studies of HMOs ignore this substantial variability in assessing HMO performance. It is important to examine the differences among HMOs to determine which service delivery models are more effective, and why.

Additional studies are needed to evaluate methods to improve the management of service utilization. More work is needed to develop techniques for analysis of provider and beneficiary claims history data to identify excessive or inappropriate service utilization. In addition, more work is needed to develop methodologies to assess the cost effectiveness and relative value of alternative utilization management interventions, such as provider education efforts, provider incentives to reduce utilization, and beneficiary-oriented interventions.

We should continue to study the relative effectiveness of capitated systems versus traditional delivery systems, especially as changing policies affect the FFS system. Equally important are studies that examine the quality of care among coordinated care systems and whether there are differences between the quality of care provided under such systems and under traditional FFS systems. Studies are needed that assess HMO internal quality assurance systems to determine how these systems focus on outcomes of care, utilize clinical data sets, and foster continuous quality improvement. Studies should also examine whether there are differences in access to and utilization of certain types of services in coordinated care systems versus traditional delivery systems. For example, what type and levels of preventive service are provided in HMOs? Are there differences in utilization rates of expensive technologies?

Further analysis is needed of the effectiveness of coordinated care approaches tailored to the unique needs of special populations, such as the frail elderly or the disabled. The existing Social/Health Maintenance Organization (S/HMO) demonstration has provided many insights into the challenges of adding services for the frail elderly to a traditional acute care benefit package. A new generation of S/HMOs, or other entities, should study how we can do a better job of integrating acute and long-term care services under one health care umbrella. A geriatric clinical management model may be feasible that includes preventive services, more anticipatory and aggressive management to reduce the number of acute care episodes as well as their severity, and improved decision making related to the use of acute, postacute, and long-term care services.

Research is needed on how beneficiaries can better understand and utilize managed care systems. Increasingly beneficiaries have been asked to make choices, but the information needed to help them make those choices has not kept pace. We need to find ways to compare health plan alternatives (including FFS alternatives) in an understandable way, and we need to provide this information in an unbiased way to beneficiaries. Complex operational data will, of course, be demanded by employers, insurers, and other major purchasers of health care. But information on such issues as average waiting room time, accessibility to a personal physician, and other consumer-oriented matters will become increasingly important.

The ongoing controversy over the AAPCC is an indication of the future research potential of improving or replacing the current payment methodology. Some approaches, such as a special working-aged adjuster, await the development of valid data but are conceptually straightforward. Others, such as risk adjusters, require substantial methodological development as well, but may ultimately yield a resource allocation tool with applications beyond managed care. Breaking the payment methodology link to FFS costs ultimately will be required, at least in areas where HMOs come to dominate their local markets. Studies are needed to explore the degree of HMO penetration at which FFS comparisons begin to fail, and to develop alternatives (such as the competitive bidding strategy espoused by Dowd).

Other approaches to payment involve reconsidering the nature of the Medicare risk contract. Studies could examine new payment methods that include partial, rather than full, risk on the part of managed care providers. Another concept worth considering is providing multi-year contracts to managed care providers in which payment rates could be fixed for the total contract period (or adjusted in some predictable way).

Managed care models also involve providers paid on a FFS basis, such as PPO networks and providers affected by various utilization or case management systems. Studies are of interest which develop cost-effective payment methods for FFS-based managed care models. Important issues include the potential role of incentive payment arrangements for organizations that manage managed care systems (such as PPOs or case management organizations), and approaches for establishing cost-effective FFS payments to providers through negotiated discounts, bundled payments, or incentive arrangements.

As managed care systems expand, we expect to see a proliferation of new service delivery models. Studies of these new risk-based approaches will reveal their applicability to the Medicare population. Some of these alternatives include:

- Direct payment capitation for physicians who are willing to assume all responsibility and risk for some (e.g., ambulatory services) or all care for beneficiaries.
- Open-ended HMOs and nonenrollment point-of-service models.
- Diagnosis-based managed care models that define benefit packages and capitated payment rates for services commonly provided in an episode or longer continuum of care for individuals with selected chronic conditions.
- Payment methods that include a combination of capitation and reinsurance for individual or aggregate expenses above threshold limits.

Conclusion

Over 2.3 million Medicare beneficiaries are enrolled in a prepaid Medicare contract, two-thirds of whom are in risk HMOs. The 30 million Medicare beneficiaries remaining in traditional FFS represent a substantial potential market for managed care plans, which offer the opportunity for more cost-efficient use of health resources, expanded choices of health service delivery systems for consumers, and better health outcomes through effective care management. Research can lead to the development of new approaches to managed care that may better meet the needs for cost-effective and efficient services for the elderly.

Health care reform efforts for the under-65 population will also shape how plans will deal with this population in the coming decade. If a managed competition approach ultimately is adopted, we may well witness the birth of scores of natural experiments, conducted by health insurance sponsors in the course of providing coverage to their members. Research is needed to aid in our understanding of the successes and failures of managed care systems, so that these systems may successfully adapt to the challenges of health care reform.

Acknowledgments

Comments by James Hadley, Thomas Kickham, Mary Kenesson, and William Clark are appreciated. This paper represents the views of the author, and does not necessarily reflect the policies of the Health Care Financing Administration.

Reference

Retchin, S. M., R. S. Brown, et al. *National Medicare Competition Evaluation: An Evaluation of the Quality of the Process of Care.* RFP number HCFA-83-ORD-29/CP. Contract number 500-83-0047. Richmond, VA: Medical College of Virginia, 1983.

Chapter 14

Medicare Risk Contracting: Policy or Market Failure?

Mark C. Hornbrook

The papers and discussions presented at this conference allow us to draw the following four important conclusions for policymakers and researchers:

- **First,** the Medicare TEFRA risk-contracting program has not yet succeeded in reaching the desired policy targets with respect to overall enrollment rates, beneficiary access, quality of care, and program cost savings. The risk program represents only a small proportion of total Medicare beneficiaries and outlays, and serious concerns have been expressed regarding perverse effects on these policy goals.

- **Second,** much more work on risk-assessment models is needed for aged populations, to support both risk payment and, more importantly, care management for frail beneficiaries. The poor performance of current risk adjustment procedures has enabled HMOS to gain excessive Medicare payments for the relatively healthier beneficiaries they have enrolled.

- **Third,** policymakers and researchers have been focusing primarily on whether HMOS are being overpaid by Medicare for the amount of risk they are willing to underwrite rather than on developing policies to stimulate HMOs to realize the inherent efficiencies of managed care for the sickest beneficiaries.

- **Fourth,** complex organizations, like group and staff model HMOs, are difficult for consumers (and policymakers) to understand and use, as revealed by several beneficiary satisfaction studies. This is no reason, however, to give up on efforts to improve managed care systems.

Specific findings from the research papers presented at this conference reveal that HMOs:

- are a relatively small segment of Medicare;
- are more efficient than fee-for-service (FFS) providers;
- provide the same or better quality of care than FFS providers;
- provide better access to basic health care services relative to FFS providers;
- stimulate competition and efficiency in the FFS sector;
- skim healthier beneficiaries;
- are overpaid by the AAPCC;
- produce less satisfaction for their enrolled beneficiaries compared to FFS beneficiaries;
- are risk averse and exit from the TEFRA risk program when financial margins become too tight; and
- ration care to Medicare beneficiaries, especially costly services and complex treatments.

In sum, we are presented with a mixed review of the risk program. HMOs are complex, multidimensional organizations, however, and one should expect to observe variation in their behavior and performance. These observations are not meant to criticize the contributions of any of the conference papers published in this volume. Indeed, the papers present an excellent summary of current research on risk assessment, selection bias, quality of care, beneficiary satisfaction, and competition under Medicare. The conference provides an excellent foundation for developing future research and policy priorities for the Medicare program.

Overreliance on financial (cost) incentives, without consideration of output policies and system structures has created some perverse manifestations of Medicare risk contracting. The apparent failure of the risk contracting program stems from a misspecification of the policy strategy: the number of policy goals has been greater than the number of policy instruments. Capitation payment, by itself, cannot produce desired performance on multiple domains of cost, quality, and access. Each independent policy target requires a separate policy instrument. A comprehensive "managed care" policy must include more than a payment mechanism; it should incorporate the appropriate structured and process elements as well (Hornbrook and Goodman 1991).

The AAPCC has been viewed strictly as an actuarial tool (which it is in its current form), with no attention given to classifying risk to inform

HMO managers, physicians, and nurses about care requirements for their members. Risk assessment models should represent an important tool for allocating resources in managed care systems, in addition to serving as a policy tool to assure efficient and equitable payment to risk contractors. We ought to direct our efforts to exploiting the comparative advantages of group, staff, and network HMOs for improving care for frail, chronically ill populations. The data on quality of care and outcomes of HMOs relative to the FFS sector are optimistic, but much more work is needed to develop and test models of care for frail and chronically ill populations. Rather than condemning HMOs for exploiting consumer ignorance and inertia, we ought to be working on ways to help consumers, policymakers, and clinicians understand how complex management tools and delivery systems can improve outcomes, cost-effectiveness, and equity of health care. Most HMOs can provide a level of service that meets the expectations of their members, if it is a top priority for all physicians, nurses, and other staff. Development of health care models based on population-based clinical practice requires major reform of medical education (Greenlick 1992), delivery systems, benefit structures, and payment systems (Enthoven 1987; Enthoven and Kronick 1989).

Purpose and Goals of the Medicare Risk Program

To place this conference in the proper context, we should return to the first point made in the first paper, by Brown and Hill, regarding the size and scope of the Medicare risk program, which has grown from the eight-HMO Prospective Payment Demonstration Project in 1980 to 83 health plans serving nearly 1.4 million beneficiaries in 1992. On the one hand, this is an important accomplishment for a program that was initially legislated to support fee-for-service payment for physicians and cost-based payment for hospitals. On the other hand, the risk program only covers 4 percent of beneficiaries and only 9 percent of those who could have selected a risk contract (paper by Rossiter, Chiu, and Chen), and the number of risk contractors has declined from a high of 134 (Brown and Hill). Moreover, risk enrollment is highly concentrated, with a few plans and a few cities accounting for more than half of the risk contact enrollment (Brown and Hill).

Rossiter, Chiu, and Chen suggest that HMOs may not have made the necessary investment in learning how to care efficiently for the elderly, so exit is higher as they learn the cost implications of caring for frail beneficiaries. Another factor at play here may be that the Medigap burden to HMOs—copayments, deductibles, preventive services, and extended benefits for home health care, drugs, vision, and hearing—may be more than many plans can manage.

Medicare's risk program, therefore, has not succeeded in giving a majority of beneficiaries the choice of an integrated Medicare/Medigap HMO plan. It has not mirrored HMO market penetration in employer groups (about 20 percent), which means that most employed HMO members are required to switch to a different type of health plan when they become eligible for Medicare. To counter resistance to development and entry of nonprofit HMOs in many large metropolitan areas, new policy initiatives are required.

HMO Effects on Use, Quality, and Outcomes

Patterns of use

Brown and Hill find that Medicare risk contractors did not reduce hospital admission rates but did reduce lengths of stay relative to FSS providers. HMOs increased access to physician services, but restricted frequent visits to physicians by Medicare beneficiaries. The same effects were observed for skilled nursing facility (SNF) admissions and home health visits. Brown and Hill interpreted these patterns as showing increased efficiency of HMOs relative to FFS, confirming the results of other studies of HMO care of nonaged populations.

Quality of care

The results of the two quality of care studies presented at this conference confirm previous research. Specifically, the paper by Carlisle et al. showed that HMOs perform better on process quality of care criteria than FFS hospitals in treating acute myocardial infarction (AMI) patients. Retchin, Clement, and Brown found no significant differences between HMO and FFS stroke patients on mortality rates, hospital readmission rates, or functional status at discharge.

One minor methodological concern arises in the Carlisle et al. study, where Carlisle describes the research design as a comparison between a random sample of 369 AMI cases treated in HMO hospitals and a random sample of 1,119 AMI cases treated in FFS hospitals. However, the HMO cases are clustered in 3 HMOs and the FFS cases are clustered in 297 hospitals. This raises a question of the true unit of analysis—the patient, the physician, or the practice? In any intervention study, the degrees of freedom are likely to be established by the organizational structure of the HMO, if sufficiently large, or by the number of HMOs, because the critical decision maker with respect to quality of care is the physician or, perhaps, even the medical group.

One implication of Carlisle et al.'s study is that managed care systems can better conform to process criteria than independent, unmanaged practitioners are able to. Moreover, they demonstrated that the real issue for policy and research is the variability in criterion conformance within both HMO and FFS sectors because it is much larger than the between-sector variance. Carlisle points out that substantial variation characterizes compliance with individual process criteria within HMO groups. It does not describe the organizational structure of the three study HMOs nor the number of different physicians are involved in the care of the study cases. The same applies to the FFS cases, albeit one suspects that the hospitals were not so clustered as to create a high probability of multiple medical staff appointments for physicians appearing in the sample. To succeed, an HMO must create a management structure, operating policies, and procedures to control medical care process and outcomes. To the extent that the study HMOs were successful in achieving this, we would expect better conformance to process criteria than independent FFS physicians would show.

The scores on Carlisle's technical diagnostic scale appear to result from rather poor performance by two of the HMOs and above-average performance by the other HMO. This suggests a structural pattern in the way that these two HMOs admit chest pain cases that undermines conformity with the diagnostic criteria. Carlisle et al.'s paper does not demonstrate that these HMOs were engaged in a self-diagnostic search for the causes of these poor scores.

To illustrate this latter point, if we look at the rankings of the three HMOs on the various process scales, we see that HMO3 had four first places and one second place, while HMO1 had only two first places, two second places, and a third place, yet ranked first overall. The results seem to be particularly sensitive to HMO1's high standing on the technical diagnostic criterion. Thus, HMO3 could have improved its overall standing markedly if it had received some help in examining its diagnostic workup procedures for AMI patients. HMO3's overall excellence is further supported by its top ranking on normal last lab results and rechecking abnormal lab values. We have, in essence, a method for stimulating and reinforcing excellence in standards of practice. Moreover, HMO2's consistent low ranking indicates an overall low standard of quality that should undergo reevaluation by top management in the health plan and medical group. It would be very interesting to know something about the structure of these HMOs. Are they group or staff models or IPAs? How large are they? How many hospitals were involved in the study? How many different physicians? Geographic considerations are crucial:

a well-developed emergency medical services system in a community may be an HMO's first defense against high AMI mortality. If this risk factor is not included in the mortality prediction models, the quality of care measures will be confounded.

Retchin, Clement, and Brown provide an intriguing insight into variations in the processes of caring for stroke patients. They found clear differences in length of stay between HMO and FFS stroke patients, but when stratified by severity, the difference narrowed considerably for ICU days for high severity patients. The pattern of care appears to be more aggressive speech therapy and quicker discharges to nursing homes for stroke patients in HMOs. This seems to result in higher levels of speech deficits persisting at discharge. Long-term follow-up was not conducted to determine whether the FFS-HMO differences persisted at three and six months postdischarge.

A significant implication of Retchin's study is that HMOs seem to be willing to explore rationing of services when efficacy has not been demonstrated. This reinforces the need for good outcome studies to examine whether prevailing standards of care call for unnecessary services. Another implication is that when hospital services are conserved, emphasis shifts to alternative modes of managing cases, including home care, nursing home care, and foster home care. With good management systems and supports, HMOs may be able to realize the same or better outcomes than FFS at low costs. This is especially true in the case of very frail patients, such as those with strokes who have multiple functional deficits that require careful integration of medical and social management. These cases require a safety net to avoid adverse events; the patients require careful monitoring, emotional support, and access advocacy to sustain their quality of life. HMOs should develop participatory care management systems (also known as shared decision-making programs (Kasper, Mulley, and Wennberg 1992) that empower patients to set limits on their own demands (which may relate, in no small way, to their fears about pain, disability, and death).

Three of the studies—Carlisle et al.; Retchin, Clement, and Brown; and Wisner, Feldman, and Dowd—reinforce the findings of previous research that HMOs provide care of better or comparable quality to urban FFS providers. Given the strong anti-HMO flavor on the favorable selection issue, a finding that HMOs were treating their patients worse than FFS standards could have been the final push toward a Canadian style single-payment system in the health care reform debate.

Competitive Effects of HMOs on Medicare Outlays

Brown and Hill's paper found evidence of favorable selection by Medicare risk contractors and estimated that HCFA paid HMOs about 5.7

percent more than would have been paid had those risk beneficiaries stayed in the FFS sector. Wisner, Feldman, and Dowd (1992) showed no differences in physical functioning between HMO and FFS beneficiaries in the Twin Cities area, but HMOs were associated with better perceived health status among older beneficiaries (age greater than 88). In contrast, Welch derives an intriguing finding from an econometric analysis of Medicare payments at the MSA level, namely, that HMOs decreased Medicare expenditures, despite other research suggesting strong favorable selection. By law, the cost savings from TEFRA risk contracts should be 5 percent if the AAPCC risk adjustment model is unbiased. Welch estimated the cost savings produced by the risk program at 1.2 percent in the short run and up to 3.9 percent in the long run.

Welch's paper suggests that HMOs can increase Medicare costs by attracting lower-cost beneficiaries and leaving a small pool of higher-cost beneficiaries in the FFS sector. An unbiased risk adjustment model should capture this effect, however. That is, a good model should leave risk contractors and HCFA indifferent regarding beneficiary choice of risk or FFS option. Thus, cost increases caused by selection bias reflect failure of the risk adjustment model. This is pertinent to HCFA's decisions regarding funding for research on risk adjustment. The favorable selection results seem to be interpreted as a condemnation of HMO enrollment practices, rather than a need to invest in development of better models. Neither the HMOs nor the beneficiaries should be viewed as being biased. Rather, the models are biased, and if HCFA is overpaying HMOs, it has the AAPCC to blame, not the HMOs. Of course, if all low-cost patients are removed from the FFS sector, it is not easy to obtain unbiased estimates of their relative risks through extrapolation from high-cost FFS beneficiaries (Hornbrook, Bennett, and Greenlick 1989). This is another reason for developing alternative methods for setting Medicare capitation rates.

Development of Risk Adjustment Models

Performance criteria for risk assessment model

Rossiter, Chiu, and Chen give a useful historical perspective on the development of performance criteria for risk assessment models, with the major point being that the estimation R^2 is a poor summary measure of model performance. The appropriate criterion is how well a model predicts for groups, not for individuals. We agree and have developed a useful strategy for assessing performance of prediction models at each stage of the development process (Table 14.1).

Risk adjustment models should relate to the underlying permanent health status of Medicare beneficiaries. Therefore, risk should relate

Table 14.1   Performance Measures for Risk-Assessment Models

Criterion	*Measure*
Derivation of Prediction Model	
Face validity	Predictors assess only enrollees' permanent health status and use propensity
Separability/Parsimony	Statistical significance of risk coefficients in multiple split samples
Construct validity	Overall F-ratio; R^2 of observed expense
Validation of Model on an Independent Unbiased Dataset	
Accuracy	Average prediction error in multiple split samples
Policy relevance	Standard deviation of predicted values
Goodness-of-fit	Intercept, slope, and R^2 of regression of predicted on actual expenses
Model bias	Regression of prediction errors on: gender, age, employment status, prior use, and functional and perceived health status
Validation of Model on Multiple Biased and Unbiased Validation Datasets	
Bias and stability	Average performance on above criteria in multiple datasets drawn from FFS and HMO experiences
Validation of Model on Health Plan Payments	
Acceptability	Gaming behavior by health plans and beneficiaries Health plan entry and exit
Over-/Underpayment	Estimate complete models of health plan choice to assess selection bias

to future valid needs for medical care regardless of which system or plan enrolls a beneficiary. A risk adjustment scheme is a taxonomy of health plan outputs. If health plans are using output-based budgeting and management, then risk classification should be applied to internal planning and management of care. That is, risk classes should be iso-resource classes, with only stochastic variation in actual resource use. They are prospectively defined classes that set relative resource intensity for managing access and planning care for persons in each class.

Strategies for validating risk assessment models should employ bootstrapping and other advanced statistical techniques to reduce the effects of outliers and random noise. Moreover, risk coefficients need to be derived from efficient, representative practice patterns (Table 14.1).

Rossiter, Chiu, and Chen pose the the "TEFRA HMO conundrum" as "why does research show that the plans should make excess profits through biased selection alone, yet the plans [complain] that payments are too low, and many HMOs avoid the market entirely?" (Chapter 11, page 252). Either the premium is not high enough to overcome risk evasion or the research on selection bias has drawn the wrong conclusions. One part of the answer might be in how Medigap is treated in selection bias studies.

Plans with adverse selection among their Medicare risk membership will tend to leave the risk contracting program because it is the only way to cope with an AAPCC biased against them. Thus, with a biased risk adjustment model one should expect favorable selection overall as plans self-select out of the program. We should not be surprised by the research results on favorable selection. With an unbiased model, however, sampling variation is expected to be small for HMOs with memberships over 50,000 and would average out over time; only small HMOs would face survival problems from random adverse selection. For this, we need a reinsurance program.

Prior use models

Rossiter, Chiu, and Chen recommend that payments to HMOs not be risk adjusted because this mechanism may present perverse incentives for efficiency. That is, if prior use is incorporated into a risk adjustment scheme, payment under such a scheme would reward greater service intensity, thereby becoming analogous to cost reimbursement and individual experience rating. A high-cost person in one year qualifies for a higher rate the next year as a payback to protect the health plans' financial position, assuming the beneficiary does not switch to another plan. This could represent a potential benefit of prior-use models—rather than dumping high-risk members, health plans could face incentives to keep them! Risk models produce truncated prediction distributions, however, and never approach the observed levels of outlier costs. Also, the highest-cost cases tend to be terminally ill beneficiaries who do not survive to qualify for higher payment. Prior use is a good predictor of future expense, to be sure, and in a transition period it could be considered as one of the options for risk adjustment. In the long run, however, the market will perform better if risk contractors face relative capitation rates that reflect underlying health status rather than use patterns per se.

SEGA risk model

Brown and Hill come to the preferred conclusion in their study of biased selection under Medicare risk contracts: improve the AAPCC risk assessment formula by including measures of serious chronic diseases. Rossiter, Chiu, and Chen recommend the six-equation group adjustment (SEGA) model, which includes such health status adjusters as ADLs and chronic health problems. The major contribution of the SEGA model is that its complex structure helps cope with the highly skewed distribution of medical care expenses. It does not, however, help our understanding of health risk determinants—who are the persons likely to require higher than average levels of care next year, and what services will they require? This understanding requires that our models incorporate the epidemiology of disease, injury, and frailty, including such factors as aging, exposure to environmental hazards, genetics, behavioral risks, immune system function, and physiologic reserve.

Feasible risk measures

Development of unbiased risk adjustment models for Medicare capitation payment is required for two equally important reasons: to alleviate the problem of market failure caused by risk avoidance strategies and to develop basic tools to assist health plans to deliver more cost-effective, higher-quality care to their members. That is, under population-based clinical practice, providers should operate on a prospective mode, seeking ways to improve access to prevention, early diagnosis, and the most appropriate treatment. Rather than always waiting until patients cross the threshold, plans need to pursue outreach efforts focused on prognostic patient classes that identify those most likely to benefit from various types of interventions. A risk taxonomy provides the foundation for primary, secondary, and tertiary prevention activities and enables providers to analyze the cost-effectiveness of alternative treatment regimens (by correcting for severity differences). Thus, the feasibility constraints that are often offered as justification for not employing clinical or functional health status measures for risk adjustment should not apply. Just because HMOs do not collect or automate health risk data is not sufficient justification to close off that approach. If a clinician should know something about a beneficiary in order to plan the most cost-effective care management plan, that health status variable should be available for risk adjustment as well. Conversely, if certain variables are shown to be a stable, accurate, and valid predictor of health status next year, HMOs ought to be routinely collecting those data to help them focus intervention efforts on the patients who can benefit the most.

Policy and research are pointed in the wrong direction: finding fault with HMO's Medicare enrollment patterns. Rather we should be focusing our efforts on making vertically integrated health care systems work better. Policy should push HMOs to collect better risk data, to measure access and queue lengths, and to measure outcomes. These data should help HMOs better serve Medicare beneficiaries. Ultimately, HMOs should develop dynamic member health status monitoring systems based on automated clinical information systems and periodic health screening. Formal cost-effectiveness analyses should inform decisions regarding indications for high-cost procedures and intensive care regimens. HMOs should be induced to collect beneficiary health status as a part of routine clinical practice so that a risk-adjustment policy need not involve overlay of another costly data collection system. Such a system will probably include diagnoses and perceived health and functional status. Prior use can be used within an HMO to allocate resources when managers are confident that practice styles are relatively homogeneous, but this method carries perverse incentives when applied across widely varying technologies.

Beneficiary Satisfaction

The study by Clement, Retchin, and Brown on beneficiary satisfaction with access and quality of care in HMO and FFS settings seems to reinforce the notion that managed care systems impose strong "hassle" burdens on Medicare beneficiaries. This is particularly salient in the areas of the patient-physician relationship (e.g., explanations, attention to the patient, amount of preventive advice, personal interest in the patient, and respect and privacy issues), access to care (seeing one's physician of choice, telephone access, and appointment lags), and perceived quality of care (perceived accuracy of the diagnosis and thoroughness of the treatment). The Clement, Retchin, and Brown paper suggests that Medicare's use of managed care as a cost-containment measure should be viewed with caution because beneficiaries are being asked to make sacrifices, assuming that they made allowances for the out-of-pocket cost of risk enrollment in rating the satisfaction on other dimensions. The authors do not present breakdowns by type of HMO or by length of membership in the health plans.

An alternative interpretation of this finding is that HMOs need to pay much greater attention to the consumer orientation of total quality management. In the past, the internal operations of group and staff HMOs have been structured to recruit physicians; by structuring physicians' workdays, reducing on-call duty, and increasing educational and annual leave, HMOs have offered physicians fewer patient contact hours per week. The trade-off is that physicians' appointment schedules are centrally controlled, leaving them less discretion in setting the pace of work. In addition, administrative duties pull many physicians out of the clinic. Thus, HMO beneficiaries may be correct in their perceptions that physicians are harried, unavailable, and unlikely to take sufficient time for explanations. However, this is not an indictment of managed care, but a description of a management problem. Reducing the length of physician workweeks and trying to increase visit productivity is a recipe for dissatisfaction and alienation of the medical group. The issue is how to make physicians more productive and increase member satisfaction at the same time. This is especially critical for older members whose multiple chronic health problems and declining social support systems present nearly overwhelming demands on physicians.

The Social/HMOs' extended benefits reduced disenrollment and increased member retention relative to aged FFS and HMO beneficiaries (Newcomer, Harrington, and Preston). S/HMO members with acute and chronic health conditions, as well as those with functional disabilities are more likely to disenroll than healthy members. One important finding of this study is the sensitivity of S/HMO members to cost issues, especially in the mature plans. The S/HMO impaired members are the least satisfied with their plans. This could relate to the fact that they present difficult challenges to physicians who must help them cope with the limitations of medical technology in curing the diseases of aging.

The study by Newcomer, Harrington, and Preston is disappointing within the context of this conference. As a satisfaction study, it represents an important contribution. However, this is the only paper on the Social/HMO concept and its sole focus on beneficiary satisfaction and disenrollment trivializes the salient contributions of the S/HMO demonstration to health services research and policy. Reform of primary care delivery systems should receive top priority for Medicare. We need to focus on benefit creativity and organizational flexibility to meet the care needs of the elderly.

We should develop a geriatric care model that includes outreach, access screening, assessment, and care planning and management. HMOs provide the logical foundation for population-based preventive services and disease screening. Medicare beneficiaries should have access to a geriatrically enhanced care model that integrates medical, long-term care, and social support services within the primary care module. Continuity of care with the same team of providers should be assured. The primary care team should incorporate medicine, nursing, pharmacy, social work, nutrition, physical therapy, and mental health. Frail and chronically ill beneficiaries should have a case manager who works with caregivers to ensure that all of the patient's needs are being met. Computerized clinical information systems should provide assurance that the patient's care plan is immediately available at any point at which the patient accesses the system, including out-of-plan providers for emergency services. With the aging of the population, research should focus on developing technological and social systems to sustain quality of life for functionally impaired beneficiaries, whether aging, disabled, or with end-stage renal disease. This will require an exploration of creative linkages between social welfare, long-term care, and medical care systems. This can be facilitated by Medicare benefit design and pooling of financing sources. Research and policy should focus on how to make the best use of existing resources to improve the quality of care, caring, and life for older persons.

Market Failure

A critical failure of the current health insurance system is highlighted in passing by Newcomer, Harrington, and Preston:

> This [narrow] tolerance for dissatisfaction among the functionally unim-paired has important health policy implications. Plans have the potential of improving their operations to meet the expectations of these members, or of selectively reducing benefits to stimulate the departure of "high-cost" or "high-risk" cases. (Chapter 5, pages 134–135).

Reinforcing this point, Wisner, Feldman, and Dowd show that the oldest, poorest, and sickest beneficiaries are found in the basic Medicare FSS sector in the Twin Cities area. Medical underwriting for Medigap policies means that poor persons with serious chronic disease or frailty are likely to face premiums they cannot afford. This relates primarily to older persons who are unable to obtain guaranteed supplemental coverage through their former employers or retirement systems. To deal with this problem, Wisner, Feldman, and Dowd propose reforming the Medicare market to require annual open enrollment periods, limits on switching between open seasons, and uniform premiums.

Why should health plans even have the option of skimming via benefit manipulation or medical underwriting for individuals? Health policy should work to remove the correlation between risk and benefits by mandating coverage that meets the health care needs set by community standards for all persons. Any coverage above this level should be for services deemed discretionary and should be paid entirely by premium contribution. One of the problems in the current Medicare risk market is that Medicare benefits are so inadequate that Medigap coverage has become the driving competitive force. Rather than competing on the basis of efficiencies in providing defined benefits, health plans have been able to use strategies to enroll the healthiest beneficiaries and disenroll the bad risks.

AAPCC Reforms

Three immediate reforms in the AAPCC suggested by the papers at this conference merit comment—the geographic factor, an outlier risk pool, and working-aged adjustment.

AAPCC geographic factor

Large and apparently random variations in the AAPCC over adjacent counties indicate a poor match between the program design and the structural characteristics of risk contractors. HMO beneficiaries who live in adjacent counties are likely to be treated in the same hospitals and medical offices by the same physicians and ancillary providers, yet their AAPCC rates can differ substantially. HMOs should face a single rate structure because their costs do not vary significantly by county within their service areas. As Rossiter, Chiu, and Chen recommend, the geographic factor in the AAPCC formula should receive high priority for immediate reform. The county as a geographic unit was established for HCFA's convenience rather than to reflect the structure of an HMO's service area.

Outlier risk pool

Rossiter, Chiu, and Chen suggest development of an outlier risk pool to handle problems of selection bias and instability. Two alternative policies should also receive consideration: (1) development of a risk-adjustment model that incorporates high-cost disease groups so that prospective payment rates can be established for annual episode phases; and (2) a reinsurance program for small HMOs. Large HMOs do not really need outlier protection—a large membership base protects them from large shifts in risk exposure from year to year. Indeed, most health plans perceive a continuity of risk that includes both market share shifts and risk selection. Outliers tend to result from serious and terminal acute and chronic disease that should be incorporated into a risk model. Diabetes, chronic obstructive pulmonary disease, congestive heart failure, HIV/AIDS, and end-stage renal disease are good examples of risk classes that are feasible, easy to measure, and understandable by all involved.

Prospective payment rates for these disease classes would avoid the problem of detailed financial audits to establish when a particular case crossed the outlier threshold. Reinsuring small Medicare risk HMOs would allow them to work in the same manner as their major line of business. (Wisner, Feldman, and Dowd document the mergers and consolidations in the Twin Cities market that, in effect, represent creation of larger risk pools.)

Working-aged adjustment

Adjustment for working-aged beneficiaries is important because it relates to correcting bias in the AAPCC. Persons who are still working after they reach age 65 are generally healthier than nonworking older persons (which includes all those persons who have retired because of poor health). Thus, even if we adjust for the fact that Medicare is a secondary payer, working-aged persons will cost less than other persons in their same age-gender cell.

Implications for Research and Policy

Despite being major participants in the Medicare risk program, prepaid group practice, staff, and network HMOs have not been fully implemented under the Medicare risk program. Payment policies and the medical culture do not stimulate contractors to fully exploit their comparative advantages in population-based clinical practice (Greenlick 1992). Medicare should promulgate a care model for its beneficiaries that includes health promotion and disease prevention; periodic disease screening; outreach and managed access to medical care; comprehensive assessment of frail and chronically ill patients; care planning; shared decision making among physician, care receiver, and caregiver; and care management to assure continuity. Reliance on episodic intervention within 15-minute office visits is not sufficient to meet the needs of frail, multiply compromised beneficiaries.

In sum, risk contracting still carries substantial promise for improving access, cost-effectiveness, and quality of care, but payment policy cannot carry the burden of achieving all of these goals. Health policymakers and researchers must focus on the organizational structure and processes of managed care plans. The medical and long-term care needs of our aging population have the potential to overwhelm the economy. The challenge for the risk contracting program is to develop and rigorously evaluate innovative care models that will stretch current Medicare outlays to provide the services listed here to persons who can best benefit from them.

Disclaimer

The statements contained in this report are solely those of the author and do not necessarily reflect the view or policies of the Kaiser Foundation Health Plan.

References

Enthoven, A. C. *Theory and Practice of Managed Competition in Health Care Finance.* Professor Dr. F. de Vries Lectures in Economics, Rotterdam School of Economics, Erasmus University, Rotterdam, The Netherlands, 1987.

Enthoven, A. C., and R. Kronick. "A Consumer-Choice Health Plan for the 1990s." *The New England Journal of Medicine* 320, no. 1 (1989): 29–37, 94–101.

Greenlick, M. R. "Educating Physicians for Population-Based Clinical Practice." *Journal of the American Medical Association* 267, no. 12 (1992): 1645–48.

Hornbrook, M. C., and M. J. Goodman. "Managed Care: Penalties, Autonomy, Risk, and Integration." In *Primary Care Research: Theory and Methods*, edited by H. Hibbing, P. A. Nutting, and M. L. Grade. Rockville, MD: Agency for Health Care Policy and Research, Public Health Service, U.S. Department of Health and Human Services, 1991, pp. 107–26.

Hornbrook, M. C., M. D. Bennett, and M. R. Greenlick. "Adjusting the AAPCC for Selectivity and Selection Bias under Medicare Risk Contracts." In *Advances in Health Economics and Health Services Research, Vol. 10*, edited by R. M. Sheffler and L. F. Rossiter. Greenwich, CT: JAI Press, Inc., 1989, pp. 111–49.

Kasper, J. F., A. B. Mulley, Jr., and J. E. Wennberg. "Developing Shared Decision-Making Programs to Improve Quality of Health Care." *Quality Review Bulletin* 18 (1992): 183–90.

Chapter 15

Summing Up

Harold S. Luft

When this conference was being developed, the organizers and participants had high hopes for both the quality of the research and its relevance for policymakers. It is my belief that the papers and discussions exceeded these expectations. The papers included not only several from the recently completed assessment of HMO enrollees under the Medicare TEFRA risk contracts but other recently completed and complementary studies. While the basic topics to be covered by the authors were known when they were asked to participate, we did not discuss their findings in detail. Thus, the contrasts and similarities in findings are all the more striking. Many of these issues were then highlighted in the ensuing discussion which helps to place the papers in context.

Research is rarely done in a vacuum; instead, it builds upon prior work. The brief background literature review is customary in research papers. Less customary, however, is a reconciliation of conflicting findings. This is understandable because the methods, data, settings, and precise questions asked may differ from study to study. Thus, it is acceptable merely to indicate differences in findings and conclusions, and many authors do not even go that far. From the perspective of a policymaker, however, conflicting findings cannot be so easily ignored. One can always merely select research that supports a preconceived view, but this incurs the short-run risk of being challenged by others with contrary viewpoints and the long-run risk of having made the wrong policy decision. Thus, reconciliation of conflicting findings is important.

Reconciliation sometimes involves the assessment that one set of results is simply superior to another in terms of its methods or quality of data. These instances are unusual. More frequently, differences in findings arise from subtle differences in study designs and execution. It is also difficult to "prove" what accounts for differences. Speculating on the reasons for differences may, however, lead to further work that eventually reconciles the findings. It is important to note that such a resolution is far more likely to show that each viewpoint is valid, from its own perspective, or with respect to the specific situation examined, than it is to declare one viewpoint correct and the other wrong. Even without such a resolution, speculation on potential reasons for conflict will alert policymakers to the hazards of merely choosing one set of results.

It is also important to consider the extent to which research findings are based on too limited a base to be generalizable for policy purposes. For example, even though many of the studies reported on at the conference relate to all Medicare beneficiaries in TEFRA risk contracts, several attendees pointed out that almost one-third of Medicare beneficiaries are in HMOs without risk contracts, and this proportion has been increasing. The researchers' focus on the risk contract HMOs is understandable, but the larger picture must also be understood.

The major sections of the conference each raise important larger questions concerning selection bias, quality of care, consumer and patient satisfaction, and the appropriateness of the AAPCC as a method of paying HMOs. Each of these areas will be discussed in turn, but it is important to note that some issues are cross-cutting, making compartmentalization difficult.

Selection Bias

To some extent, selection may be at the heart of many problems we face in assessing HMO performance. Yet, since the alternative of forced assignment of people into specific health plans is not politically viable, we must learn how to interpret evidence and differences in performance in the context of selection. Furthermore, it is important to recognize that selection occurs at many levels, only some of which are explicitly addressed in the usual research study.

There is selection of providers into health plans, HMOs in particular, and this varies across the nation in nonrandom ways. That is, some states have many HMOs, with varying organizational forms, while others still have no HMOs. When HMOs are present, it is safe to assume that physicians are selectively attracted to work in such settings, while others stay in fee-for-service practice. Thus, HMOs reflect not just economic and organizational characteristics, but also the professionals they attract. At the same time that HMOs are unevenly distributed across the nation, the willingness of HMOs to contract with the Medicare program is also uneven. Some parts of the country with substantial HMO enrollment among the working age population have relatively few Medicare enrollees, often because plans are unwilling to contract with Medicare at the rates based on the adjusted average per capita cost (AAPCC). Then, given the availability of an HMO willing to enroll the Medicare population, the attractiveness of the HMO relative to FFS will depend on a wide range of factors. Thus, one should be surprised by evidence of an absence of selection, rather than by its presence.

The papers by Brown and Hill and Wisner, Feldman, and Dowd appear to offer quite different findings with respect to selection. Reconciliation of these differences is difficult, but there are enough differences in the methods and settings to account for the conflicting findings. First, it is important to note that within each paper one could find statements suggesting no selection problem and other statements suggesting important problems. The authors are neither confused nor deliberately misleading. Rather, each paper addresses multiple issues and draws different conclusions on each issue.

Brown and Hill state that in their sample of FFS and enrollees in TEFRA risk contract HMOs, their statistical tests indicate that "estimates from the simpler model are not biased by self-selection of beneficiaries." It is important to note that this refers to the potential of selection to affect their estimated equations. Furthermore, these equations already include a substantial number of enrollee health status and attitudinal variables. When only the variables normally included in the AAPCC are used, their results suggest that HCFA payments would be above the predicted costs of these enrollees had they been in FFS. This implies favorable selection of about 5.7 percent, after adjusting for the AAPCC factors, but not adjusting for the other variables Brown and Hill find to be important predictors of use. One should recall, however, that the cost and utilization figures refer to the period prior to the enrollee survey, so some of these risk factors may be "post-dictors," rather than predictors.

Wisner, Feldman, and Dowd, in contrast, find that the AAPCC risk factors account for most of the differences in risk across plans in the Twin Cities area and that there is little additional selectivity. Again, this is based on statistical models that may not necessarily reflect the likely cost and utilization experience of enrollees. On the other hand, they find that the actual Medicare claims for the sampled population indicates an average reimbursement of $1,435 per beneficiary, in contrast to a weighted average AAPCC payment of $3,221. If true, this would imply no selection across plans within the Twin Cities, but substantial selection of the Twin Cities relative to the AAPCC.

An alternative explanation is that the model may not have been sufficiently detailed to capture important differences among plans. One key finding of the authors is the marked differences in health status and other measures for those in the FFS sector with and without supplemental insurance policies. Those without supplemental policies tend to be poorer and sicker, reflecting the frequently seen connection between the two variables and the fact that both FFS and HMO plans in the Twin Cities used risk screening. When the authors attempted to test for this, they had difficulty estimating their model, so it is difficult to rule out a selection effect.

The large difference between estimated and observed expenditures is likely to reflect several factors. Perhaps the most important is that the sample of 1,446 FFS beneficiaries used in the study may have been too small to assure a reasonable number of the very high cost cases which tend to dominate the Medicare expenditures. The study design used a 12-month follow-up period after the questionnaire, thereby assuring prediction rather than post-diction. However, this also meant that some people may not have filed claims due to their not having met the deductible—only 686 of these people had any reimbursements. This observation underscores the difficulty in designing research projects; the survey approach used by Brown and Hill avoided this problem of claims filing, but introduced the problem of post-diction. No methodology is simultaneously perfect, timely, and inexpensive.

Patient Satisfaction

The two studies of patient satisfaction are consistent in that both report relatively more dissatisfaction among HMO enrollees along most of the dimensions measured. The key exception is cost, in which HMO enrollees are typically more satisfied. Here again, selection issues are important for understanding the results. By definition, in every location in which one observes HMO enrollees, they have made a positive decision to be in the HMO rather than in FFS. In many cases, but not all, they have obtained more comprehensive coverage and better benefits, often at little or no out-of-pocket cost. (Roughly 50 percent of the HMO enrollees in the Clement, Retchin, and Brown study were in HMOs that required no additional premium and that also covered copayments and deductibles.) Their counterparts in FFS Medicare would typically have to pay additional amounts for supplemental coverage—unless their former employers offered such coverage as a benefit for retirees.

The Newcomer, Harrington, and Preston study of Social/HMO enrollees shows a similar pattern, but it is even more complex, because these people all had the choice of being in FFS, a traditional HMO, or an HMO (sometimes a traditional one) with additional long-term care coverage. Thus, there is the potential for selection not only between FFS and HMO coverage, but also between HMO plans with and without the extra-cost long-term care coverage. Not surprisingly, patient assessments of various dimensions are sensitive to the level of the patient's impairment, and thus their need for selected services and coverage.

Various comments by the attendees highlighted the notion that one must consider not only how people assess plans along various dimensions, such as access, waiting times, quality, and cost, but how they weigh these various dimensions in arriving at an overall assessment. For example, some people find the filing of claims a major burden, so they would rate highly that dimension and prefer an HMO, other things being equal. Other people might actually prefer to know exactly what was ordered for them and find the provision of such information in a claims form a desirable feature of FFS, rather than a negative. Likewise, the assessments of health plans one might elicit from someone with a bothersome chronic condition might be quite different from the assessments of someone who is generally healthy and only needs care for occasional acute, but potentially serious problems.

It is also important to combine measures of satisfaction with behavioral indicators. Even though the overall satisfaction measures were lower for the HMO enrollees, they still chose to remain enrolled. That is, on balance, they must have preferred the HMO over the always-available FFS option. This is not to say that dissatisfaction should be ignored. In fact, several commentators suggested that HMOs should use such information to assess and improve their own performance.

The Newcomer, Harrington, Preston study also demonstrated the importance of local market and HMO factors on measures of satisfaction *across* plans. In particular, it appeared that in some instances, where there were few alternatives with as comprehensive benefits as the S/HMO, disenrollment rates were lower and dissatisfaction was higher. This is consistent with the notion that people make complex decisions weighing various factors, and may be quite dissatisfied with a choice, yet prefer it to the alternative. While some might consider this a typical market situation, it is also one likely to lead to political action to improve the options.

Quality of Care

The two papers on quality of care were quite consistent in suggesting that quality was certainly no worse, and perhaps somewhat better in the HMOs than in FFS. The Carlisle et al. paper compares the quality of care for AMI patients in each of three HMOs to that of FFS beneficiaries in five states. Thus, the relatively better performance of the HMOs may actually be a reflection of the standards of care in their localities, relative to that of the five-state average. Beyond this point, however, Carlisle shows that quality of care was similar in two of the HMOs and markedly worse in one. This finding reinforces the importance of plan-specific assessments and the fallacy of assuming that all HMOs are comparable. Of course, one should likewise not assume that all physicians and hospitals in FFS are offering equal quality of care. The various quality review organizations well understand this, but the point is often lost on those who praise or criticize HMOs based on findings of one or two organizations.

Given this concern, the Retchin, Clement, and Brown study has the major advantage of being a representative sample of Medicare beneficiaries in risk contract HMOs. This, however, is also a disadvantage since enrollees are highly concentrated in a small number of HMOs, largely in southern California and south Florida. Their care was compared with that of FFS beneficiaries in the same counties as the HMO enrollees, so we are unable to know much about the overall performance of HMOs. It is also impossible to determine from the results presented whether there are differences in outcomes among patients in the different HMOs in their sample.

Two underlying problems remain, even with these carefully done studies. One problem is that assessments of quality of care still tend to take FFS as the "gold standard," particularly in determining what tests and procedures ought to be undertaken. Many aspects incorporated in the "standards" have not been well tested and may be either unnecessary or actually harmful. While better measures of quality are always desirable, this critique is particularly bothersome since it suggests that current measures have a bias against HMOs and thus may not be fair.

A second problem is that most of the quality assessment focus has been on the process and outcomes of care for hospitalized patients, yet most people are not hospitalized for serious problems. Thus, many more studies are needed of how various delivery systems deal with the more common chronic and minor acute problems, where death is rarely an outcome, but quality of life and the patient's perception of the process of care are important. Just as consumers do not assess cars only on their safety in a collision, quality assessments need to concentrate less on life-threatening problems.

Paying the HMOs: The Adequacy of the AAPCC

Perhaps more than any other issue, assessing the adequacy of the current AAPCC mechanism is dependent on one's perspective. Given the broad nature of this question, it is not surprising that throughout the conference speakers repeatedly touched on this problem.

As is usually the case when major conflicts arise over the interpretation of research, both methodological and ideological issues are at play.

The methodological issues arise within the context of the intent of the law requiring development of the AAPCC, that is, that Medicare should pay its risk-based contractors 95 percent of what their enrollees would have cost under the fee-for-service system sponsored by Medicare. The current approach combines data on the county's relative costs under FFS with the relative cost weights for Medicare beneficiaries in various age-gender-risk cells. HMOs are then offered premiums based on 95 percent of this figure, weighted by their actual mix of Medicare enrollees.

There is substantial controversy over how well this formula accounts for the actual costs these enrollees would have incurred under FFS. That is, many argue that HMOs typically experience favorable selection, even after the AAPCC adjustments. The evidence on this, however, is not uniform; even the two papers presented here disagree. Some of these arguments arise from differences in methods, for example, whether one uses risk factors to (prospectively) predict use (as in the Wisner, Feldman, and Dowd paper) or to (retrospectively) explain use (as in the Brown and Hill paper). Much of the focus is on whether there are a small number of relatively objective variables that, if added to the formula, would make it more accurate. Others, such as Rossiter, Chiu, and Chen, suggest that more work needs to be done on the modeling techniques, in order to approximate more closely the very skewed distribution of expenditures. This is not just an econometric exercise; since a large portion of Medicare expenditures are attributable to a small number of individuals, accurately characterizing these people and their risk is extraordinarily important in attempting to improve the AAPCC.

A different viewpoint is offered by those who step back from the issue of whether enrollees in HMOs have favorable selection and focus on why there might be favorable selection. This relates back to a point raised earlier: HMOs have the option of participating in the Medicare risk-based market. While the derivation of the AAPCC formula is complex, it is relatively easy for an HMO to approximate how much it will be paid for its enrollees. It must then decide whether to actively seek Medicare beneficiaries, a decision that will reflect a series of factors not often included in studies of selection bias. For example, the real-world market for Medicare enrollees has to take into account the role of Medicare supplemental insurance. This insurance reduces or eliminates the coinsurance and deductibles, which help constrain FFS use under Medicare. Thus, in areas with extensive "Medigap" coverage, FFS Medicare use will tend to be higher, and thus the AAPCC will tend to be higher, making market entry for HMOs more attractive. The HMOs, however, tend to bundle the benefits and coverage of a supplemental plan in with their base premium, and sometimes this is offered at no additional cost. In other instances, there may be an extra premium. Whether this premium is partially or fully covered by the enrollee's former employer can also have a major impact on selection. Both the Brown and Hill and Wisner, Feldman, and Dowd studies attempted to include some of these measures in their enrollee studies, but neither were designed to explore the interaction of the HMO decisions and those of the local populations.

Further confounding the analytic problem are several aspects of economies of scale. While people do not suddenly change their medical care needs when they turn 65, the contractual relationships between HMOs and sponsors, such as employers and Medicare, are quite different. Employers typically offer a limited number of health plan options, with an annual open enrollment season and little direct marketing to the enrollees. Medicare, however, allows its beneficiaries to switch plans on a monthly basis and offers no group marketing or enrollment support. Furthermore, Medicare has a complex set of contracting, consumer complaint, and quality assurance requirements. Even if the latter are no more stringent than those used by the HMO for its "regular business," the rules are usually different. This means that the administrative costs associated with having a small number of Medicare enrollees will be substantial. Thus, it is not surprising that the national Medicare market is dominated by a small number of HMOs with large enrollments. Since marketing and administrative costs often exhibit substantial economies of scale, potential new entrants may only be likely when the AAPCC is unusually high or if there are opportunities for favorable selection. These incentives are reinforced by the ability of HMOs to continue to cover their enrollees who age into Medicare under cost-based or other nonrisk contracts.

A final view on the AAPCC is that its underlying goal is wrong. That is, if the growth and development of HMOs has a beneficial effect on the system as a whole, then they should be encouraged even if it requires payments to HMOs above those that would have been required for the same people under FFS. There are at least two components to this viewpoint. One is that HMOs offer more to their enrollees than does the FFS system, so even if the Medicare program does not save its full 5 percent (as required under the AAPCC formula), there is a net social gain. That is, if the HMOs are able to incorporate many of the benefits included under a Medicare supplemental plan with little or no additional premium, then there are clear advantages for enrollees. Of course, assessing whether this is truly the case has to go beyond simple examination of the use and costs of medical care and incorporate quality and patient assessment measures. The inability of HCFA to recapture these potential savings is similar to the complaints of employers that HMO premiums do not save them money relative to FFS, even though their employees are enjoying additional benefits and lower out-of-pocket costs. In theory, at least, these additional benefits may reduce the pressure for higher wages or Social Security payments.

The second aspect takes an even broader view of the effects of HMOs. If they are able to engender a competitive response by FFS providers that leads to changes in practice patterns that lower the cost of medical care for everyone, then the presence of HMOs has a beneficial effect on the whole "system" even though they may be "subsidized" by an inaccurate AAPCC. Put another way, if this argument is true, not having HMOs would lead to higher costs for everyone. Welch makes this intriguing point, but the reliability and validity of the data he uses were questioned by some conference participants. Given the importance of this argument, and its relevance for policies concerning managed competition, it is well worth additional examination.

Thus, even though the current debate about health reform is focusing on coverage and cost-containment efforts for the nonelderly population, this conference is relevant in at least two ways. First, much of what we know today about HMO performance is drawn from experience with Medicare populations. Some of those findings will be generalizable to the nonelderly population. For example, it is difficult to believe that HMOs providing high-quality care for their Medicare enrollees with heart attacks do not provide similarly high-quality care for their under-65 enrollees with AMIs. Other findings may not be directly generalizable, such as the overall assessments of patient satisfaction by HMO and FFS beneficiaries, but the methodologies and underlying lessons, such as the importance of the competitive environment in assessing performance, offer important insights to our examination of managed care plans. Both the positive and negative lessons of risk adjustment under Medicare will be very important for the design of a workable managed competition model.

The second major benefit of this conference is that we can be sure that even if health care reform incorporates only minimal direct changes for Medicare, there will be enormous indirect effects. If managed competition is encouraged for the nonelderly population, this will alter substantially the availability and willingness of HMOs and similar plans to contract for the elderly population. Furthermore, each year a new cohort of Medicare beneficiaries will be used to dealing with managed care plans, bringing with them expectations and preferences quite different from previous cohorts who were used to only FFS. Substantial "spillovers" in methods of assessment and quality improvement will flow from the Medicare to the non-Medicare side, and vice versa. Continued work on assessing the use of HMOs by the elderly will yield benefits for all parties.

Index

About the Editor

Harold S. Luft, Ph.D., is Acting Director and Professor of Health Economics at the Institute for Health Policy Studies, University of California, San Francisco. Prior to coming to UCSF in 1978, he was a member of the faculty of the Stanford University Health Services Research Program. His interest in HMOs began in the mid-1970s with a review for the Brookings Institution about what was known about HMO performance. That report led to new research and was markedly expanded and published in 1981 as *Health Maintenance Organizations: Dimensions of Performance.* One of the key findings of that book was the need to be attentive to issues of biased selection and the competitive effects of HMOs. Professor Luft has been working on these issues for the last decade. Recently, he has returned to reviewing the current literature on HMO performance with his colleague, Robert Miller.

In addition to his work on HMOs and managed care systems, Professor Luft has undertaken extensive research on the relationship between hospital volumes and patient outcomes. This work led to an interest in outcomes and the development of models using routinely collected administrative data to adjust for differences in patient risk factors in assessing quality of care. This line of research came together with the work on HMOs to examine competitive behavior of hospitals and patients in the context of geographic markets. Throughout his career, Professor Luft has maintained a strong interest in the need to make research relevant and accessible to policymakers.

Other Publications From
Health Administration Press

▼▼▼▼▼▼▼▼▼▼▼▼▼▼▼▼▼▼▼▼▼

HEALTH POLICY ISSUES:
An Economic Perspective on Health Reform
By Paul J. Feldstein

In this issue-oriented book the author explores topics in healthcare policy from an economic perspective. This book is written primarily for non-economists – both students and professionals – to help them understand the political aspects of financing and delivering health services.

Feldstein, a professor and FHP Foundation Distinguished Chair in Health Care Management at the University of California, Irvine, discusses health policy from the point of view that the most effective solutions to economic problems will be those that continue to rely on market incentives to control costs.

Chapters cover such topics as: the rise in medical expenditures, how much should be spent on medical care, how much insurance should everyone have, rationing of medical services, competition among hospitals, the new Medicare payment system, vertically integrated healthcare organizations and employer mandated national health insurance.

Softbound, 321 pages, September 1994, $34.00, Order No. 0949, ISBN 1-56793-019-0. An AUPHA/ HAP Book.

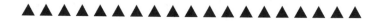

MANAGED CARE IN MEDICAID:
Lessons for Policy and Program Design
By Robert E. Hurley, Deborah A. Freund, and John E. Paul

This important book chronicles and explores a decade of Medicaid reform initiatives–specificallly those relating to primary care case management (PCCM). The authors evaluate three sets of managed care programs likely to be adopted. One set reimburses the provider on a fee-for-service basis, another utilizes networks of physicians at financial risk, and the third involves the enrollment of Medicaid beneficiaries in HMOs.

Softbound, 215 pages, 1993, $35.00, Order No. 0930 ISBN 0-910701-95-4. An AHSR/HAP Book.

HEALTH POLICYMAKING IN THE UNITED STATES
By Beaufort B. Longest, Jr.

This new book presents a basic model of the healthcare policymaking process that integrates the various and sometimes competing interests of our society. The author illustrates how policies are formulated, implemented, and modified.

The book covers the following topics: the definition of health policy and the way policies affect the health of our society, political dimensions of the policymaking process, the formulation of policy and the legislative process, how policies are implemented and changed, and the political interests of various parties in the policymaking process. The author also discusses how future healthcare policy is likely to be affected by the political marketplace and the U.S. economy.

Hardbound, 215 pages, August 1994, $38.00, Order No. 0947, ISBN 1-56793-017-4. An AUPHA/HAP Book.

A Health Administration Press Journal

▼▼▼▼▼▼▼▼▼▼▼▼▼▼▼▼▼▼▼▼

FRONTIERS OF HEALTH SERVICES MANAGEMENT

The ideal guide for busy executives, each quarterly issue is a collection of forecasts and perspectives on one of today's emerging healthcare topics. Past issues have discussed regional hospital systems, effective governance in the 1990s, universal health insurance, trends in hospital–physician relationships, future health personnel issues, strategic alliance management, and total quality management.

Subscriptions: $65.00/year in the U.S.; $75.00 in Canada and all other countries. ISSN 0748-8157.

BOOK ORDERING INFORMATION

All Health Administration Press Publications are sent on a 30-day approval. To order call, (708) 450-9952, or send your order to The Foundation of the American College of Healthcare Executives, Order Processing Center, Dept. LU94, 1951 Cornell Avenue, Melrose Park, IL 60160-1001.

JOURNAL SUBSCRIPTION INFORMATION

Health Administration Press offers a money-back guarantee on all journal subscriptions. If you are not completely satisfied, simply write and cancel your subscription, you will receive a refund on all unmailed issues. Multi-year subscriptions are not available.

Please send checks made payable to the name of the publication for subscriptions. Current rates expire on December 31, 1995. Address orders to: The Foundation of the American College of Healthcare Executives, Order Processing Center, Dept. LU94, 1951 Cornell Avenue, Melrose Park, IL 60160-1001. Or for more information, call: (708) 450-9952.

▼▼▼▼▼▼▼▼▼▼▼▼▼▼▼▼▼▼▼▼